Medical Statistics

A Guide to SPSS, Data Analysis and Critical Appraisal

Medical Statistics

A Guide to SPSS, Data Analysis and Critical Appraisal

Second Edition

Belinda Barton
Children's Hospital Education Research Institute, The Children's Hospital at Westmead, Sydney, Australia

Jennifer Peat
Honorary Professor, Australian Catholic University and Research Consultant, Sydney, Australia

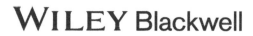

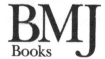

This edition first published 2014 © 2014 by John Wiley & Sons Ltd.
BMJ Books is an imprint of BMJ Publishing Group Limited, used under licence by John Wiley & Sons.

First edition © 2005 by Blackwell Publishing Ltd.

Registered office: John Wiley & Sons, Ltd, The Atrium, Southern Gate, Chichester, West Sussex, PO19 8SQ, UK

Editorial offices: 9600 Garsington Road, Oxford, OX4 2DQ, UK
    The Atrium, Southern Gate, Chichester, West Sussex, PO19 8SQ, UK
    111 River Street, Hoboken, NJ 07030-5774, USA

For details of our global editorial offices, for customer services and for information about how to apply for permission to reuse the copyright material in this book please see our website at www.wiley.com/wiley-blackwell

Library of Congress Cataloging-in-Publication Data

Peat, Jennifer K., author.
  Medical statistics : a guide to SPSS, data analysis, and critical appraisal / Belinda Barton, Jennifer Peat. – Second edition.
      p. ; cm.
  Author's names reversed on the first edition.
  Includes bibliographical references and index.
  ISBN 978-1-118-58993-9 (pbk.)
  I. Barton, Belinda, author. II. Title.
  [DNLM: 1. Statistics as Topic–methods. 2. Research Design. WA 950]
  R853.S7
  610.285'555–dc23
                                                                              2014020556

A catalogue record for this book is available from the British Library.

Wiley also publishes its books in a variety of electronic formats. Some content that appears in print may not be available in electronic books.

Typeset in 9.5/12pt Meridien & Frutiger by Laserwords Private Limited, Chennai, India

1   2014

Contents

Introduction

Statistical thinking will one day be as necessary a qualification for efficient citizenship as the ability to read and write.
H.G. WELLS

Anyone who is involved in medical research should always keep in mind that science is a search for the truth and that, in doing so, there is no room for bias or inaccuracy in statistical analyses or interpretation. Analyzing the data and interpreting the results are the most exciting stages of a research project because these provide the answers to the study questions. However, data analyses must be undertaken in a careful and considered way by people who have an inherent knowledge of the nature of the data and of their interpretation. Any errors in statistical analyses will mean that the conclusions of the study may be incorrect.[1] As a result, many journals may require reviewers to scrutinize the statistical aspects of submitted articles, and many research groups include statisticians who direct the data analyses. Analyzing data correctly and including detailed documentation so that others can reach the same conclusions are established markers of scientific integrity. Research studies that are conducted with integrity bring personal pride, contribute to a successful track record and foster a better research culture, advancing the scientific community.

In this book, we provide a step-by-step guide to the complete process of analyzing and reporting your data – from creating a file to entering your data to how to report your results for publication. We provide a guide to conducting and interpreting statistics in the context of how the participants were recruited, how the study was designed, the types of variables used, and the interpretation of effect sizes and *P* values. We also guide researchers, through the processes of selecting the correct statistic, and show how to report results for publication. Each chapter includes worked research examples with real data sets that can be downloaded and used by readers to work through the examples.

We have included the SPSS commands for methods of statistical analysis, commonly found in the health care literature. We have not included all of the tables from the SPSS output but only the most relevant SPSS output information that is to be interpreted. We have also included the commands for obtaining graphs using SigmaPlot, a graphing software package that is frequently used. In this book, we use SPSS version 21 and SigmaPlot version 12.5, but the messages apply equally well to other versions and other statistical packages.

We have written this book as a guide from the first principles with explanations of assumptions and how to interpret results. We hope that both novice statisticians and seasoned researchers will find this book a helpful guide.

In this era of evidence-based health care, both clinicians and researchers need to critically appraise the statistical aspects of published articles in order to judge the implications and reliability of reported results. Although the peer review process goes a long way to improving the standard of research literature, it is essential to have the skills to decide whether published results are credible and therefore have implications for current clinical practice or future research directions. We have therefore included critical appraisal guidelines at the end of each chapter to help researchers to evaluate the results of studies.

Features of this book

- Easy to read and step-by-step guide
- Practical
- Limited use of computational or mathematical formulae
- Specifies the assumptions of each statistical test and how to check the assumptions
- Worked examples and corresponding data sets that can be downloaded from the book's website
- SPSS commands to conduct a range of statistical tests
- SPSS output displayed and interpreted
- Examples on how to report your results for publication
- Commands and output on how to visually display results using SPSS or SigmaPlot
- Critical appraisal checklists that can be used to systematically evaluate studies and research articles
- Glossary of terms
- List of useful websites such as effect size and sample size on-line calculators, free statistical packages and sources of statistical help.

New to this edition

In this second edition, the significant changes include updating all the IBM Statistics SPSS commands and output using version 21. As the versions of SPSS are very similar, the majority of the commands are applicable to previous and future versions. Similarly, we have updated the commands and the output for SigmaPlot to version 12.5. We have also included additional sections and discussions on statistical power, the sample size required and the different measures of effect size and their interpretations.

There is an additional chapter on the analysis of longitudinal data, where the outcome is measured repeatedly over time for each participant. We have included both statistical methods that can be used to analyze these types of data – repeated measures and linear mixed models. In Chapter 12 on survival analysis, we have included a section on Cox's regression, which provides an estimate of survival time while adjusting for the effects of other explanatory or predictor variables.

In reporting study findings, it is important that they are presented clearly and contain the necessary information to be interpreted by readers. Although disciplines and journals may differ slightly in the information that require to be reported, we provide examples of how to report the information required for most publications, both in a written and in a tabular format, as well as visually such as by graphs. Finally, we have updated the glossary and the links to useful websites and resources.

There is a saying that 'everything is easy when you know how' – we hope that this book will provide the 'know how' and make statistical analysis and critical appraisal easy for all researchers and health care professionals.

Belinda Barton
Head of Children's Hospital Education Research Institute (CHERI) and Psychologist, The Children's Hospital at Westmead, Sydney, Australia

Jennifer Peat
Honorary Professor, Australian Catholic University and Research Consultant, Sydney, Australia

Reference

1. Altman DG. *Statistics in medical research*. In: *Practical statistics for medical research*. Chapman and Hall: London, 1996.

Acknowledgements

We extend our thanks to our colleagues, hospitals and universities for supporting us. We also thank all of the researchers and students who attend our classes and consultations and provide encouragement and feedback. Mostly, we will always be eternally grateful to our friends and our families who inspired us and supported whilst we were revising this book.

About the companion website

This book is accompanied by a companion website:

www.wiley.com/go/barton/medicalstatistics2e

The website includes:
- Original data files for SPSS

CHAPTER 1

Creating an SPSS data file and preparing to analyse the data

There are two kinds of statistics, the kind you look up and the kind you make up.
REX STOUT

Objectives

The objectives of this chapter are to explain how to:
- create an SPSS data file that will facilitate straightforward statistical analyses
- ensure data quality
- manage missing data points
- move data and output between electronic spreadsheets
- manipulate data files and variables
- devise a data management plan
- select the correct statistical test
- critically appraise the quality of reported data analyses

1.1 Creating an SPSS data file

Creating a data file in SPSS and entering the data is a relatively simple process. In the SPSS window located on the top left-hand side of the screen is a menu bar with headings and drop-down options. A new file can be opened using the *File → New → Data* commands located on the top left-hand side of the screen. The SPSS IBM Statistics Data Editor has two different screens called the 'Data View' and 'Variable View'. You can easily move between the two views by clicking on the tabs located at the bottom left-hand side of the screen.

1.1.1 Variable View screen

Before entering data in Data View, the features or attributes of each variable need to be defined in Variable View. In this screen, details of the variable names, variable types and labels are stored. Each row in Variable View represents a new variable and each

---

Medical Statistics: A Guide to SPSS, Data Analysis and Critical Appraisal, Second Edition.
Belinda Barton and Jennifer Peat.
Companion website: www.wiley.com/go/barton/medicalstatistics2e

column represents a feature of the variable such as type (e.g. numeric, dot, string, etc.) and measure (scale, ordinal or nominal). To enter a variable name, simply type the name into the first field and default settings will appear for almost all of the remaining fields, except for *Label* and *Measure*.

The Tab, arrow keys or mouse can be used to move across the fields and change the default settings. In Variable View, the settings can be changed by a single click on the cell and then pulling down the drop box option that appears when you double click on the domino on the right-hand side of the cell. The first variable in a data set is usually a unique identification code or a number for each participant. This variable is invaluable for selecting or tracking particular participants during the data analysis process.

Unlike data in Excel spreadsheets, it is not possible to hide rows or columns in either Variable View or Data View in SPSS and therefore, the order of variables in the spreadsheet should be considered before the data are entered. The default setting for the lists of variables in the drop-down boxes that are used when running the statistical analyses are in the same order as the spreadsheet. It can be more efficient to place variables that are likely to be used most often at the beginning of the spreadsheet and variables that are going to be used less often at the end.

Variable names

Each variable name must be unique and must begin with an alphabetic character. Variable names are entered in the column titled *Name* displayed in Variable View. The names of variables may be up to 64 characters long and may contain letters, numbers and some non-punctuation symbols but should not end in an underscore or a full stop. Variable names cannot contain spaces although words can be separated with an underscore. Some symbols such as @, # or $ can be used in variable names but other symbols such as %, > and punctuation marks are not accepted. SPSS is case sensitive so capital and lower case letters can be used.

Variable type

In medical statistics, the most common types of data are numeric and string. Numeric refers to variables that are recorded as numbers, for example, 1, 115, 2013 and is the default setting in Variable View. String refers to variables that are recorded as a combination of letters and numbers, or just letters such as 'male' and 'female'. However, where possible, variables that are a string type and contain important information that will be used in the data analyses should be coded as categorical variables, for example, by using 1= male and 2 = female. For some analyses in SPSS, only numeric variables can be used so it is best to avoid using string variables where possible.

Other data types are comma or dot. These are used for large numeric variables which are displayed with commas or periods delimiting every three places. Other options for variable type are scientific notation, date, dollar, custom currency and restricted numeric.

Width and decimals

The width of a variable is the number of characters to be entered for the variable. If the variable is numeric with decimal places, the total number of characters needs to include the numbers, the decimal point and all decimal places. The default setting is 8 characters which is sufficient for numbers up to 100,000 with 2 decimal places.

Decimals refers to the number of decimal places that will be displayed for a numeric variable. The default setting is two decimal places, that is, 51.25. For categorical variables, no decimal places are required. For continuous variables, the number of decimal places must be the same as the number that the measurement was collected in. The decimal setting does not affect the statistical calculations but does influence the number of decimal places displayed in the output.

Labels

Labels can be used to name, describe or identify a variable and any character can be used in creating a label. Labels may assist in remembering information about a variable that is not included in the variable name. When selecting variables for analysis, variables will be listed by their variable label with the variable name in brackets in the dialogue boxes. Also, output from SPSS will list the variable label. Therefore, it is important to keep the length of the variable label short where possible. For example, question one of a questionnaire is 'How many hours of sleep did you have last night?'. The variable name could be entered as q1 (representing question 1) and the label to describe the variable q1 could be 'hrs sleep'. If many questions begin with the same phrase, it is helpful to include the question number in the variable label, for example, 'q1: hrs sleep'.

Values

Values can be used to assign labels to a variable, which makes interpreting the output from SPSS easier. Value labels are most commonly used when the variable is categorical or nominal. For example, a label could be used to code 'Gender' with the label 'male' coded to a value of 1 and the label 'female' coded to a value of 2. The SPSS dialogue box *Value Labels* can be obtained by single clicking on the Values box, then clicking on the grey domino on the right-hand side of the box. Within this box, the buttons *Add*, *Change* and *Remove* can be used to customize and edit the value labels.

Missing

Missing can be used to assign user system missing values for data that are not available for a participant. For example, a participant who did not attend a scheduled clinical appointment would have data values that had not been measured and which are called missing values. Missing values are not included in the data analyses and can sometimes create pervasive problems. The seriousness of the problem depends largely on the pattern of missing data, how much is missing and why it is missing.[1]

For a full stop to be recognized as a system missing value, the variable type must be entered as numeric rather than a string variable. Other approaches to dealing with missing data will be discussed later in this chapter.

Columns and align

Columns can be used to define the width of the column in which the variable is displayed in the Data View screen. The default setting is 8 and this is generally sufficient to view the name in the Variable View and Data View screens. Align can be used to specify the alignment of the data information in Data View as either right, left or centre justified within cells.

Measure

In SPSS, the measurement level of the variable can be classified as nominal, ordinal or scale under the *Measure* option. The measurement scales used which are described below determine each of these classifications.

Nominal variables

Nominal scales have no order and are generally categories with labels that have been assigned to classify items or information. For example, variables with categories such as male or female, religious status or place of birth are nominal scales. Nominal scales can be string (alphanumeric) values or numeric values that have been assigned to represent categories, for example 1 = male and 2 = female.

Ordinal variables

Values on an ordinal scale have a logical or ordered relationship across the values and it is possible to measure some degree of difference between categories. However, it is usually not possible to measure a specific amount of difference between categories. For example, participants may be asked to rate their overall level of stress on a five-point scale that ranges from no stress, mild, moderate, severe or extreme stress. Using this scale, participants with severe stress will have a more serious condition than participants with mild stress, although recognizing that self-reported perception of stress may be subjective and is unlikely to be standardized between participants. With this type of scale, it is not possible to say that the difference between mild and moderate stress is the same as the difference between moderate and severe stress. Thus, information from these types of variables has to be interpreted with care.

Scale variables

Variables with numeric values that are measured by an interval or ratio scale are classified as scale variables. On an interval scale, one unit on the scale represents the same magnitude across the whole scale. For example, Fahrenheit is an interval scale because the difference in temperature between $10\,°F$ and $20\,°F$ is the same as the difference in temperature between $40\,°F$ and $50\,°F$. However, interval scales have no true zero point. For example, $0\,°F$ does not indicate that there is no temperature. Because interval scales have an arbitrary rather than a true zero point, it is not possible to compare ratios.

A ratio scale has the same properties as ordinal and interval scales, but has a true zero point and therefore ratio comparisons are valid. For example, it is possible to say that a person who is 40 years old is twice as old as a person who is 20 years old and that a person is 0 years old at birth. Other common ratio scales are length, weight and income.

Role

Role can be used with some SPSS statistical procedures to select variables that will be automatically assigned a role such as input or target. In Data View, when a statistical procedure is selected from *Analyze* a dialogue box opens up and variables to be analysed must be selected such as an independent or dependent variable. If the role of the variables has been defined in Variable View, the variables will be automatically displayed in the destination list of the dialogue box. Role options for a variable are input (independent variable), target (dependent variable), both (can be an input or an output variable), none (no role assignment), partition (to divide the data into separate samples) and split (this option is only used in SPSS Modeler). The default setting for *Role* is input.

1.1.2 Saving the SPSS file

After the information for each variable has been defined, the variable details entered in the Variable View screen can be saved using the commands shown in Box 1.1. When the file is saved, the name of the file will replace the word *Untitled* at the top left-hand side of the Data View screen. The data can then be entered in the Data View screen and also saved using the commands shown in Box 1.1. The data file extension is *.sav*. When there is only one data file open in the Data Editor, the file can only be closed by exiting the SPSS program. When there is more than one data file open, the SPSS commands *File → Close* can be used to close a data file.

Box 1.1 SPSS commands for saving a file

SPSS Commands

Untitled – SPSS IBM Statistics Data Editor
        File → Save As
Save Data As
        Enter the name of the file in File name
Click on Save

1.1.3 Data View screen

The Data View screen displays the data values and is similar to many other spreadsheet packages. In general, the data for each participant should occupy one row only in the spreadsheet. Thus, if follow-up data have been collected from the participants on one or more occasions, the participants' data should be an extension of their baseline data row and not a new row in the spreadsheet. However, this does not apply for studies in which controls are matched to cases by characteristics such as gender or age or are selected as the unaffected sibling or a nominated friend of the case and therefore the data are paired. The data from matched case–control studies are used as pairs in the statistical analyses and therefore it is important that matched controls are not entered on a separate row but are entered into the same row in the spreadsheet as their matched case. This method will inherently ensure that paired or matched data are analysed correctly and that the assumptions of independence that are required by many statistical tests are not violated. Thus, in Data View, each column represents a separate variable and each row represents a single participant, or a single pair of participants in a matched case–control study, or a single participant with follow-up data. This data format is called 'wide format'. For some longitudinal modelling analyses, the data may need to be changed to 'long format', that is, each time a point is represented on a separate row. This is discussed in Chapter 6.

In Data View, data can be entered and the mouse, tab, enter or cursor keys can be used to move to another cell of the data sheet. In Data View, the value labels button which is displayed at the top of the spreadsheet (17th icon from the left-hand side), with an arrow pointing to '1' and another arrow pointing to 'A' can be used to switch between displaying the values or the value labels that have been entered.

1.2 Opening data from Excel in SPSS

Data can be entered in other programs such as Excel and then imported into the SPSS Data View sheet. Many researchers use Excel or Access for ease of entering and managing the data. However, statistical analyses are best executed in a specialist statistical package such as SPSS in which the integrity and accuracy of the statistics are guaranteed.

Opening an Excel spreadsheet in SPSS can be achieved using the commands shown in Box 1.2. In addition, specialized programs are available for transferring data between different data entry and statistics packages (see Section Useful Websites).

Box 1.2 SPSS commands for opening an Excel data file

SPSS Commands

Untitled – SPSS IBM Statistics Data Editor
File → Open → Data
Open Data
      Click on Files of type to show Excel (*.xls, *.xlsx,*xlsm)
      Look in: find and click on your Excel data file
      Click Open
Opening Excel Data Source
      Check that the correct Worksheet within the file is selected
      Tick 'Read variable names from the first row of data' (default setting)
      Click OK

If data are entered in Excel or another database before being exported into SPSS, it is a good idea to use variable names that are accepted by SPSS to avoid having to rename the variables. For numeric values, blank cells in Excel are converted to the system missing value, that is a full stop, in SPSS.

Once in the SPSS spreadsheet, features of the variables can be adjusted in Variable View, for example, by changing column widths, entering the labels and values for categorical variables and checking that the number of decimal places is appropriate for each variable. Once data quality is ensured, a back-up copy of the database should be archived at a remote site for safety. Few researchers need to resort to their archived copies but, when they do, they are an invaluable resource.

The spreadsheet that is used for data analyses should not contain any information that would contravene ethics guidelines by identifying individual participants. In the working data file, names, addresses and any other identifying information that will not be used in data analyses should be removed. Identifying information that is required can be recoded and de-identified, for example, by using a unique numerical value that is assigned to each participant.

1.3 Categorical and continuous variables

While variables in SPSS can be classified as scale, ordinal or nominal values, a more useful classification for variables when deciding how to analyse data is as categorical variables (ordered or non-ordered) or continuous variables (scale variables). These clas-sifications are essential for selecting the correct statistical test to analyse the data and are not provided in Variable View by SPSS. Categorical variables have discrete categories, such as male and female, and continuous variables are measured on a scale, such as height which is measured in centimetres.

Categorical values can be non-ordered or ordered. For example, gender which is coded as 1 = male and 2 = female and place of birth which is coded as 1 = local, 2 = regional and 3 = overseas are non-ordered variables. Categorical variables can also be ordered, for example, if the continuous variable length of stay was recoded into categories of 1 = 1–10 days, 2 = 11–20 days, 3 = 21–30 days and 4 = >31 days, there is a progression in magnitude of length of stay. A categorical variable with only two possible outcomes such as yes/no or disease present/disease absent is referred to as a binary variable.

1.4 Classifying variables for analyses

Before conducting any statistical tests, a formal, documented plan that includes a list of hypotheses to be tested and identifies the variables that will be used should be drawn up. For each question, a decision on how each variable will be used in the analyses, for example, as a continuous or categorical variable or as an outcome or explanatory variable, should be made.

Table 1.1 shows a classification system for variables and how the classification influ-ences the presentation of results. An outcome or dependent variable is a variable is generally the outcome of interest in the study that has been measured, for example, cholesterol levels or blood pressure may be measured in a study to reduce cardiovascu-lar risk. An outcome variable is proposed to be changed or influenced by an explanatory variable. An explanatory or independent variable is hypothesized to affect the outcome variable and is generally manipulated or controlled experimentally. For example, treat-ment status defined as whether participants receive the active drug treatment or inactive treatment (placebo) is an independent variable.

A common error in statistical analyses is to misclassify the outcome variable as an explanatory variable or to misclassify an intervening variable as an explanatory variable. It is important that an intervening variable, which links the explanatory and outcome

Table 1.1   Names used to identify variables

Variable name	Alternative name/s	Axis for plots, data analysis and tables
Outcome variables	Dependent variables (DVs)	y-axis, columns
Intervening variables	Secondary or alternative outcome variables	y-axis, columns
Explanatory variables	Independent variables (IVs) Risk factors Exposure variables Predictors	x-axis, rows

variable because it is directly on the pathway to the outcome variable, is not treated as an independent explanatory variable in the analyses.[2] It is also important that an alternative outcome variable is not treated as an independent risk factor. For example, hay fever cannot be treated as an independent risk factor for asthma because it is a symptom that is a consequence of the same allergic developmental pathway.

In part, the classification of variables depends on the study design. In a case–control study in which disease status is used as the selection criterion, the explanatory variable will be the presence or absence of disease and the outcome variable will be the exposure. However, in most other observational and experimental studies such as clinical trials, cross-sectional and cohort studies, the disease will be the outcome and the exposure or the experimental group will be an explanatory variable.

1.5   Hypothesis testing and *P* values

Most medical statistics are based on the concept of hypothesis testing and therefore an associated *P* value is usually reported. In hypothesis testing, a 'null hypothesis' is first specified, that is a hypothesis stating that there is no difference, for example, there is no difference in the summary statistics of the study groups (placebo and treatment). The null hypothesis assumes that the groups that are being compared are drawn from the same population. An alternative hypothesis, which states that there is a difference between groups, can also be specified. The *P* value is then calculated, that is, the probability of obtaining a difference as large as or larger than the one observed between the groups, assuming the null hypothesis is true (i.e. no difference between groups).

A *P* value of less than 0.05, that is a probability of less than 1 chance in 20, is usually accepted as being statistically significant. If a *P* value is less than 0.05, we accept that it is unlikely that a difference between groups has occurred by chance if the null hypothesis was true. In this situation, we reject the null hypothesis and accept the alternative hypothesis, and therefore conclude that there is a statistically significant difference between the groups. On the other hand, if the *P* value is greater than or equal to 0.05 and therefore the probability with which the test statistic occurs is greater than 1 chance in 20, we accept that the difference between groups has occurred by chance. In this case, we accept the null hypothesis and conclude that the difference is not attributed to sampling.

In accepting or rejecting a null hypothesis, it is important to remember that the *P* value only provides a probability value and does not provide absolute proof that the null hypothesis is true or false. A *P* value obtained from a test of significance should only be interpreted as a measure of the strength of evidence against the null hypothesis. The smaller the *P* value the stronger the evidence against the null hypothesis.

1.6   Choosing the correct statistical test

Selecting the correct test to analyse data depends not only on the study design but also on the nature of the variables collected. Tables 1.2–1.5 show the types of tests that can be selected based on the nature of variables. It is of paramount importance that the correct test is used to generate *P* values and to estimate a size of effect. Using an incorrect test will inviolate the statistical assumptions of the test and may lead to inaccurate or biased *P* values.

Table 1.2   Choosing a statistic when there is one outcome variable only

Type of variable	Number of times measured in each participant	Statistic	SPSS menu
Binary	Once	Incidence or prevalence and 95% confidence interval (95% CI)	Descriptive statistics; Frequencies
	Twice	McNemar's chi-square; Kappa	Descriptive statistics; Crosstabs
Continuous	Once	Tests for normality	Non-parametric tests; One sample; Kolmogorov–Smirnov Descriptive statistics; Explore; Plots; Normality plots with tests
		One-sample *t*-test	Compare means; One-sample *t*-test
		Mean, standard deviation (SD) and 95% CI	Descriptive statistics; Explore
		Median (Mdn) and inter-quartile (IQR) range	Descriptive statistics; Explore
	Twice	Paired *t*-test	Compare means; Paired-samples *t*-test
		Mean difference and 95% CI	Compare means; Paired-samples *t*-test
		Measurement error	Compare means; Paired-samples *t*-test
		Mean-versus-differences plot	Graphs; Legacy Dialogs; Scatter/Dot
		Intra-class correlation coefficient	Scale; Reliability Analysis
	Three or more	Repeated measures ANOVA	General linear model; Repeated measures

Table 1.3 Choosing a statistic when there is one outcome variable and one explanatory variable

Type of outcome variable	Type of explanatory variable	Number of levels of the categorical variable	Statistic	SPSS menu
Categorical	Categorical	Both variables are binary	Chi-square	Descriptive statistics; Crosstabs
			Odds ratio or relative risk	Descriptive statistics; Crosstabs
			Logistic regression	Regression; Binary logistic
			Sensitivity and specificity	Descriptive statistics; Crosstabs
			Likelihood ratio	Descriptive statistics; Crosstabs
		At least one of the variables has more than two levels	Chi-square	Descriptive statistics; Crosstabs
			Chi-square trend	Descriptive statistics; Crosstabs
			Kendall's correlation	Correlate; Bivariate
Categorical	Continuous	Categorical variable is binary	ROC curve	ROC curve
			Survival analyses	Survival; Kaplan–Meier
		Categorical variable is multi-level and ordered	Spearman's correlation coefficient	Correlate; Bivariate
Continuous	Categorical	Explanatory variable is binary	Independent samples t-test	Compare means; Independent samples t-test
			Mean difference and 95% CI	Compare means; Independent samples t-test
		Explanatory variable has three or more categories	Analysis of variance	Compare means; One-way ANOVA
Continuous	Continuous	No categorical variables	Regression	Regression; Linear
			Pearson's correlation	Correlate; Bivariate

1.7 Sample size requirements

The sample size is one of the most critical issues in designing a research study because it affects all aspects of interpreting the results. The sample size needs to be large enough so that a definitive answer to the research question is obtained. This will help to ensure

Table 1.4 Choosing a statistic for one or more outcome variables and more than one explanatory variable

Type of outcome variable/s	Type of explanatory variable/s	Number of levels of categorical variable	Statistic	SPSS menu
Continuous – only one outcome	Both continuous and categorical	Categorical variables are binary	Multiple regression	Regression; Linear
	Categorical	At least one of the explanatory variables has three or more categories	Two-way analysis of variance	General linear model; Univariate
	Both continuous and categorical	One categorical variable has two or more levels	Analysis of covariance	General linear model; Univariate
Continuous – outcome measured more than once	Both continuous and categorical	Categorical variables can have two or more levels	Repeated measures analysis of variance	General linear model; Repeated measures Mixed Models; Linear
No outcome variable	Both continuous and categorical	Categorical variables can have two or more levels	Factor analysis	Dimension reduction: Factor

Table 1.5 Parametric and non-parametric equivalents

Parametric test	Non-parametric equivalent	SPSS menu
Mean and standard deviation	Median and inter-quartile range	Descriptive statistics; Explore
Pearson's correlation coefficient	Spearman's or Kendall's correlation coefficient	Correlate; Bivariate
One-sample sign test	Wilcoxon signed rank test	Non-parametric tests; One Sample
Two sample t-test	Sign test or Wilcoxon matched pair signed rank test	Non-parametric tests; Related samples
Independent t-test	Mann–Whitney U	Non-parametric tests; Independent samples
Analysis of variance	Kruskall–Wallis one-way test	Non-parametric tests; Independent samples
Repeated measures analysis of variance	Friedman's two-way ANOVA test	Non-parametric tests; Related samples

generalizability of the results and precision around estimates of effect. However, the sample has to be small enough so that the study is practical to conduct. In general, studies with a small sample size, say with less than 30 participants, can usually only provide imprecise and unreliable estimates.

P values are strongly influenced by the sample size. The larger the sample size the more likely a difference between study groups will be statistically significant. Box 1.3 provides a definition of type I and type II errors and shows how the size of the sample can contribute to these errors, both of which have a profound influence on the interpretation of the results. In addition, type I and II error rates are inversely related because both are influenced by sample size – when the risk of a type I error is reduced, the risk of a type II error is increased. Therefore, it is important to carefully calculate the sample size required prior to the study commencing and also consider the sample size when interpreting the results of the statistical tests.

Box 1.3 Type I and type II errors

Type I errors

- are false positive results
- occur when a statistical significant difference between groups is found but no clinically important difference exists
- the null hypothesis is rejected in error
- usually occur when the sample size is very large

Type II errors

- are false negative results
- a clinical important difference between groups does exist but does not reach statistical significance
- the null hypothesis is accepted in error
- usually occur when the sample size is small

1.8 Study handbook and data analysis plan

The study handbook should be a formal documentation of all of the study details that is updated continuously with any changes to protocols, management decisions, minutes of meetings and so on. This handbook should be available for anyone in the team to refer to at any time to facilitate considered data collection and data analysis practices. Suggested contents of data analysis log sheets that could be kept in the study handbook are shown in Box 1.4.

Box 1.4 Data analysis log sheets

Data analysis log sheets should contain the following information:
- Title of proposed paper, report or abstract
- Author list and author responsible for data analyses and documentation
- Specific research questions to be answered or hypotheses to be tested
- Outcome and explanatory variables to be used
- Statistical methods
- Details of database location and file storage names
- Journals and/or scientific meetings where results will be presented

Data analyses must be planned and executed in a logical and considered sequence to avoid errors or misinterpretation of results. In this, it is important that data are treated carefully and analysed by people who are familiar with their content, their meaning and the interrelationship between variables.

Before beginning any statistical analyses, a data analysis plan should be agreed upon in consultation with the study team. The plan can include the research questions or hypotheses that will be tested, the outcome and explanatory variables that will be used, the journal where the results will be published and/or the scientific meeting where the findings will be presented.

A good way to handle data analyses is to create a log sheet for each proposed paper, abstract or report. The log sheets should be formal documents that are agreed to by all stakeholders and that are formally archived in the study handbook. When a research team is managed efficiently, a study handbook is maintained that has up-to-date documentation of all details of the study protocol and the study processes.

1.9 Documentation

Documentation of data analyses, which allows anyone to track how the results were obtained from the data set collected, is an important aspect of the scientific process. This is especially important when the data set will be accessed in the future by researchers who are not familiar with all aspects of data collection or the coding and recoding of the variables.

Data management and documentation are relatively mundane processes compared to the excitement of statistical analyses but are essential. Laboratory researchers document every detail of their work as a matter of course by maintaining accurate laboratory books. All researchers undertaking clinical and epidemiological studies should be equally diligent and document all of the steps taken to reach their conclusions.

Documentation can be easily achieved by maintaining a data management book with a log sheet for each data analysis. In this, all steps in the data management processes are recorded together with the information of names and contents of files, the coding and names of variables and the results of the statistical analyses. Many funding bodies and ethics committees require that all steps in data analyses are documented and that in addition to archiving the data, the data sheets, the output files and the participant records are kept for 5 years or up to 15 years after the results are published.

1.10 Checking the data

Prior to beginning statistical analysis, it is essential to have a thorough working knowledge of the nature, ranges and distributions of each variable. Although it may be tempting to jump straight into the analyses that will answer the study questions rather than spend time obtaining descriptive statistics, a working knowledge of the descriptive statistics often saves time by avoiding analyses having to be repeated for example because outliers, missing values or duplicates have not been addressed or groups with small numbers are not identified.

When entering data, it is important to crosscheck the data file with the original records to ensure that data has been entered correctly. It is important to have a high standard of data quality in research databases at all times because good data management practice is a hallmark of scientific integrity. The steps outlined in Box 1.5 will help to achieve this.

Box 1.5 Data organization

The following steps ensure good data management practices:
- Crosscheck data with the original records
- Use numeric codes for categorical data where possible
- Choose appropriate variable names and labels to avoid confusion across variables
- Check for duplicate records and implausible data values
- Make corrections
- Archive a back-up copy of the data set for safe keeping
- Limit access to sensitive data such as names and addresses in working files

---

It is especially important to know the range and distribution of each variable and whether there are any outliers or extreme values (see Chapter 2) so that the statistics that are generated can be explained and interpreted correctly. Describing the characteristics of the sample also allows other researchers to judge the generalizability of the results. A considered pathway for data management is shown in Box 1.6.

Box 1.6 Pathway for data management before beginning statistical analysis

The following steps are essential for efficient data management:
- Obtain the minimum and maximum values and the range of each variable
- Conduct frequency analyses for categorical variables
- Use box plots, histograms and other tests to ascertain normality of continuous variables
- Identify and deal with missing values and outliers
- Recode or transform variables where necessary
- Rerun frequency and/or distribution checks
- Document all steps in a study handbook

1.11   Avoiding and replacing missing values

Missing values must be omitted from the analyses and not inadvertently included as data points. This can be achieved by proper coding that is recognized by SPSS as a system missing value. The default character to indicate a missing value is a full stop. This is preferable to using an implausible value such as 9 or 999 which was commonly used in the past. If these values are not accurately defined as discrete missing values in Missing column displayed in Variable View, they are easily incorporated into the analyses, thus producing erroneous results. Although these values can be predefined as system missing, this coding scheme is discouraged because it is inefficient, requires data analysts to be familiar with the coding scheme and has the potential for error. If missing values are

Table 1.6 Classification of variables in the file surgery.sav

Variable label	Type	SPSS measure	Classification for analysis decisions
ID	Numeric	Scale	Not used in analyses
Gender	String	Nominal	Categorical/non-ordered
Place of birth	String	Nominal	Categorical/non-ordered
Birth weight	Numeric	Scale	Continuous
Gestational age	Numeric	Ordinal	Continuous
Length of stay	Numeric	Scale	Continuous
Infection	Numeric	Scale	Categorical/non-ordered
Prematurity	Numeric	Scale	Categorical/non-ordered
Procedure performed	Numeric	Nominal	Categorical/non-ordered

required in an analysis, for example to determine if people with missing data have the characteristics as people with complete data, the missing values can easily be recoded to a numeric value in a new variable.

The file **surgery.sav**, which contains the data from 141 babies who underwent surgery at a paediatric hospital, can be opened using the *File → Open → Data* commands. The classification of the variables as shown by SPSS and the classifications that are needed for statistical analysis are shown in Table 1.6.

In the spreadsheet, the variable for 'place of birth' is coded as a string variable. The command sequences shown in Box 1.7 can be used to obtain frequency information of this variable, where L = local, O = overseas and R = regional.

Box 1.7 SPSS commands for obtaining frequencies

SPSS Commands

surgery.sav – SPSS IBM Statistics Data Editor
> *Analyze → Descriptive Statistics → Frequencies*
Frequencies
> *Highlight Place of birth and click into Variable(s)*
> *Click OK*

Frequency table

Place of Birth

		Frequency	Per cent	Valid per cent	Cumulative per cent
Valid		9	6.4	6.4	6.4
	L	90	63.8	63.8	70.2
	O	9	6.4	6.4	76.6
	R	33	23.4	23.4	100.0
	Total	141	100.0	100.0	

The nine children with no information of birthplace are included in the valid and cumulative percentages shown in the Frequency table. If the variable had been defined as numeric, the missing values would have been omitted.

When collecting data in any study, it is essential to have methods in place to prevent missing values in, say, at least 95% of the data set. Methods such as restructuring questionnaires in which participants decline to provide sensitive information or training research staff to check that all fields are complete at the point of data collection are invaluable in this process. In large epidemiological and longitudinal data sets, some missing data may be unavoidable. However, in clinical trials, it may be unethical to collect insufficient information about some participants so that they have to be excluded from the final analyses.

If the number of missing values is small and the missing values occur randomly throughout the data set, the cases with missing values can be omitted from the analyses. This is the default option in most statistical packages and the main effect of this process is to reduce statistical power, that is the ability to show a statistically significant difference between groups when a clinically important difference exists. Missing values that are scattered randomly throughout the data are less of a problem than non-random missing values that can affect both the power of the study and the generalizability of the results. For example, if people in higher income groups selectively decline to answer questions about income, the distribution of income in the population will not be known and analyses that include income will not be generalizable to people in higher income groups. When analysing data, it is important to determine whether data is missing completely at random, missing at random, or missing not at random.[3]

In some situations, it may be important to replace a missing value with an estimated value that can be included in analyses. In longitudinal clinical trials, it has become common practice to use the last score obtained from the participant and carry it forward for all subsequent missing values – this is commonly called last observation carried forward (LOCF) or last value carried forward (LVCF). In other studies, a mean value (if the variable is normally distributed) or a median value (if the variable is non-normal distributed) may be used to replace missing values. This can be undertaken in SPSS using the commands *Transform* ⟶ *Replace Missing Values*.

These simple imputation solutions are not ideal – for example, LOCF can result in reducing the variance of the sample and can also lead to biased results.[3] Other more complicated methods for replacing missing values have been described and should be considered.[4]

1.12   SPSS data management capabilities

SPSS has many data management capabilities which are listed in the *Data* and *Transform* menus. A summary of some of the commands that are widely used in routine data analyses are shown in Table 1.7. How to use the commands to select a subset of variables and recode variables is shown below. Also, the use of these commands is demonstrated in more detail in the following chapters.

Table 1.7   Data management capabilities in SPSS

Menu	Command	Purpose
Data menu	Identify duplicate cases	Labels primary and duplicate cases as defined by specified variables.
	Sort cases	Sorts the data set into ascending or descending order using one or more variables.
	Merge files	Allows the merge of one or more data files using a variable common to both sets. Additional cases or variables can be added.
	Restructure	Changes data sets from wide format (one line per subject) to long format (multiple lines per subject, for example, when there are multiple time points), and vice versa.
	Split file	Separates the file into separate groups for analysis.
	Select cases	By using conditional expressions, a subgroup of cases can be selected for analysis based on one or more variables. Arithmetic operators and functions can also be used in the expression.
Transform menu	Compute	Creates a new variable based on transformation of existing variables or by using mathematical functions.
	Recode	Reassigns values or collapses ranges into the same or a new variable.
	Visual binning	A categorical variable can be created from a scale variable. Variables can be grouped into 'bins' or interval cut off points such as quantiles or tertiles.
	Date and time wizard	Used to create a date/time variable, to add or subtract dates and times. The result is presented in a new variable in units of seconds and needs to be back converted to hours or days.
	Replace missing values	Replaces missing values with an option to use various methods of imputation.

1.12.1   Using subsets of variables

When conducting an analysis, it is common to want to use only a few of the variables. A smaller subset of variables to be used in analyses can be selected as shown in Box 1.8. When using a subset, only the variables selected are displayed in the data analysis dialogue boxes. This can make analyses more efficient by avoiding having to search up and down a long list of variables for the ones required. Using a subset is especially useful when working with a large data set and only a few variables are needed for a current analysis. To see the whole data set again simply use the SPSS commands *Utilities → Show All Variables*.

Box 1.8 SPSS commands for defining variable sets

SPSS Commands

surgery.sav – IBM SPSS Statistics Data Editor
    Utilities → Define Variable Sets
Define variable sets
    Enter Set Name e.g. Set_1
    Highlight Variables required in the analyses and click them into Variables in Set
    Click on Add Set
    Click Close
surgery.sav – IBM SPSS Statistics Data Editor
    Utilities → Use Variable Sets
    Click Uncheck all
    Tick Set 1
    Click OK

1.12.2   Recoding variables and using syntax

In the frequency statistics conducted above, place of birth was coded as a string variable and the missing values were treated as valid values and included in the summary statistics. To remedy this, the syntax shown in Box 1.9 can be used to recode place of birth from a string variable into a numeric variable.

Box 1.9 Recoding a variable into a different variable

SPSS Commands

surgery.sav – SPSS IBM Statistics Data Editor
    Transform → Recode → Into Different Variables
Recode into Different Variables
    Highlight Place of birth and click into Input Variable → Output Variable
    Enter Output Variable Name as place2,
    Enter Output Variable Label as Place of birth recoded/ Click Change
    Click Old and New Values
Recode into Different Variables: Old and New Values
    Old Value → Value=L, New Value → Value=1/Click Add
    Old Value → Value =R, New Value → Value =2/Click Add
    Old Value → Value=0, New Value → Value=3/Click Add
    Click Continue
Recode into Different Variables
    Click OK (or Paste/Run → All)

The paste command is a useful tool to provide automatic documentation of any changes that are made. The paste commands writes the recoding to a Syntax screen that can be saved or printed for documentation and future reference. Using the *Paste* command for the above recode provides the following documentation.

RECODE place ('L'=1) ('R'=2) ('O'=3) INTO place2.
VARIABLE LABELS place2 'Place of birth recoded'.
EXECUTE.

After recoding, the value labels for the three new categories of place2 that have been created can be added in the Variable View window. In this case, place of birth needs to be defined as 1 = Local, 2 = Regional and 3 = Overseas. This can be added by clicking on the Values cell and then double clicking on the grey domino box on the right of the cell to add the value labels. Similarly, gender which is also a string variable can be recoded into a numeric variable (gender2) with Male = 1 and Female = 2. After recoding variables, it is important to check that the number of decimal places is correct. This process will ensure that the number of decimal places is appropriate on the SPSS data analysis output.

1.12.3 Dialog recall

A useful function in SPSS to repeat recently conducted commands is the *Dialog Recall* button. This button recalls the most recently used SPSS commands. The *Dialog Recall* button is the fourth icon at the top left-hand side of the Data or Variable View screen or the sixth icon in the top left-hand side of the SPSS Output Viewer screen.

Using the *Dialog Recall* button to obtain *Frequencies* for place 2, which is labelled 'Place of birth recoded', the following output is produced.

Frequencies

Place of Birth Recoded

		Frequency	Per cent	Valid per cent	Cumulative per cent
Valid	Local	90	63.8	68.2	68.2
	Regional	33	23.4	25.0	93.2
	Overseas	9	6.4	6.8	100.0
	Total	132	93.6	100.0	
Missing	System	9	6.4		
Total		141	100.0		

The frequency of place of birth shown in the Frequencies table show that the recoding sequence was executed correctly. When the data are recoded as numeric, the nine babies who have missing data for birthplace are correctly omitted from the valid and cumulative percentages.

1.12.4 Displaying names or labels

There are options to change how variables are viewed when running the analyses or how to display the variable names on SPSS output. By using the command *Edit → Options → General* you can select whether variables will be displayed by their variable names or their labels in the dialog command boxes. There is also an option to select whether variables are presented in alphabetical order, in the order they are entered in the file or in measurement level. Under the command *Edit → Options → Output*, there are options to select whether the variable and variable names will be displayed as labels, values or both on the output.

1.13   Managing SPSS output

1.13.1   Formatting SPSS output

There are many output formats in SPSS. The format of the frequencies table obtained previously can easily be changed by double clicking on the table and using the commands *Format → TableLooks*. To obtain the output in the format below, which is a classical academic format with no vertical lines and minimal horizontal lines that is used by many journals, highlight *Academic* under *TableLooks*. The column widths, font and other features can also be changed using the commands *Format → Table Properties*. By clicking on the table and using the commands *Edit → Copy*, or by clicking on the table and right clicking the mouse and selecting '*Copy*', the table can be copied and pasted into a word file.

Place of birth (recoded)

		Frequency	Per cent	Valid per cent	Cumulative per cent
Valid	Local	90	63.8	68.2	68.2
	Regional	33	23.4	25.0	93.2
	Overseas	9	6.4	6.8	100.0
	Total	132	93.6	100.0	
Missing	System	9	6.4		
Total		141	100.0		

1.13.2   Exporting output and data from SPSS

Output can be saved in SPSS and printed directly from SPSS. However, output sheets can also be exported from SPSS into many different programs including Excel, Word or .pdf format using the commands shown in Box 1.10. A data file can also be exported to Excel using the *File → Save as → Save as type: Excel* commands.

Box 1.10 Exporting SPSS output into an Excel, Word, PowerPoint or PDF document

SPSS Commands

Output – SPSS IBM Statistics Viewer
　　　File → Export
Export Output

*Objects to Export: Click All, All visible or Selected to indicate part of output to export
Document: Click on Type to select output file type; File Name: enter the file name;
click Browse to select the directory to save the file*
Click OK

1.14   SPSS help commands

SPSS has two levels of extensive help commands. By using the commands *Help* → *Topics* → *Index*, the index of help topics appears in alphabetical order. By typing in a keyword, followed by enter, a topic can be displayed. At the end of the *Help* options, the next major heading is *Tutorial*, which is a step by step guide how to perform certain SPSS procedures such as 'using the data editor', 'working with output', or 'working with syntax'. There is also the 'Statistics Coach', which displays the SPSS commands to be used for some statistical tests and corresponding example outputs.

There is also another level of help that explains the meaning of the statistics shown in the output. For example, help can be obtained for the above frequencies table by doubling clicking on the left-hand mouse button to outline the table with a hatched border and then single clicking on the right-hand mouse button on any of the statistics labels. This produces a dialog box with *What's This?* at the top. Clicking on *What's This?* provides an explanation of the highlighted statistical term. Clicking on *Cumulative Percent* opens up a dialog box providing the explanation that this is 'The percentage of cases with non-missing data that have values less than or equal to a particular value'.

1.15   Golden rules for reporting numbers

Throughout this book the results are presented using the rules that are recommended for reporting statistical analyses in the literature.[5–7] Numbers are usually presented as digits except in a few special circumstances as indicated in Table 1.8. When reporting data, it is important not to imply more precision than actually exists, for example, by using too many decimal places. Results should be reported with the same number of decimal places as the measurement, and summary statistics should have no more than one extra decimal place. A summary of the rules for reporting numbers and summary statistics is shown in Table 1.8.

1.16   Notes for critical appraisal

When critically appraising statistical analyses reported in the literature, that is when applying the rules of science to assess the validity of the results from a study, it is important to ask the questions shown in Box 1.11. Results from studies in which outliers are treated inappropriately, in which the quality of the data is poor or in which an incorrect statistical test has been used are likely to be biased and to lack scientific merit. The CONSORT, which stands for Consolidated Standards of Reporting Trials

Table 1.8   Golden rules for reporting numbers

Rule	Correct expression
In a sentence, numbers less than 10 are words	In the study group, eight participants did not complete the intervention
In a sentence, numbers 10 or more are numbers	There were 120 participants in the study
Use words to express any number that begins a sentence, title or heading. Try and avoid starting a sentence with a number	Twenty per cent of participants had diabetes
Numbers that represent statistical or mathematical functions should be expressed in numbers	Raw scores were multiplied by 3 and then converted to standard scores
In a sentence, numbers below 10 that are listed with numbers 10 and above should be written as a number	In the sample, 15 boys and 4 girls had diabetes
Use a zero before the decimal point when numbers are less than 1	The P value was 0.013
Do not use a space between a number and its per cent sign	In total, 35% of participants had diabetes
Use one space between a number and its unit	The mean height of the group was 170 cm
Report percentages to only one decimal place if the sample size is larger than 100	In the sample of 212 children, 10.4% had diabetes
Report percentages with no decimal places if the sample size is less than 100	In the sample of 44 children, 11% had diabetes
Do not use percentages if the sample size is less than 20	In the sample of 18 children, 2 had diabetes
Do not imply greater precision than the measurement instrument	Only use one decimal place more than the basic unit of measurement when reporting statistics (means, medians, standard deviations, 95% confidence interval, inter-quartile ranges, etc.), for example, mean height was 143.2 cm
For ranges use 'to' or a comma but not '-' to avoid confusion with a minus sign. Also use the same number of decimal places as the summary statistic	The mean height was 162 cm (95% CI 156 to 168) The mean height was 162 cm (95% CI 156, 168) The median was 0.5 mm (inter-quartile range −0.1 to 0.7) The range of height was 145–170 cm
P values >0.05 should be reported with two decimal places	There was no significant difference between groups ($P = 0.35$)
P values between 0.001 and 0.05 should be reported to three decimal places	There was a significant difference in blood pressure between the two groups ($t = 3.0$, $df = 45$, $P = 0.004$)
P values shown on output as 0.000 should be reported as <0.0001	Children with diabetes had significantly lower levels of insulin than control children without diabetes ($t = 5.47$, $df = 78$, $P < 0.0001$)

developed by the CONSORT Group also provides a useful checklist to determine whether appropriate study information for a randomized controlled trial (RCT) has been reported (see http://www.consort-statement.org/home/).

Box 1.11 Questions for critical appraisal

Answers to the following questions are useful for checking the integrity of statistical analyses:

- Have details of the methods and statistical packages used to analyse the data been reported?
- Are the variables classified correctly as outcome and explanatory variables?
- Are any intervening or alternative outcome variables mistakenly treated as explanatory variables?
- Are missing values and outliers treated appropriately?
- Is the sample size large enough to avoid type II errors?

References

1. Tabachnick BG, Fidell LS. *Using multivariate statistics*, 4th edn. Allyn and Bacon: Boston, MA, 2001.
2. Peat JK, Mellis CM, Williams K, Xuan W. *Health science research. A handbook of quantitative methods*. Allen and Unwin: Crows Nest, Australia, 2001.
3. Bell ML, Fairclough DL. Practical and statistical issues in missing data for longitudinal patient reported outcomes. *Stat Methods Med Res*. Published online before print February 19, 2013, doi: 10.1177/0962280213476378.
4. Fairclough DL. *Design and analysis of quality of life studies in clinical trials*, 2nd edn. Chapman & Hall/CRC: Boca Raton, FL, 2010.
5. Stevens J. *Applied multivariate statistics for the social sciences*, 3rd edn. Lawrence Erlbaum Associates: Mahwah, NJ, 1996.
6. Peat JK, Elliott E, Baur L, Keena V. *Scientific writing: easy when you know how*. BMJ Books: London, 2002.
7. Lang TA, Secic M. *How to report statistics*. American College of Physicians: Philadelphia, PA, 1977.

CHAPTER 2
Descriptive statistics

It is wonderful to be in on the creation of something, see it used, and then walk away and smile at it.

LADY BIRD JOHNSON, U.S. FIRST LADY

Objectives

The objectives of this chapter are to explain how to:
- assess whether a continuous variable has a normal distribution
- decide whether to use a parametric or non-parametric test
- present summary statistics for continuous variables
- decide whether parametric tests have been used appropriately in the literature

---

Before beginning the statistical analyses of a continuous variable, it is essential to examine the distribution of the variable for skewness (symmetry), kurtosis (peakedness), spread (range of the values) and outliers (data values that are extreme compared to the rest of the data). If a variable has significant skewness or kurtosis or has univariate outliers, or any combination of these, it will not be normally distributed, that is, the distribution histogram will not conform to a bell shape. Information about each of these characteristics determines whether parametric or non-parametric tests need to be used and ensures that the results of the statistical analyses can be accurately explained and interpreted. A description of the characteristics of the sample also allows other researchers to judge the generalizability of the results. A typical pathway for beginning the statistical analysis of continuous data variables is shown in Box 2.1.

Box 2.1 Data analysis pathway for continuous variables

The pathway for conducting the data analysis of continuous variables is as follows:
- check the range (minimum and maximum values) of each variable
- check for the presence and pattern of any missing data
- check for the presence of univariate/multivariate outliers: deal with outliers
- conduct checks of normality

Medical Statistics: A Guide to SPSS, Data Analysis and Critical Appraisal, Second Edition.
Belinda Barton and Jennifer Peat.
© 2014 John Wiley & Sons, Ltd. Published 2014 by John Wiley & Sons, Ltd.
Companion website: www.wiley.com/go/barton/medicalstatistics2e

- transform variables with non-normal distributions or recode into categorical variables, for example, quartiles or quintiles
- rerun distribution checks for transformed variables
- document all steps in the study handbook

2.1 Parametric and non-parametric statistics

Statistical tests can be either parametric or non-parametric. Parametric tests assume that the continuous variable being analysed has a normal distribution in the population. To check this assumption, the distribution of the variable for a sample, which is an estimate of the population, must be examined. In general, parametric tests can be used if a continuous variable is normally distributed variable. Other assumptions that may also be specific to a parametric test must also be checked before analysis.

In general, parametric tests are preferable to non-parametric tests because a larger variety of tests are available and, as long as the sample size is not very small, they provide approximately 5% more power than non-parametric rank tests to show a statistically significant difference between groups.[1] For non-parametric tests or distribution free tests no assumptions are made about the distribution of data. Results from non-parametric tests can be a challenge to present in a clear and meaningful way because summary statistics such as ranks are not intuitive to interpret as are the summary statistics from parametric tests. Summary statistics from parametric tests such as the mean (average value of the sample) and standard deviation are always more readily understood and more easily communicated than the equivalent median (a data value which half of the highest values lie above and half of the lowest values lie below), inter-quartile range or the rank statistics from non-parametric tests.

2.2 Normal distribution

A normal distribution such as the distribution shown in Figure 2.1 is classically a bell-shaped curve that is bilaterally symmetrical. If a variable is normally distributed, then the mean and the median values will be approximately equal. A standard normal distribution has a mean value equal to 0 and a standard deviation equal to 1. A standard deviation is a measure of spread or dispersion from the mean value. The larger the standard deviation, the more dispersion or variability there is within the sample.

If a normal distribution is divided into quartiles, that is, four equal parts, the exact position of the cut-off values for the quartiles is at 0.68 standard deviation above and below the mean. Other features of a normal distribution are that the area of one standard deviation on either side of the mean as shown in Figure 2.1 contains 68% of the values in the sample and the area of 1.96 standard deviations on either side of the mean contains 95% of the values. These properties of a normal distribution are critical for understanding and interpreting the output from parametric tests.

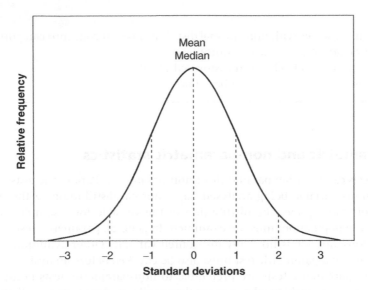

Figure 2.1 Characteristics of a normal distribution.

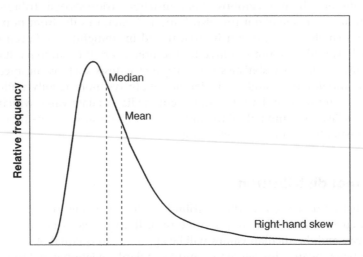

Figure 2.2 Characteristics of a skewed distribution.

2.3 Skewed distributions

If a variable has a skewed distribution, the mean will be a biased estimate of the centre of the data as shown in Figure 2.2. A variable that has a classically skewed distribution is length of stay in hospital because many patients have a short stay and few patients have a very long stay. When a variable has a skewed distribution, it can be difficult to predict where the centre of the data lies or the range in which the majority of data values fall.

For a variable that has a positively skewed distribution with a tail to the right, the mean will usually be larger than the median as shown in Figure 2.2. For a variable with a negatively skewed distribution with a tail to the left, the mean will usually be lower than the median because the distribution will be a mirror image of the curve shown in Figure 2.2. These features of non-normal distributions are helpful in estimating the direction of bias in critical appraisal of studies in which the distribution of the variable has not been taken into account when selecting the statistical tests.

Typically, the median and inter-quartile range are used to describe data that are skewed or data from very small sample sizes. The data of the distribution is divided into four sections or quartiles. The median is the second quartile, with 50% of the measurements having a larger value than this point and 50% of the measurements having a smaller value than this point. The lower bound for the inter-quartile range is the first quartile, where 25% of the measurements are below this point. The upper bound for the inter-quartile range is the third quartile, where 75% of the measurements are below this point. Therefore, the inter-quartile range is the range or distance between the first and third quartile.

Exploratory analyses

The file **surgery.sav** contains data from 141 babies who were referred to a paediatric hospital for surgery. The distributions of three continuous variables in the data set, that is, birth weight, gestational age and length of stay can be examined using the commands shown in Box 2.2.

Box 2.2 SPSS commands to obtain descriptive statistics and plots

SPSS Commands

surgery – SPSS IBM Statistics Data Editor
    Analyze → Descriptive Statistics → Explore
Explore
    Highlight variables Birth weight, Gestational age, and Length of stay and click into
        Dependent List
    Display: tick Both (default)
    Click on Statistics
Explore: Statistics
    Click on Descriptives (default), Confidence Interval for Mean: 95% (default)
    Click on Outliers
    Click Continue
Explore
    Click on Plots
Explore: Plots
    Boxplots – select Factor levels together (default)

> *Descriptive – untick Stem and leaf (default), tick Histogram and tick Normality plots*
>   *with tests*
>   *Click Continue*
> *Explore*
>   *Click on Options*
> *Explore: Options*
>   *Missing values – tick Exclude cases pairwise, Click Continue*
> *Explore*
>   *Click OK*

In the Options menu in Box 2.2, *Exclude cases pairwise* is selected. This option provides information about each variable independently of missing values in the other variables and is the option that is used to describe the entire sample. The default setting for Options is *Exclude cases listwise* but this will exclude a case from the data analysis if there are missing data for any one of the variables entered into the *Dependent List*. The option *Exclude cases listwise* for the data set **surgery.sav** shows that there are 126 babies with complete information for all three continuous variables and 15 babies with missing information for one or more of the three variables. Multivariate statistics refers to the analysis of multiple variables at the same time. Therefore, the information for these 126 babies would be important for describing the sample if multivariate statistics that only include babies without missing data are planned. The characteristics of these 126 babies would be used to describe the generalizability of a multivariate model but not the generalizability of the sample.

The Case Processing Summary table with the *Exclude cases pairwise* option shows that two of the 141 babies have missing birth weights, eight babies have missing gestational age and nine babies have missing length of stay data. This information is important if bivariate statistics (when only two variables are analysed at the same time) will be used in which as many cases as possible are included. The Descriptives table shows the summary statistics for each variable. In the table, all statistics are in the same units as the original variables, that is, grams for birth weight, weeks for gestational age and days for length of stay. The exceptions are the variance, which is in squared units, and the skewness and kurtosis values, which are in units that are relative to a normal distribution.

Case Processing Summary

	Cases					
	Valid		Missing		Total	
	N	Per cent	*N*	Per cent	*N*	Per cent
Birth weight	139	98.6	2	1.4	141	100.0
Gestational age	133	94.3	8	5.7	141	100.0
Length of stay	132	93.6	9	6.4	141	100.0

Descriptives

			Statistic	Std. error
Birth weight	Mean		2463.99	43.650
	95% confidence interval for mean	Lower bound	2377.68	
		Upper bound	2550.30	
	5% trimmed mean		2452.53	
	Median		2425.00	
	Variance		264,845.695	
	Std. deviation		514.632	
	Minimum		1150	
	Maximum		3900	
	Range		2750	
	Inter-quartile range		755	
	Skewness		0.336	0.206
	Kurtosis		−0.323	0.408
Gestational age	Mean		36.564	0.1776
	95% confidence interval for mean	Lower bound	36.213	
		Upper bound	36.915	
	5% trimmed mean		36.659	
	Median		37.000	
	Variance		4.195	
	Std. deviation		2.0481	
	Minimum		30.0	
	Maximum		41.0	
	Range		11.0	
	Inter-quartile range		2.0	
	Skewness		−0.590	0.210
	Kurtosis		0.862	0.417
Length of stay	Mean		38.05	3.114
	95% confidence interval for mean	Lower bound	31.89	
		Upper bound	44.21	
	5% trimmed mean		32.79	
	Median		27.00	
	Variance		1280.249	
	Std. deviation		35.781	
	Minimum		0	
	Maximum		244	
	Range		244	
	Inter-quartile range		22	
	Skewness		3.212	0.211
	Kurtosis		12.675	0.419

2.4   Checking for normality

There are several ways of checking whether a continuous variable is normally distributed. Many measurements such as height, weight and blood pressure may be normally distributed in the community but may not be normally distributed if the study has a selected sample or a small sample size. In practice, several checks of normality need

Table 2.1 Comparisons between mean and median values

Variable	Mean − median	Per cent difference	Interpretation
Birth weight	2464.0 − 2425.0 = 39.0 g	1.5%	Values almost identical, suggesting a normal distribution
Gestational age	36.6 − 37.0 = −0.4 month	1.1%	Values almost identical, suggesting a normal distribution
Length of stay	38.1 − 27.0 = 11.1 days	29.1%	Discordant values, with the mean higher than the median indicating skewness to the right

to be undertaken to obtain a good understanding of the shape of the distribution of each variable in the study sample. It is also important to identify the position of any outliers to gain an understanding of how they may influence the results of any statistical analyses.

The proximity of the mean to the median can indicate possible skewness. A quick informal check of normality is to examine whether the mean and the median values are close to one another. From the Descriptives table, the differences between the median and the mean can be summarized as shown in Table 2.1. The percent difference is calculated as the difference between the mean and the median as a percentage of the mean.

In Table 2.1, the differences between the mean and median values of birth weight and gestational age are small, thereby suggesting a normal distribution but the large difference between the mean and median values for length of stay suggests that this variable has a non-normal distribution.

2.4.1 Using the standard deviation to check for normality

An inherent feature of a normal distribution is that 95% of the data values lie between −1.96 standard deviation and +1.96 standard deviations from the mean as shown in Figure 2.1. That is, most data values should lie in the area that is approximately two standard deviations above and below the mean. A good approximate check for normality is to double the standard deviation of the variable and then subtract and also add this amount to the mean value. This will give an estimated range in which 95% of the values should lie. The estimated range should be slightly within the actual range of data values, that is the minimum and maximum values. The estimated 95% range for each variable is shown in Table 2.2.

For birth weight and gestational age, the estimated 95% range is within or close to the minimum and maximum values from the Descriptives table. However, for length of stay, the estimated 95% range is not a good approximation of the actual range. The estimated lower value is invalid because it is negative and the estimated upper value is significantly below the maximum value. This is a classical indication of a skewed distribution. If the two estimated values are lower than the actual minimum and maximum values, as in this case, the distribution is usually skewed to the right, indicating positive skewness. If the two estimated values are much higher than the actual minimum and maximum values, the distribution is usually skewed to the left indicating negative skewness.

Table 2.2 Calculation of 95% range of variables

Variable	Calculation of range (mean ± 2 SD)	Estimated 95% range	Minimum and maximum values
Birth weight	2464 ± (2 × 514.6)	1434 to 3493	1150 to 3900
Gestational age	36.6 ± (2 × 2.0)	32.6 to 40.6	30.0 to 41.0
Length of stay	38.1 ± (2 × 35.8)	−33.5 to 109.7	0 to 244

A rule of thumb is that a variable with a standard deviation that is larger than one half of the mean value is non-normally distributed, assuming that negative values are impossible.[2] Thus, the mean length of stay of 38.1 days with a standard deviation almost equal to its mean value is an immediate alert to evidence of non-normality.

2.4.2 Skewness

Further information about the distribution of the variable can be obtained from the skewness and kurtosis statistics in the Descriptives table. A perfectly standard normal distribution has skewness and kurtosis values equal to zero. Skewness values that are positive indicate a tail to the right and skewness values that are negative indicate a tail to the left. Values between −1 and +1 indicate an approximate bell-shaped curve and values from −1 to −3 or from +1 to +3 indicate that the distribution is tending away from a bell shape with >1 indicating moderate skewness and >2 indicating severe skewness. Any values above +3 or below −3 are a good indication that the variable is not normally distributed.

The Descriptives table shows that the skewness values for birth weight and gestational age are between −1 and +1 suggesting that the distributions of these variables are within the limits of a normal distribution. However, the high skewness value of 3.212 for length of stay confirms a non-normal distribution with a tail to the right.

2.4.3 Kurtosis

A kurtosis value above 1 indicates that the distribution tends to be peaked and a value below 1 indicates that the distribution tends to be flat. As for skewness, a kurtosis value between −1 and +1 indicates normality and a value between −1 and −3 or between +1 and +3 indicates a tendency away from normality. Values below −3 or above +3 strongly indicate non-normality. For birth weight and gestational age, the kurtosis values are small and are not a cause for concern. However, for length of stay the kurtosis value is 12.675, which indicates that the distribution is peaked in a way that is not consistent with a bell-shaped distribution.

2.4.4 Critical values

Further tests of normality are to divide skewness and kurtosis values by their standard errors as shown in Table 2.3. In practice, dividing a value by its standard error produces

Table 2.3 Using skewness and kurtosis statistics to test for a normal distribution

	Skewness (SE)	Critical value (skewness/SE)	Kurtosis (SE)	Critical value (kurtosis/SE)
Birth weight	0.336 (0.206)	1.63	−0.323 (0.408)	−0.79
Gestational age	−0.590 (0.210)	−2.81	0.862 (0.417)	2.07
Length of stay	3.212 (0.211)	15.22	12.675 (0.419)	30.25

a critical value that can be used to judge probability. A critical value that is outside the range of −1.96 to +1.96 indicates that a variable is not normally distributed. The critical values in Table 2.3 suggest that birth weight has a normal distribution with critical values for both skewness and kurtosis within the critical range of ±1.96 and gestational age is deviating from a normal distribution with values outside the critical range. Length of stay is not normally distributed with large critical values of 15.22 and 30.25.

Extreme Values

			Case number	Value
Birth weight	Highest	1	5	3900
		2	54	3545
		3	16	3500
		4	50	3500
		5	141	3500
	Lowest	1	4	1150
		2	103	1500
		3	120	1620
		4	98	1680
		5	38	1710
Gestational age	Highest	1	85	41.0
		2	11	40.0
		3	26	40.0
		4	50	40.0
		5	52	40.0[a]
	Lowest	1	2	30.0
		2	79	31.0
		3	38	31.0
		4	4	31.0
		5	117	31.5
Length of stay	Highest	1	121	244
		2	120	211
		3	110	153
		4	129	138
		5	116	131
	Lowest	1	32	0
		2	33	1
		3	12	9
		4	22	11
		5	16	11

[a]Only a partial list of cases with the value 40.0 are shown in the table of upper extremes.

2.4.5 *Extreme values*

By requesting outliers as shown in Box 2.2, the five largest and five smallest values of each variable and the corresponding case numbers or data base rows are obtained and are shown in the Extreme Values table. It is important to identify outliers and extreme values that cause skewness. However, the values in the Extreme Values table are the minimum and maximum values in the data set and these may not be influential outliers.

2.4.6 *Outliers*

Outliers are data values that are extreme when compared to the other values in the data set. There are two types of outliers: univariate outliers and multivariate outliers. A univariate outlier is a data point that is very different to the rest of the data for one variable. An outlier is measured by its distance from the remainder of the data in units of the standard deviation, which is a standardized measure of the spread of the data. For example, an IQ score of 150 would be a univariate outlier because the mean IQ of the population is 100 with a standard deviation of 15. Thus, an IQ score of 150 is 3.3 standard deviations away from the mean, whereas the next closest value may be only 2 standard deviations away from the mean resulting in a significant gap between the two data points.

A multivariate outlier is a case that is an extreme value on a combination of variables. For example, a boy aged 8 years with a height of 155 cm and a weight of 45 kg is very unusual and would be a multivariate outlier. It is important to identify values that are univariate and/or multivariate outliers because they can have a substantial influence on the distribution and mean of the variable and can influence the results of analyses and thus the interpretation of the findings.

Univariate outliers are easier to identify than multivariate outliers. For a continuously distributed variable with a normal distribution, about 99% of scores are expected to lie within three standard deviations above and below the mean value. Data points outside this range are classified as univariate outliers. Sometimes a case, that is, a univariate outlier for one variable will also be a univariate outlier for another variable. Potentially, these cases may be multivariate outliers. Multivariate outliers can be detected by inspecting the residuals around a model or by using statistics called leverage values or Cook's distances, which are discussed in Chapter 5, or Mahalanobis distances, which are discussed in Chapter 7.

There are many reasons why outliers occur. Outliers may be errors in data recording, incorrect data entry values that can be corrected, or genuine values. When outliers are from participants from another population with different characteristics to the intended sample, they are called contaminants. This happens, for example, when a participant with a well-defined illness is inadvertently included as a healthy participant. Occasionally, outliers can be excluded from the data analyses if they are contaminants or biologically implausible values. However, deleting values simply because they are outliers is usually unacceptable and it is preferable to find a way to accommodate the values without causing undue bias in the analyses.

The methods for dealing with outliers are summarized in Table 2.4. Identifying and dealing with outliers is discussed further throughout this book. It is important that the methods used to accommodate outliers are reported so that the generalizability of the results is clear.

Table 2.4   Methods for dealing with outliers

Method	Outcome
Exclude	Subjective judgement that reduces the generalizability of the results
Code closer to data	Reduces influence while maintaining the full data set
Transform the data	A transformation, for example, taking logarithms, may reduce outliers
Retain	Use non-parametric analyses

2.4.7   Statistical tests of normality

By requesting normality plots in *Analyze* → *Descriptive Statistics* → *Explore* (Box 2.2), the following tests of normality are obtained:

Tests of Normality

	Kolmogorov–Smirnov[a]			Shapiro–Wilk		
	Statistic	df	Sig.	Statistic	df	Sig.
Birth weight	0.067	139	0.200*	0.981	139	0.056
Gestational age	0.151	133	0.000	0.951	133	0.000
Length of stay	0.241	132	0.000	0.643	132	0.000

*This is a lower bound of the true significance.
[a]Lilliefors significance correction.

The Tests of Normality table provides the results of two tests: a Kolmogorov–Smirnov statistic with a Lilliefors significance correction and a Shapiro–Wilk statistic. A limitation of the Kolmogorov–Smirnov test of normality without the Lilliefors correction is that it is very conservative and is sensitive to extreme values that cause tails in the distribution. The Lilliefors significance correction makes this test a little less conservative. The Shapiro–Wilk test has more statistical power to detect a non-normal distribution than the Kolmogorov–Smirnov test.[3] The Shapiro–Wilk test is often used when the sample size is less than 50 but can also be used with larger sample sizes. The Shapiro–Wilk test is based on the correlation between the data and the corresponding normal scores. The values of the Shapiro–Wilk statistic range between zero, which indicates non-normality of the data and a value of one which indicates normality.

A distribution that passes these tests of normality provides extreme confidence that parametric tests can be used. However, variables that do not pass these tests may not be so non-normally distributed that parametric tests cannot be used, especially if the sample size is large. This is not to say that the results of these tests can be ignored but rather that a considered decision using the results of all the available checks of normality needs to be made.

For both the Shapiro–Wilk and Kolmogorov–Smirnov tests, a *P* value less than 0.05 provides evidence that the distribution is significantly different from normal. The *P* values are shown in the column labelled Sig. in the Tests of Normality table. Birth weight marginally fails the Shapiro–Wilk test but the *P* values for gestational age and length of stay show that they have potentially non-normal distributions. The Kolmogorov–Smirnov test shows that the distribution of birth weight is not significantly different from a normal distribution with a P value greater than 0.2. However, the Kolmogorov–Smirnov test indicates that the distributions of both gestational age and length of stay are significantly different from a normal distribution at $P < 0.0001$.

These tests of normality do not provide any information about why a variable is not normally distributed and therefore, it is always important to obtain skewness and kurtosis values using *Analyze → Descriptive Statistics → Explore* and to request plots in order to visually inspect the distribution of data and identify any reasons for non-normality.

2.4.8 Histograms and plots

A histogram shows the frequency of measurements and the shape of the data and therefore provides a visual judgement of whether the distribution approximates to a bell shape. Histograms also show whether there are any gaps in the data which is common in small data sets, whether there are any outlying values and how far any outlying values are from the remainder of the data.

The normal Q–Q plot shows each data value plotted against the value that would be expected if the data came from a normal distribution. The values in the plot are the quantiles of the variable distribution plotted against the quantiles that would be expected if the distribution was normal. If the variable was normally distributed, the points would fall directly on the straight line. Any deviations from the straight line indicate some degree of non-normality.

The detrended normal Q–Q plots show the deviations of the points from the straight line of the normal Q–Q plot. If the distribution is normal, the points will cluster randomly around the horizontal line at zero with an equal spread of points above and below the line. If the distribution is non-normal, the points will be in a pattern such as J or an inverted U distribution and the horizontal line may not be in the centre of the data.

The box plot shows the median as the black horizontal line inside the box and the inter-quartile range as the length of the box. The inter-quartile range indicates the 25th to 75th percentiles, that is, the range in which the central 25–75% (50%) of the data points lie. The whiskers are the lines extending from the top and bottom of the box. The whiskers represent the minimum and maximum values when they are within 1.5 times above or below the inter-quartile range. If values are outside this range, they are plotted as outlying values (circles) or extreme values (asterisks).

Any outlying values that are between 1.5 and 3 box lengths from the upper or lower edge of the box are shown as open circles, and are identified with the corresponding number of the data base row. Extreme values that are more than three box lengths from the upper or lower edge of the box are shown as asterisks. Extreme and/or outlying values should be checked to see whether they are univariate outliers. If there are several extreme values at either end of the range of the data or the median is not in the centre of the box, the variable will not be normally distributed. If the median is closer to the bottom end of the box than to the top, the data are positively skewed. If the median is closer to the top end of the box, the data are negatively skewed.

Finally, from the commands in Box 2.2, descriptive and normality plots were requested for each variable. All of the plots should be inspected because each plot provides different information. In Figure 2.3 the histogram for birth weight shows that this distribution is not strictly bell shaped but the normal Q–Q plot follows an approximately normal distribution apart from the tails, and the box plot is symmetrical with no outlying or extreme values. These features indicate that the mean value will be an accurate estimate of the centre of the data and that the standard deviation will accurately describe the spread.

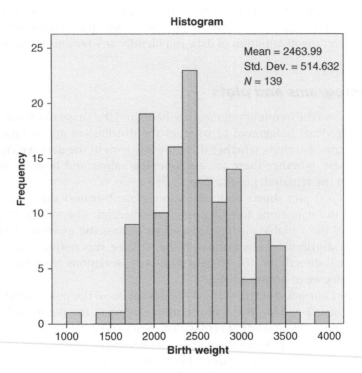

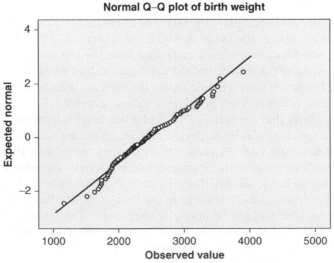

Figure 2.3 Histogram and plots of birth weight.

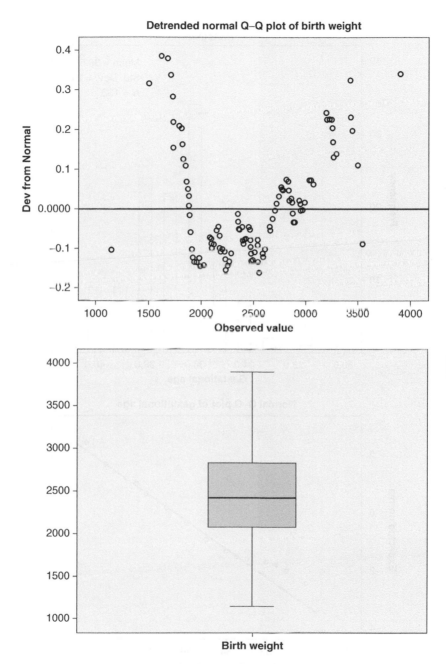

Figure 2.3 (*continued*)

In Figure 2.4 the histogram for gestational age shows that this distribution has a small tail to the left and only deviates from normal at the lower end of the normal Q–Q plot. The box plot for this variable appears to be symmetrical but has a few outlying values at the lower end of the data values.

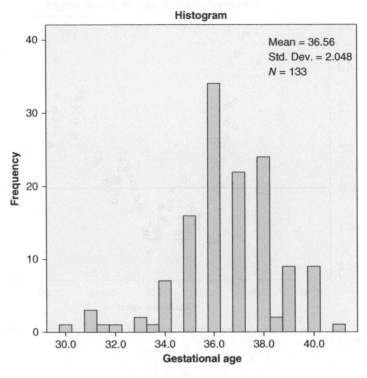

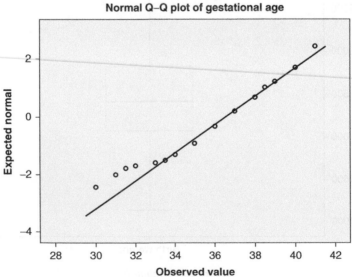

Figure 2.4 Histogram and plots of gestational age.

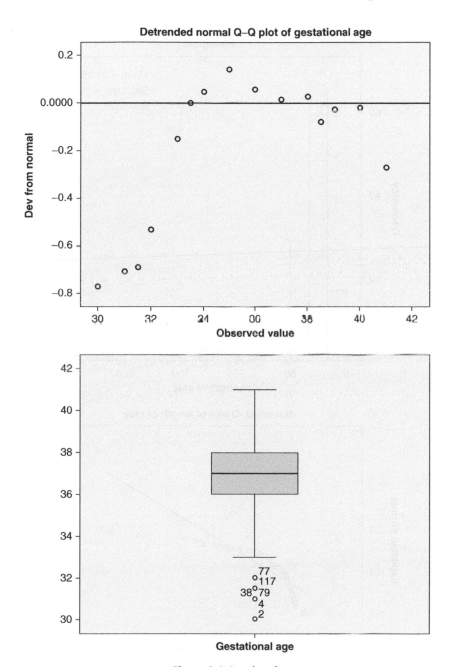

Figure 2.4 (*continued*)

In contrast, in Figure 2.5 the histogram for length of stay has a marked tail to the right so that the distribution deviates markedly from a straight line on the normal Q–Q plot. On the detrended normal Q–Q plot, the pattern is similar to a U shape. The box plot shows some outlying values and many extreme values at the upper end of the distribution. The outliers and/or extreme values can be identified by their ID or case number.

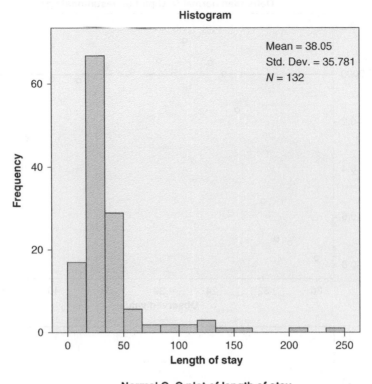

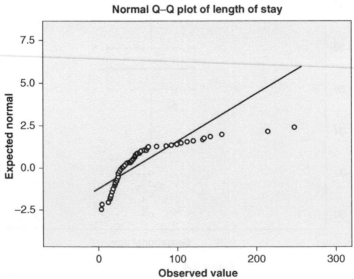

Figure 2.5 Histogram and plots of length of stay.

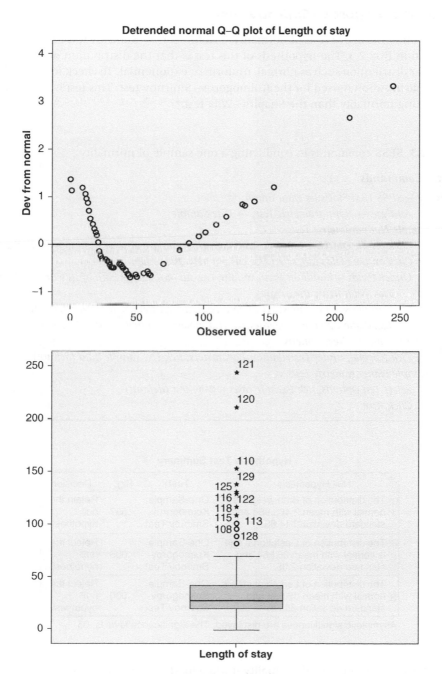

Figure 2.5 (*continued*)

2.4.9 Kolmogorov–Smirnov test

In addition to the above tests of normality, a Kolmogorov–Smirnov test can be obtained as shown in Box 2.3. The hypothesis of this test is that the distribution of the data is a particular distribution such as normal, uniform or exponential. To check for normality, a normal distribution is used for the Kolmogorov–Smirnov test. This test is less powerful in detecting normality than the Shapiro–Wilk test.[4]

Box 2.3 SPSS commands to conducting a one sample of normality

SPSS Commands

surgery – SPSS IBM Statistics Data Editor
    Analyze → Nonparametric Tests → One Sample
One-Sample Nonparametric Tests
    Click on the Objective tab, tick Automatically compare observe data to hypothesized
    Click on the Fields tab, select Use custom field assignments
    Under Fields – highlight Birth weight, Gestational age, Length of stay and click into
        Test Fields using the arrow
    Click on the Settings tab, select Choose Tests, tick Customize tests, tick Test observed
        distribution against hypothesized (Kolmogorov-Smirnov test), click on Options
Kolmogorov-Smirnov Test Options
    Tick Normal, under Distribution Parameters, tick Use sample data (default), click OK
One-Sample Nonparametric Tests
    Select Test Options, tick Exclude cases test-by-test (default)
    Click Run

Hypothesis Test Summary

	Null Hypothesis	Test	Sig.	Decision
1	The distribution of Birth weight is normal with mean 2,463.986 and standard deviation 514.63.	One-Sample Kolmogorov-Smirnov Test	.557	Retain the null hypothesis.
2	The distribution of Gestational age is normal with mean 36.564 and standard deviation 2.05.	One-Sample Kolmogorov-Smirnov Test	.005	Reject the null hypothesis.
3	The distribution of Length of stay is normal with mean 38.053 and standard deviation 35.78.	One-Sample Kolmogorov-Smirnov Test	.000	Reject the null hypothesis.

Asymptotic significances are displayed. The significance level is .05.

The P values for the test of normality in the One-Sample Kolmogorov–Smirnov Test table are different from Kolmogorov–Smirnov P values obtained in *Analyze → Descriptive Statistics → Explore* because the one-sample test shown here is without the Lilliefors correction. Without the correction applied this test, which is based on slightly different assumptions about the mean and the variance of the normal distribution being tested for fit, is extremely conservative. Once again, the P values suggest that birth weight is

Table 2.5 Summary of whether descriptive statistics and plots indicate a normal distribution

	Mean − median	Mean ± 2 SD	Skewness and kurtosis	Critical values	K–S test	Plots	Overall decision
Birth weight	Probably	Yes	Yes	Yes	Yes	Probably	Yes
Gestational age	Yes	Yes	Yes	No	No	Probably	Yes
Length of stay	No	No	No	No	No	No	No

normally distributed ($P = 0.557$) but gestational age and length of stay have P values that are statistically significant at less than 0.05 providing evidence that these variables do not have a normal distribution.

2.4.10 Deciding whether a variable is normally distributed

The information from the descriptive statistics and normality plots can be summarized as shown in Table 2.5. In this table, 'Yes' indicates that the check for normality provides evidence that the data follows an approximately normal distribution and 'No' indicates that the check for normality provides evidence that the data does not have a normal distribution.

Clearly, the results of tests of normality are not always in agreement. By considering all of the information together, a decision can be made about whether the distribution of each variable is approximately normal to justify using parametric tests or whether the deviation from normal is so marked that non-parametric or categorical tests need to be used. These decisions, which sometimes involve subjective judgements, should be based on all processes of checking for normality.

Table 2.5 shows that parametric tests are appropriate for analysing birth weight because of checks of normality provide very strong evidence that this variable is normally distributed. The variable gestational age is approximately normally distributed with some indications of a small deviation. However, the mean value is a good estimate of the centre of the data. Parametric tests are robust to some deviations from normality if the sample size is large, say greater than 100 as is this sample. If the sample size had been small, say less than 30, then this variable would have to be perfectly normally distributed rather than approximately normally distributed before parametric tests could be used.

Length of stay is clearly not normally distributed and therefore this variable needs to be either transformed to normality to use parametric tests, analysed using non-parametric tests or transformed to a categorical variable. There are a number of factors to consider in deciding whether a variable should be transformed. Parametric tests generally provide more statistical power than non-parametric tests. However, if a parametric test does not have a non-parametric equivalent then transformation is essential.

2.5 Transforming skewed variables

Transformation of a variable may allow parametric statistics to be used if the transformed variable follows a normal distribution. However, difficulties arise sometimes in interpreting the results because few people think naturally in transformed units. For example, if length of stay is transformed by calculating its square root, the results of parametric tests will be presented in units of the square root of length of stay and will be more difficult to interpret and to compare with results from other studies.

Various mathematical formulae can be used to transform a skewed distribution to normality. When a distribution has a marked tail to the right-hand side, a logarithmic transformation of scores is often effective.[5] The advantage of logarithmic transformations is that they provide interpretable results after being back transformed into original units.[6] Other common transformations include square roots and reciprocals.[7] When data are transformed and differences in transformed mean values between two or more groups are compared, the summary statistics will not apply to the means of the original data but will apply to the medians of the original data.[6]

Length of stay can be transformed to logarithmic values using the commands shown in Box 2.4. The transformation *LG10* can be clicked in from the Functions box and the variable can be clicked in from the variable list. Either base e or base 10 logarithms can be used but base 10 logarithms are a little more intuitive in that $0 = 1$ (10°), $1 = 10$ (10^{1}), $2 = 100$ (10^{2}), and so on and are therefore a little easier to interpret and communicate. Since logarithm functions are defined only for values greater than zero, any values that are zero in the data set will naturally be declared as invalid and registered as missing values in the transformed variable.

Box 2.4 SPSS commands for computing a new variable

SPSS Commands

surgery – SPSS IBM Statistics Data Editor
    Transform → Compute Variable
Compute Variable
    Target Variable = LOS2
    Select Arithmetic for Function group and Select Lg10 for Functions and Special Variables
    Click on the arrow located to the left hand side of Functions and Special Variables to enter LG10 as Numeric Expression
    Click Length of stay into Numeric Expression using the arrow to insert between the brackets so LG10(lengthst)
    Click OK

On completion of the logarithmic transformation, an error message will appear in the output viewer of SPSS specifying any case numbers that have been set to system missing. In this data set, case 32 has a value of zero for length of stay and has been transformed to a system missing value for logarithmic length of stay. To ensure that all cases are included, for cases that have zero or negative values, a constant can be added to each value to ensure that the logarithmic transformation can be undertaken.[8] For example, if the minimum value is −2.2, then a constant of 3 can be added to all values. This value can be subtracted again when the summary statistics are transformed back to original units.

Whenever a new variable is created, it should be labelled and its format adjusted. The log-transformed length of stay can be reassigned in Variable View by adding a label 'Log length of stay' to ensure that the output is self-documented. In addition, the number of decimal places can be adjusted to an appropriate number, in this case three and Measure can be changed to Scale. Once a newly transformed variable is obtained, its distribution must be checked again using the *Analyze → Descriptive Statistics → Explore* commands shown in Box 2.2, which will provide the following output.

Explore

Case Processing Summary

	Cases					
	Valid		Missing		Total	
	N	Per cent	N	Per cent	N	Per cent
Log length of stay	131	92.9	10	7.1	141	100.0

The Case Processing Summary table shows that there are now 131 valid cases for log-transformed length of stay compared with 132 valid cases for length of stay because case 32, which had a zero value, could not be transformed and has been assigned a system missing value.

Descriptives

			Statistic	Std. Error
Log length of stay	Mean		1.47250	0.026227
	95% confidence interval for mean	Lower bound	1.42061	
		Upper bound	1.52439	
	5% trimmed mean		1.46440	
	Median		1.43136	
	Variance		0.090	
	Std. deviation		0.300183	
	Minimum		0.000	
	Maximum		2.387	
	Range		2.387	
	Inter-quartile range		0.301	
	Skewness		−0.110	0.212
	Kurtosis		4.474	0.420

The Descriptives table shows that mean log length of stay is 1.4725 and the median value is 1.4314. The two values are only 0.0411 units apart, which suggests that the distribution is now much closer to being normally distributed. Also, the skewness value is now closer to zero, indicating no significant skewness. The kurtosis value of 4.474 indicates that the distribution remains peaked, although not as markedly as before. The values for two standard deviations below and above the mean value, that is, $1.4725 \pm (2 \times 0.3)$ or 0.87 and 2.07, respectively, are much closer to the minimum and maximum values of 0 and 2.39 for the variable.

Following transformation, the extreme values should be the same because the same data points are still the extreme points. However, since case 32 was not transformed and was replaced with a system missing value, this case is now not listed as a lowest extreme value and the next extreme value, case 28 has been listed.

Extreme Values

			Case number	Value
Log length of stay	Highest	1	121	2.387
		2	120	2.324
		3	110	2.185
		4	129	2.140
		5	116	2.117
	Lowest	1	33	0.000
		2	12	0.954
		3	22	1.041
		4	16	1.041
		5	28	1.079

Dividing skewness by its standard error, that is, $-0.110/0.212$, gives the critical value of -0.52, indicating a normal distribution. However, dividing the kurtosis by its standard error, that is, $4.474/0.42$, gives the critical value of 10.65, confirming that the distribution remains too peaked to conform to normality. In practice, peakness is not as important as skewness for deciding when to use parametric tests because deviations in kurtosis do not bias mean values.

Tests of Normality

	Kolmogorov–Smirnov[a]			Shapiro–Wilk		
	Statistic	df	Sig.	Statistic	df	Sig.
Log length of stay	0.097	131	0.004	0.916	131	0.000

[a]Lilliefors significance correction.

In the Tests of Normality table, the results of the Kolmogorov–Smirnov and Shapiro–Wilk tests indicate that the distribution remains significantly different from a normal distribution at $P = 0.004$ and $P < 0.0001$, respectively.

The histogram for the log-transformed variable shown in Figure 2.6 conforms to a bell-shaped distribution better than the original variable except for some outlying values in both tails and a gap in the data on the left. Such gaps are a common feature of data distributions when the sample size is small but they need to be investigated when the sample size is large as in this case. The lowest extreme value for log length of stay is a univariate outlier. Although log length of stay is not perfectly normally distributed, it will provide less biased P values than the original variable if parametric tests are used.

2.5.1 Back transformation

Care must be taken when transforming summary statistics in log units back into their original units.[6] In general, it is best to carry out all statistical tests using the transformed scale and only transform summary statistics back into original units in the final presentation of the results. Thus, the interpretation of the statistics should be undertaken using summary statistics of the transformed variable. When a logarithmic mean is anti-logged it is called a geometric mean. The standard deviation (spread)

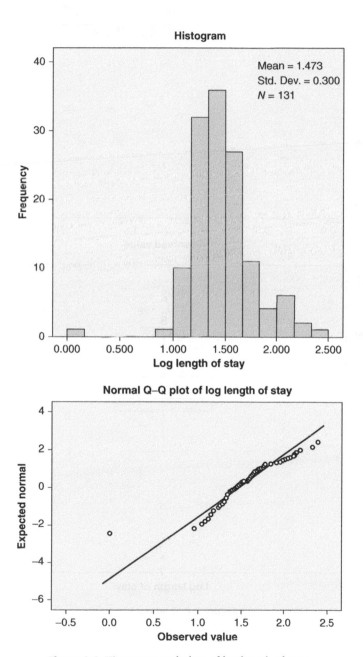

Figure 2.6 Histogram and plots of log length of stay.

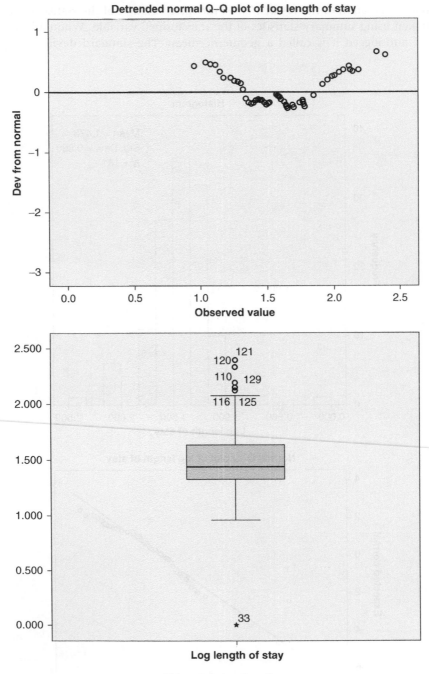

Figure 2.6 (*continued*)

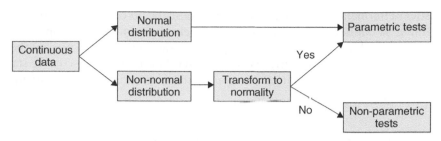

Figure 2.7 Pathway for the analysis of continuous variables.

cannot be back transformed to have the usual interpretation although the 95% confidence interval can be back transformed and will have the usual interpretation.

2.6   Data analysis pathway

The pathway for the analysis of continuous variables is shown in Figure 2.7.

Skewness, kurtosis and outliers can all distort a normal distribution. If a variable has a skewed distribution, it is sometimes possible to transform the variable to normality using a mathematical algorithm so that the data points in the tail do not bias the summary statistics and P values, or the variable can be analysed using non-parametric tests.

If the sample size is small, say less than 30, data points in the tail of a skewed distribution can markedly increase or decrease the mean value so that it no longer represents the actual centre of the data. If the estimate of the centre of the data is inaccurate, then the mean values of two groups will look more alike or more different than the central values actually are and the P value to estimate their difference will be correspondingly reduced or increased. It is important to avoid this type of bias.

2.7   Reporting descriptive statistics

In all research studies, it is important to report details of the characteristics of the study sample or study groups to describe the generalizability of the results. For this, statistics that describe the centre of the data and its spread are appropriate. Therefore, for variables that are normally distributed, the mean and the standard deviation are reported. For variables that are non-normally distributed, the median (Mdn) and the inter-quartile range (IQR) are reported.

Table 2.6   Baseline characteristics of the study sample

Characteristic	N	M (SD)
Birth weight	139	2464.0 g (514.6)
Gestational age	133	36.6 weeks (2.0)
Length of stay	132	27.0 days (21.8 days)[a]

[a] Mdn (IQR)

Statistics of normally distributed variables that describe precision, that is, the standard error and 95% confidence interval, are more useful for comparing groups or making inferences about differences between groups. Table 2.6 shows how to present the characteristics of the babies in the **surgery.sav** data set. In presenting descriptive statistics, no more than one decimal point greater than in the units of the original measurement should be used.[9]

2.8   Checking for normality in published results

When critically appraising journal articles, it may be necessary to transform a measure of spread (standard deviation) to a measure of precision (standard error of the mean), or vice versa, for comparing with results from other studies. The standard error of the mean provides an estimate of how precise the sample mean is as an estimate of the population mean.

Computing a standard deviation from a standard error, or vice versa, is simple because the formula is:

$$\text{Standard error (SE)} = \frac{\text{Standard deviation (SD)}}{\sqrt{n}}, \text{where } n \text{ is the sample size}$$

Also, by adding and subtracting two standard deviations from the mean, it is possible to roughly estimate whether the distribution of the data conforms to a bell-shaped distribution. For example, Table 2.7 shows summary statistics of lung function with the mean and standard deviation in a sample of children with severe asthma and in a sample of healthy controls. In this table, FEV_1 is forced expiratory volume in the first second of expiration, that is, how much air is exhaled during a forced breath in the first second. It is rare that this value would be below 30%, even in a child with severe lung disease.

In the active group, the lower value of the 95% range of per cent predicted FEV_1 is 37.5% − (2 × 16.0)%, which is 5.5%. Similarly, the lower value of the 95% range for the control group is 6.0%. Both of these values for predicted FEV_1 are implausible and are a clear indication that the data are skewed. Therefore, the standard deviation is not an appropriate statistic to describe the spread of the data and parametric tests should not be used to compare the groups.

If the lower estimate of the 95% range is too low, the mean will be an overestimate of the median value. If the lower estimate is too high, the mean value will be an underestimate of the median value. In Table 2.7, the variables are significantly skewed with a tail

Table 2.7 Mean lung function value of children with asthma and healthy controls

	Asthma group (n = 50)	Control group (n = 50)	
	M ± SD	M ± SD	P value
FEV₁ (% predicted value)	37.5 ± 16.0	36.0 ± 15.0	0.80

FEV_1, forced expiratory volume in 1 s.

to the right-hand side. In this case, the median and inter-quartile range would provide more accurate estimates of the centre and spread of the data and non-parametric tests would be needed to compare the groups.

2.9 Notes for critical appraisal

Questions to ask when assessing descriptive statistics published in the literature are shown in Box 2.5.

Box 2.5 Questions for critical appraisal

The following questions should be asked when appraising published results:
- Have several tests of normality been considered and reported?
- Are appropriate statistics used to describe the centre and spread of the data?
- Do the values of the mean ±2 SD represent a reasonable 95% range?
- If a distribution is skewed, has the mean of either group been underestimated or overestimated?
- If the data are skewed, have the median and inter-quartile range been reported?

References

1. Healy MJR. Statistics from the inside. 11. Data transformations. *Arch Dis Child* 1993; **68**: 260–264.
2. Lang TA, Secic M. *How to report statistics in medicine*. American College of Physicians: Philadelphia, PA, 1997.
3. Stevens J. *Applied multivariate statistics for the social sciences*, 3rd edn. Lawrence Erlbaum Associates: Mahwah, NJ, 1996.
4. Justel, A, Peña, D, Zamar, R. A multivariate Kolmogorov-Smirnov test of goodness of fit. *Stat Probabil Lett* 1997; **35**: 251–259
5. Chinn S. Scale, parametric methods, and transformations. *Thorax* 1991; **46**: 536–538.
6. Bland JM, Altman DG. Transforming data. *BMJ* 1996; **312**: 770.
7. Tabachnick BG, Fidell LS. *Using multivariate statistics*, 4th edn. Allyn and Bacon: Boston, 2001.
8. Peat JK, Unger WR, Combe D. Measuring changes in logarithmic data, with special reference to bronchial responsiveness. *J Clin Epidemiol* 1994; **47**: 1099–1108.
9. Altman DG, Bland JM. Presentation of numerical data. *BMJ* 1996; **312**: 572.

CHAPTER 3

Comparing two independent samples

Do not put faith in what statistics say until you have carefully considered what they do not say.
WILLIAM W. WATT

Objectives

The objectives of this chapter are to explain how to:
- conduct an independent two-sample, parametric or non-parametric test
- assess for homogeneity of variances
- calculate and interpret effect sizes and 95% confidence intervals
- report the results in a table or a graph
- understand sample size requirements
- critically appraise the analysis of data from two independent groups in the literature

---

3.1 Comparing the means of two independent samples

A two-sample *t*-test is a parametric test used to estimate whether the mean value of a normally distributed outcome variable is significantly different between two groups of participants. This test is also known as a Student's *t*-test or an independent samples *t*-test. Two-sample *t*-tests are classically used when the outcome is a continuous variable and when the explanatory variable is binary. For example, this test would be used to assess whether mean height is significantly different between a group of males and a group of females.

A two-sample *t*-test is used to assess whether two mean values are similar enough to have come from the same population or whether their difference is large enough for the two groups to have come from different populations. Rejecting the null hypothesis of a two-sample *t*-test indicates that the difference in the means of the two groups is large and is not due to either chance or sampling variation.

Medical Statistics: A Guide to SPSS, Data Analysis and Critical Appraisal, Second Edition.
Belinda Barton and Jennifer Peat.
© 2014 John Wiley & Sons, Ltd. Published 2014 by John Wiley & Sons, Ltd.
Companion website: www.wiley.com/go/barton/medicalstatistics2e

3.1.1 *Assumptions of a two-sample t-test*

The assumptions that must be met to use a two-sample t-test are shown in Box 3.1.

Box 3.1 Assumptions for using a two-sample t-test

The assumptions that must be satisfied to conduct a two-sample t-test are:
- the groups must be independent, that is, each participant must be in one group only
- the measurements must be independent, that is, a participant's measurement can be included in their group once only
- the outcome variable must be on a continuous (interval or ratio) scale
- the outcome variable must be normally distributed in each group
- the variances between groups are approximately equal, that is, homogeneity of variances (if data fail this assumption an adjustment to the t value is made)

The first two assumptions in Box 3.1 are determined by the study design. To conduct a two-sample t-test, each participant must be on a separate row of the spreadsheet and each participant must be included in the spreadsheet only once. In addition, one of the variables must indicate the group to which the participant belongs.

The fourth assumption that the outcome variable must be normally distributed in each group must also be met. If the outcome variable is not normally distributed in each group, a non-parametric test such a Mann–Whitney U test (described later in this chapter) or a transformation of the outcome variable will be needed. However, two-sample t-tests are fairly robust to some degree of non-normality if the sample size is large and if there are no influential outliers. The definition of a 'large' sample size varies, but there is common consensus that t-tests can be used when the sample size of each group contains at least 30–50 participants. If the sample size is less than 30 per group, or if outliers significantly influence one or both of the distributions, or if the distribution is clearly non-normal, then a two-sample t-test should not be used.

In addition to testing for normality, it is also important to inspect whether the variance in each group is similar, that is, whether there is homogeneity of variances between groups. Variance (the square of the standard deviation) is a measure of spread and describes the total variability of a sample. Data points in the sample can be described in terms of their distance (deviation) from their mean value.

If the variance is different between the two groups, there is heterogeneity of variances and the degrees of freedom and t value associated with a two-sample t-test are calculated differently. In this situation, a fractional value for degrees of freedom is used and the t-test statistic is calculated using individual group variances. In SPSS, Levene's test for equality of variances is automatically calculated as part of the two-sample t-test and the information is displayed in the SPSS output. If the Levene's test result is statistically significant ($P \leq 0.05$), this provides evidence that the data do not show homogeneity of variance and the variability of the two groups is not equal.

3.2 One- and two-sided tests of significance

When a hypothesis is tested, it is possible to conduct a one-sided (one-tailed) or a two-sided (two-tailed) test. A one-sided test is used to test an alternative hypothesis of an effect in only one direction (i.e. $mean_1 > mean_2$ or $mean_1 < mean_2$), for example, an active treatment is better than placebo. A two-sided test is used to test an alternative hypothesis of whether one mean value is smaller or larger than another mean value (i.e. $mean_1 \neq mean_2$). That is, there is a difference in either direction between the two populations from which the samples were selected.

Assuming that the null hypothesis of no difference between population means is true, in 95% of the cases the observed t values would fall within the critical t value range and differences would be due to sampling error. Observed t values that fall outside this critical range, which occurs in 5% of the cases, represent an unlikely t value to occur when the null hypothesis is true; therefore, the null hypothesis is rejected.

For two-sided tests, the probability of the test statistic occurring in either the upper or lower tail of the distribution is calculated. As shown in Figure 3.1, for a two-sided test, 2.5% of the rejection region is placed in the positive tail of the distribution (i.e. $mean_1 > mean_2$) and 2.5% is placed in the negative tail (i.e. $mean_1 < mean_2$). When a one-sided test is used, the 5% rejection region is placed only in one tail of the distribution. For example, if the hypothesis $mean_1 > mean_2$ was being tested, the 5% rejection region would be in the positive end of the tail. This means that for one-sided tests, P values on the margins of significance are reduced and the difference is more likely to be significant than a two-sided test.

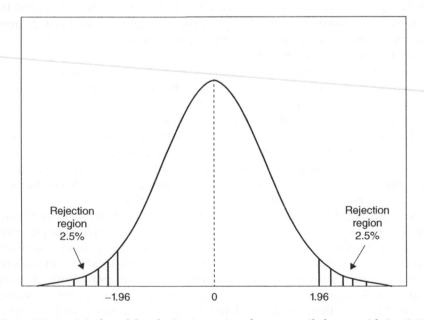

Figure 3.1 Statistical model and rejection regions for a two-tailed t-test with $P = 0.05$.

In the majority of studies, two-sided tests of significance are used. In health care research, it is important to allow for the possibility that extreme results could occur by chance and could occur equally often in either direction. In clinical trials, this would mean evidence for a beneficial or harmful effect. Two-sided tests are more conservative than one-sided tests in that the P value is higher, that is, less significant. Therefore, two-tailed tests reduce the chance that a between-group difference is declared statistically significant in error, and thus that a new treatment is incorrectly accepted as being more effective than an existing treatment.

In most clinical studies, the use of one-tailed tests is rarely justified because we should expect that a result could be in either direction. If a one-sided test is used, the direction should be specified in the study design prior to data collection. However, it is most unusual for researchers to be certain about the direction of effect before the study is conducted and, if they were, the study would probably not need to be conducted at all.[1] For this reason, one-tailed statistics are rarely used.

3.3   Effect sizes

Effect size is a term used to describe the size of the difference in mean values between two groups relative to the standard deviation. Effect sizes can be used to describe the magnitude of the difference between two groups in either experimental or observational study designs.

Effect sizes are measured in units of the standard deviation. The standard deviation around each group's mean value indicates the spread of the measurements in each group and is therefore a useful unit for describing the distance between the two mean values. The advantage of using an effect size to describe the difference between study groups is that unlike 95% confidence intervals and P values, the effect size is not related to the sample size. Effect sizes also allow comparisons across multiple outcome measures regardless of whether different measurements or scales have been used or whether there is variability between the samples.

To compare two mean values the following three effect sizes are commonly used.

3.3.1   Cohen's d

Many journals request that Cohen's d is reported because Cohen developed well-accepted interpretations of this size of the effect which help to guide understanding of the magnitude of between group differences. Cohen's d statistic is computed as the difference between two mean values divided by the population standard deviation as follows:

$$\text{Effect size} = \frac{(\text{Mean}_2 - \text{Mean}_1)}{\text{SD}} \text{ where SD denotes the standard deviation}$$

If the variances of the two groups are similar, then the standard deviation of either group can be used in calculating Cohen's d.[2] Otherwise the pooled standard deviation, which is the average of the standard deviations of the two groups, is used. The pooled standard deviation is the root mean square of the two standard deviations and

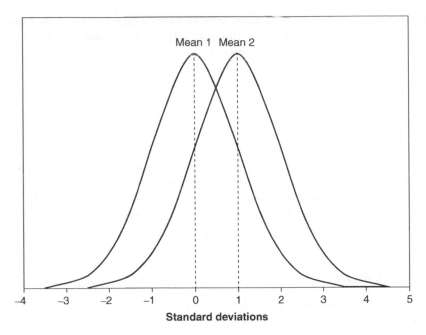

Figure 3.2 Mean values of two groups that are one standard deviation apart.

is calculated as follows:

$$\text{Pooled standard deviation} = \sqrt{\left[\frac{(\text{SD}_1^2 + \text{SD}_2^2)}{2}\right]}$$

where SD_1 is the standard deviation of group 1 and SD_2 is the standard deviation of group 2.

Cohen's d should only be used when the data are normally distributed and this statistic is most accurate when the group sizes and the group standard deviations are equal. Figure 3.2 shows the distribution of a variable in two groups that have mean values that are one standard deviation apart, that is, an effect size of 1 SD.

Table 3.1 shows the interpretation of Cohen's d and the per cent overlap between the groups for each effect size. In general, an effect size less than 0.2 is considered small,

Table 3.1 Effect sizes for Cohen's d and per cent overlap

Effect size	Cohen's d	Per cent overlap of the two groups
Small	0.20	85%
Medium	0.50	67%
Large	0.80	53%

0.3−0.5 is considered medium and 0.8 and over is considered large.[3] The classification of Cohen's d effect size should be considered a guideline and effect sizes should be evaluated in the context of the research and other similar interventions or studies. For example, effect sizes for educational research may be much smaller than that observed in medical or clinical research. A typical effect size of classroom-based educational interventions identified from a synthesis of over 300 meta-analyses on student achievement is 0.40.[4] Therefore, in this context, a classroom education intervention with an effect size equal to 0.70 may be considered to be large.

3.3.2   Hedges's g

Cohen's d can over-estimate the effect size when the sample size is small because in this situation, the estimate of the means and SDs are less representative of the true population compared to larger samples. Therefore, when the sample size is not large, an adjusted d value called Hedges's g is computed. This gives a slightly smaller, less biased estimate of the population effect size than is provided by Cohen's d. Hedges's g is also calculated from means and SDs of the two groups but is adjusted for unequal sample size or unequal SDs as follows:

$$\text{Hedges's } g = \frac{\text{mean1} - \text{mean2}}{\sqrt{((n_1-1)SD_1^2 + (n_2-1)SD_2^2)/n_1 + n_2 - 2}}$$

Alternative, Hedges's g can be estimated from Cohen's d as follows:

$$\text{Hedges's } g = \frac{d}{\sqrt{(n_1 + n_2)/(n_1 + n_2 - 2)}}$$

3.3.3   Glass's Δ (delta)

If the study has an experimental group (i.e. a group in which a treatment or intervention is being tested) and this is being compared to a control group, then the effect size Glass's should be used. This is calculated as Cohen's d but the SD of the control group is used instead of using the pooled SD from the two groups. This makes sense if the control SD is considered to be a better estimate of the population SD than the experimental group SD. If the sample size of the control group is large, the standard deviation will be an unbiased estimate of the population who have not received the new treatment or intervention. In an experimental study, Glass's gives a more reliable estimate of effect size for the population to which the results will be inferred.[5]

The effect size as estimated by Glass's can be considered the average percentile ranking of the experimental group relative to the control group. Therefore, an effect size of 1 indicates that the mean of the experimental group is at the 84th percentile of the control group.[2]

3.4   Study design

Two-sample t-tests can be used to analyse data from any type of experimental or non-experimental study design where the explanatory variable can be classified into two groups, for example, males and females, cases and controls, and intervention and non-intervention groups. For a two-sample t-test, there must be no relation or dependence between the participants in each of the two groups. Therefore, two-sample t-tests cannot be used to analyse scores from follow-up studies where data from participants are obtained on repeated occasions for the same measure or for matched case–control studies in which participants are treated as pairs in the analyses. In these types of studies, a paired t-test should be used as described in Chapter 4.

3.5   Influence of sample size

It is important to interpret significant P values in the context of the size of the difference between the groups and the sample size. The size of the study sample is an important determinant of whether a difference in means between two groups is statistically significant. Ideally, studies should be designed and conducted with a sample size that is sufficient for a clinically important difference between two groups to become statistically significant. In addition to specialized computer programs, there are a number of resources that can be used to calculate the sample size required to show that a nominated effect size is statistically significant and assess the power of a study (see Useful Websites). Power is a term that refers to the sample size required to avoid a type II error, that is, incorrectly accepting the null hypothesis of no difference when a clinically important difference between the groups exists.

If the study is expected to have small effect size and/or a lower level of significance is used (e.g. $P = 0.01$), then a large sample size will be needed to detect the effect with sufficient power.[3] In general, with power equal to 80% and a level of significance equal to 0.05, 30 participants per group are needed to show that a large effect size of 0.75 of one standard deviation is statistically significant, 64 per group for a moderate effect size of 0.5 and over 200 per group for a small effect size of less than 0.3.[6]

When designing a study, a power analysis should be conducted to calculate the sample size that is needed to detect a predetermined effect size with sufficient statistical power. If the sample size is too small, then type II errors may occur, that is, a clinically important difference between groups will not be statistically significant.

In observational studies, the two groups may have unequal sample sizes. In this situation, a two-sample t-test can still be used but in practice leads to a loss of statistical power, which may be important when the sample size is small. For example, a study with three times as many cases as controls and a total sample size of 100 participants (75 cases and 25 controls) has roughly the same statistical power as a balanced study with 76 participants (38 cases and 38 controls).[6] Thus, the unbalanced study requires the recruitment of an extra 24 participants to achieve the same statistical power.

Research question

The data file **babies.sav** contains the information of birth length, birth weight and head circumference measured at 1 month of age in 256 babies. The babies were recruited during a population study in which one of the inclusion criteria was that the babies had to have been a term birth. The research question and null hypothesis are shown below. Unlike the null hypothesis, the research question usually specifies the direction of effect that is expected. Nevertheless, a two-tailed test should be used because the direction of effect could be in either direction and if the effect is in a direction that is not expected, it is usually important to know this especially in experimental studies. Therefore, the alternate hypothesis is that there is a difference in either direction between the two populations from which the samples were selected.

In this example, all three outcome measurements (birth length, birth weight and head circumference) are continuous and the explanatory measurement (gender) is a binary group variable.

Questions:	Are males longer than females?
	Are males heavier than females?
	Do males have a larger head circumference than females?
Null hypothesis:	There is no difference between males and females in length.
	There is no difference between males and females in weight.
	There is no difference between males and females in head circumference.
Variables:	Outcome variables = birth length, birth weight and head circumference (continuous)
	Explanatory variable = gender (categorical, binary)

If the data satisfy the assumptions of *t*-tests (see Box 3.1), then the appropriate statistic that is used to test differences between groups is the *t* value. If the *t* value obtained from the two-sample *t*-test falls outside the *t* critical range and is therefore in the rejection region, the *P* value will be small and the null hypothesis will be rejected. In SPSS, the *P* value is calculated so it is not necessary to check statistical tables to obtain *t* critical values. When the null hypothesis is rejected, the conclusion is made that the difference between groups is statistically significant and did not occur by chance. It is important to remember that statistical significance not only reflects the size of the difference between groups but also the sample size. Thus, small unimportant differences between groups can be statistically significant when the sample size is large.

Before differences in outcome variables between groups can be tested, it is important that all of the assumptions specified in Box 3.1 are checked. In the data file **babies.sav**, each participant appears only once in their group, therefore the groups and the measurements are independent. In addition, all three outcome variables are on a continuous scale for each group, so the first three assumptions shown in Box 3.1 are satisfied. To check the fourth assumption, that the outcome variable is normally distributed, descriptive statistics need to be obtained for the distribution of each outcome variable in each group rather than for the entire sample. It is also important to check for univariate outliers, calculate the effect size and test the fifth assumption, homogeneity of variances. It is essential to identify univariate outliers that tend to bias mean values of groups and make them more different or more alike than median values show they are. Box 3.2 shows how to obtain the descriptive information for each group in SPSS.

The Case Processing Summary table indicates that there are 119 males and 137 females in the sample and that none of the babies have missing values for any of the variables.

The first check of normality is to compare the mean and median values provided by the Descriptives table and summarized in Table 3.2. The differences between the mean and median values are small for birth weight and relatively small for birth length and for head circumference.

Box 3.2 SPSS commands to obtain descriptive statistics

SPSS Commands

babies.sav – IBM SPSS Statistics Data Editor
    Analyze → Descriptive Statistics → Explore
Explore
    Highlight Birth weight, Birth length, and Head circumference and click
        into Dependent List
    Highlight Gender and click into Factor List
    Click on Plots
Explore: Plots
    Boxplots: select Factor levels together (default)
    Descriptive: untick Stem and leaf (default) and tick Histogram, tick Normality
        plots with tests, Spread vs Level with Levene test: select None (default)
    Click Continue
Explore
    Click on Options
Explore: Options
    Missing Values – select Exclude cases pairwise
    Click Continue
Explore
    Display: tick Both (default)
    Click OK

Case Processing Summary

		Cases					
		Valid		Missing		Total	
	Gender	*N*	Per cent	*N*	Per cent	*N*	Per cent
Birth weight (kg)	Male	119	100.0	0	0.0	119	100.0
	Female	137	100.0	0	0.0	137	100.0
Birth length (cm)	Male	119	100.0	0	0.0	119	100.0
	Female	137	100.0	0	0.0	137	100.0
Head circum-	Male	119	100.0	0	0.0	119	100.0
ference (cm)	Female	137	100.0	0	0.0	137	100.0

Information from the Descriptives table indicates that the skewness and kurtosis values are all less than or close to ± 1, suggesting that the data are approximately normally distributed. Calculations of normality statistics for skewness and kurtosis in Table 3.2 show that the critical values of kurtosis/SE for birth length for both males and females are less than -1.96 and outside the normal range, indicating that the distributions of birth length are relatively flat. The head circumference of females is negatively skewed

Descriptives

	Gender			Statistic	Std. error
Birth weight (kg)	Male	Mean		3.4430	0.03030
		95% confidence interval for mean	Lower bound	3.3830	
			Upper bound	3.5030	
		5% trimmed mean		3.4383	
		Median		3.4300	
		Variance		0.109	
		Std. deviation		0.33057	
		Minimum		2.70	
		Maximum		4.62	
		Range		1.92	
		Inter-quartile range		0.47	
		Skewness		0.370	0.222
		Kurtosis		0.553	0.440
	Female	Mean		3.5316	0.03661
		95% confidence interval for mean	Lower bound	3.4592	
			Upper bound	3.6040	
		5% trimmed mean		3.5215	
		Median		3.5000	
		Variance		0.184	
		Std. deviation		0.42849	
		Minimum		2.71	
		Maximum		4.72	
		Range		2.01	
		Inter-quartile range		0.56	
		Skewness		0.367	0.207
		Kurtosis		−0.128	0.411
Birth length (cm)	Male	Mean		50.333	0.0718
		95% confidence interval for mean	Lower bound	50.191	
			Upper bound	50.475	
		5% trimmed mean		50.342	
		Median		50.500	
		Variance		0.614	
		Std. deviation		0.7833	
		Minimum		49.0	
		Maximum		51.5	
		Range		2.5	
		Inter-quartile range		1.0	
		Skewness		−0.354	0.222
		Kurtosis		−0.971	0.440
	Female	Mean		50.277	0.0729
		95% confidence interval for mean	Lower bound	50.133	
			Upper bound	50.422	

Descriptives

Gender				Statistic	Std. error
		5% trimmed mean		50.264	
		Median		50.000	
		Variance		0.728	
		Std. deviation		0.8534	
		Minimum		49.0	
		Maximum		52.0	
		Range		3.0	
		Inter-quartile range		1.5	
		Skewness		−0.117	0.207
		Kurtosis		−1.084	0.411
Head circumference (cm)	Male	Mean		34.942	0.1197
		95% confidence interval for mean	Lower bound	34.705	
			Upper bound	35.179	
		5% trimmed mean		34.967	
		Median		35.000	
		Variance		1.706	
		Std. deviation		1.3061	
		Minimum		31.5	
		Maximum		38.0	
		Range		6.5	
		Inter-quartile range		2.0	
		Skewness		−0.208	0.222
		Kurtosis		0.017	0.440
	Female	Mean		34.253	0.1182
		95% confidence interval for mean	Lower bound	34.019	
			Upper bound	34.486	
		5% trimmed mean		34.301	
		Median		34.000	
		Variance		1.914	
		Std. deviation		1.3834	
		Minimum		29.5	
		Maximum		38.0	
		Range		8.5	
		Inter-quartile range		1.5	
		Skewness		−0.537	0.207
		Kurtosis		0.850	0.411

because the critical value of skewness/SE of −2.59 is less than −1.96 and outside the normal range. Also, the distribution of head circumference for females is slightly peaked because the critical value of kurtosis/SE for this variable is outside the normal range of +1.96.

From the Descriptives table, it is possible to also compute effect sizes and estimate homogeneity of variances as shown in Table 3.3. The effect sizes using the pooled standard deviation are small for birth weight, very small for birth length and medium for

Table 3.2   Checking whether data have a normal distribution

	Gender	Mean – median	Skewness (SE)	Skewness/SE (critical value)	Kurtosis (SE)	Kurtosis/SE (critical value)
Birth weight	Male	0.013	0.370 (0.222)	1.67	0.553 (0.440)	1.26
	Female	0.032	0.367 (0.207)	1.77	−0.128 (0.411)	−0.31
Birth length	Male	−0.167	−0.354 (0.222)	−1.59	−0.971 (0.440)	−2.21
	Female	0.277	−0.117 (0.207)	−0.57	−1.084 (0.411)	−2.64
Head circumference	Male	−0.058	−0.208 (0.222)	−0.94	0.017 (0.440)	0.04
	Female	0.253	−0.537 (0.207)	−2.59	0.850 (0.411)	2.07

Table 3.3   Effect sizes and homogeneity of variances

	Difference in means and SD	Effect size (d)	Maximum and minimum variance	Variance ratio
Birth weight	3.443 – 3.532/0.38	0.23	0.184, 0.109	1:1.7
Birth length	50.33 – 50.28/0.82	0.06	0.728, 0.614	1:1.2
Head circumference	34.94 – 34.25/1.35	0.51	1.914, 1.706	1:1.1

head circumference. The variance of birth weight for females compared to males is 0.109–0.184 or 1:1.7. This indicates that females have a wider spread of birth weight scores, which is shown by similar minimum values for males and females (2.70 vs 2.71 kg) but a higher maximum value for females (4.62 vs 4.72 kg). For birth length and head circumference, males and females have similar variances with ratios of 1:1.12 and 1:1.1, respectively.

The Tests of Normality table shows that with P values less than 0.05, the distribution of birth weight for males and females is not significantly different from a normal distribution and therefore passes these tests of normality. However, both the Kolmogorov–Smirnov and Shapiro–Wilk tests of normality indicate that birth length and head circumference for males and females are significantly different from a normal distribution.

Tests of Normality

	Gender	Kolmogorov–Smirnov[a]			Shapiro–Wilk		
		Statistic	df	Sig.	Statistic	df	Sig.
Birth weight (kg)	Male	0.044	119	0.200*	0.987	119	0.313
	Female	0.063	137	0.200*	0.983	137	0.094
Birth length (cm)	Male	0.206	119	0.000	0.895	119	0.000
	Female	0.232	137	0.000	0.889	137	0.000
Head circumference (cm)	Male	0.094	119	0.012	0.977	119	0.037
	Female	0.136	137	0.000	0.965	137	0.001

*This is a lower bound of the true significance.
[a] Lilliefors significance correction.

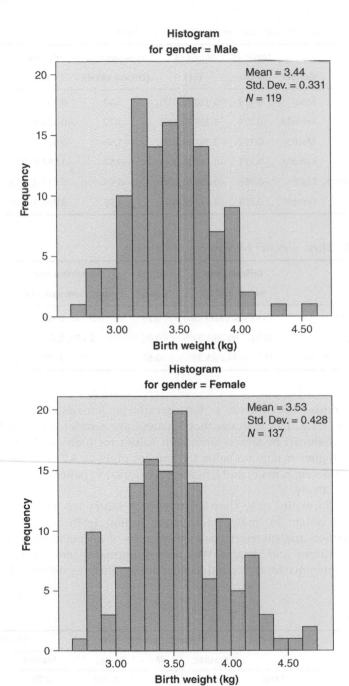

Figure 3.3 Histograms and plot of birth weight by gender.

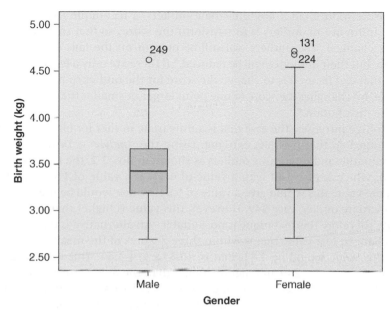

Figure 3.3 (*continued*)

The histograms shown in Figure 3.3 indicate that the data for birth weight of males and females follow an approximately normal distribution with one or two outlying values to the right hand side. The box plots shown in Figure 3.3 indicate that there is one outlying value for males and two outlying values for females that are 1.5–3 box lengths from the upper edge of the box. Both groups have outlying values at the high end of the data range that would tend to increase the mean value of each group. To check whether these outlying values are univariate outliers, the mean of the group is subtracted from the outlying value and then divided by the standard deviation of the group. This calculation converts the outlying value to a z score. If the absolute value of the z score is greater than 3, then the value is a univariate outlier. If the sample size is very small, then an absolute z score greater than 2 should be considered to be a univariate outlier.[7]

For the birth weight of males, the outlying value is the maximum value of 4.62 and is case 249. By subtracting the mean from this value and dividing by the standard deviation, that is, $((4.62 - 3.44)/0.33)$, a z value of 3.58 is obtained indicating that case 249 is a univariate outlier. This score is an extreme value compared to the rest of the data points and should be checked to ensure that it is not a transcribing or data entry error. On checking, it was found that the score was entered correctly and came from a minority ethnic group. There is only one univariate outlier and the sample size is large and therefore it is unlikely that this outlier will have a significant influence on the summary statistics. If the sample size is large, say at least 100 cases, then a few cases with z scores greater than the absolute value of 3 would be expected by chance.[7]

If there were more than a few univariate outliers, a technique that can be used to reduce the influence of outliers is to transform the scores so that the shape of the distribution is changed. The outliers will still be present on the tails of the transformed distribution, but their influence will be reduced.[8] If there are only a few outliers, another technique that can be used is to change the score for the outlier so it is not so extreme, for example, by changing the score to one point larger or smaller than the next extreme value in the distribution.[8]

For illustrative purposes, the case that is a univariate outlier for birth weight of males will be changed so that it is less extreme. Using the *Analyze → Descriptive Statistics → Explore* commands and requesting outliers as shown in Box 2.2, the next extreme value is obtained, which is case 149 with a value of 4.31. If a value of 1 were added to the next extreme value this would give a value of 5.31, which would be the changed value for the univariate outlier, case 249. However, this value is higher than the actual value of case 249, therefore this technique is not suitable. An alternative is that the univariate outlier is changed to a value that is within three z scores of the mean. For birth weight of males, this value would be 4.43, that is, $(0.33 \times 3) + 3.44$. This value is lower than the present value of case 249 and slightly higher than the next extreme value, case 149. Therefore, the value of case 249 is changed from 4.62 to 4.43. This information should be recorded in the study handbook and the adjustment of the score reported in any publications.

After the case has been changed, the Descriptives table for birth weight of males should be obtained with new summary statistics. This table shows that the new maximum value for birth weight is 4.43. The mean of 3.4414 is almost the same as the previous mean of 3.4430, and the standard deviation, skewness and kurtosis values of the group have slightly decreased, indicating a slightly closer approximation to a normal distribution.

For the birth weight of females, cases 131 and 224 are outlying values and are also from the same minority ethnic group as case 249. Case 131 is the higher of the two values and is the maximum value of the group with a value of 4.72, which is 2.77 standard deviations above the group mean and is not a univariate outlier. Therefore, case 224 is not a univariate outlier and the values of both cases 131 and 224 are retained.

Another alternative to transforming data or changing the values of univariate outliers is to omit the outliers from the analysis. If there were more univariate outliers from the same minority ethnic group, the data points could be included so that the results could be generalized to all ethnic groups in the recruitment area. Alternatively, all data points from the minority group could be omitted regardless of outlier status although this would limit the generalizability of the results.

The decision of whether to omit or include outlying values is always difficult. If the sample was selected as a random sample of the population, omission of some participants from the analyses should not be considered.

The histograms shown in Figure 3.4 indicate that birth length of males and females does not follow a classic normal distribution and explains the kurtosis statistics for males and females in the Descriptives table. The birth length of both males and females has a narrow range of only 49 to 52 cm as shown in the Descriptives table. The histograms show that birth length is recorded to the nearest 0.5 of a centimetre for both male and female babies males (Figure 3.4). This rounding of birth length may be satisfactory for obstetric records but it would be important to ensure that observers measure length to an exact standard in a research study. Since birth length has only been recorded to the nearest centimetre, summary statistics for this variable should be reported using no more than one decimal place.

Descriptives

	Gender			Statistic	Std. error
Birth weight (kg)	Male	Mean		3.4414	0.02982
		95% confidence	Lower bound	3.3824	
		Interval for mean	Upper bound	3.5005	
		5% trimmed mean		3.4383	
		Median		3.4300	
		Variance		0.106	
		Std. deviation		0.32525	
		Minimum		2.70	
		Maximum		4.43	
		Range		1.73	
		Inter-quartile range		0.4700	
		Skewness		0.235	0.222
		Kurtosis		0.028	0.440
	Female	Mean		3.5316	0.03661
		95% confidence	Lower bound	3.4592	
		Interval for mean	Upper bound	3.6040	
		5% trimmed mean		3.5215	
		Median		3.5000	
		Variance		0.184	
		Std. deviation		0.42849	
		Minimum		2.71	
		Maximum		4.72	
		Range		2.01	
		Inter-quartile range		0.5550	
		Skewness		0.367	0.207
		Kurtosis		−0.128	0.411

The box plots shown in Figure 3.4 confirm that females have a lower median birth length than males but have a wider absolute range of birth length values as indicated by the length of the box. This suggests that the variances of each group may not be homogeneous.

The histograms for head circumference shown in Figure 3.5 indicate that the data are approximately normally distributed although there is a slight tail to the left for females. This is confirmed by the box plot in Figure 3.5 that shows a few outlying values at the lower end of the distribution, indicating that a few female babies have a head circumference that is smaller than most other babies in the group. The smallest value is case 184 with a head circumference of 29.5, which has a z score of 3.44 and is a univariate outlier. The next smallest value is case 247 with a value of 30.2, which has a z score of 2.93. There is only one univariate outlier, which is expected in this large sample as part of normal variation. It is unlikely that this one outlier will have a significant impact on summary statistics, so it is not adjusted and is included in the data analyses. The maximum value for head circumference of females is case 108 with a value of 38, which has a z value of 2.71 and is not a univariate outlier.

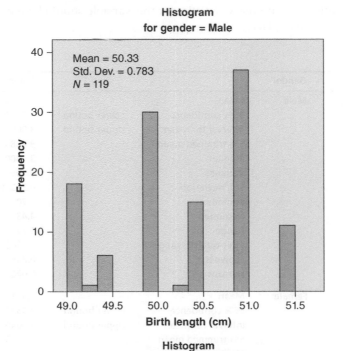

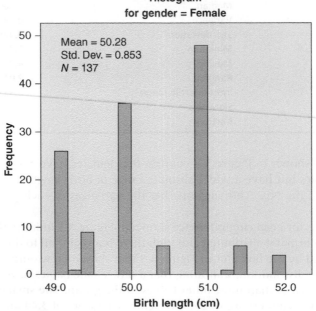

Figure 3.4 Histograms and plot of birth length by gender.

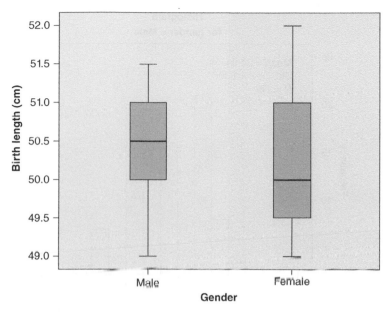

Figure 3.4 (*continued*)

Table 3.4   Summary of whether descriptive statistics indicates a normal distribution in each group

		Mean – median	Skewness	Kurtosis	K–S test	Plots	Overall decision
Birth weight	Males	Yes	Yes	Yes	Yes	Yes	Yes
	Females	Yes	Yes	Yes	Yes	Yes	Yes
Birth length	Males	Yes	Yes	No	No	No	Yes
	Females	Probably	Yes	No	No	No	Yes
Head circumference	Males	Yes	Yes	Yes	No	Yes	Yes
	Females	Probably	No	No	No	Yes	Yes

Finally, after the presence of outliers has been assessed and all tests of normality have been conducted, the tests of normality can be summarized as shown in Table 3.4. In the table, 'Yes' indicates that the distribution is within the normal range and 'No' indicates that the distribution is outside the normal range.

Based on all checks of normality, the birth weight of males and females is normally distributed so a two-sample *t*-test can be used. The distribution of birth length of males and females has a flat shape but does not have any outliers. While birth length of both males and females has some kurtosis, this has less impact on summary statistics than if the data were skewed. The variable head circumference is normally distributed for males but for females has some slight skewness caused by a few outlying values. However, the mean and median values for females are not largely different. Also, in the female group there is only one outlier and the number of outlying values is small and the sample size is large, and a *t*-test will be robust to these small deviations from normality. Therefore, the distribution of each outcome variable is approximately

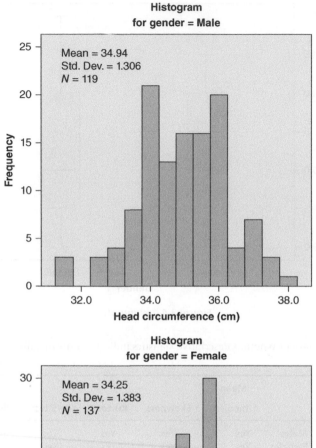

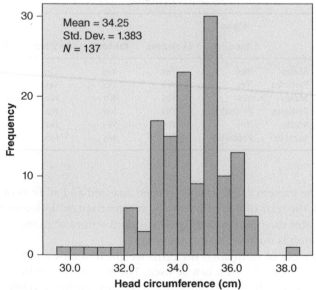

Figure 3.5 Histograms and plot of head circumference by gender.

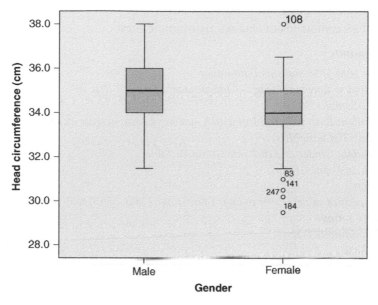

Figure 3.5 (*continued*)

normally distributed for both males and females, and a two-sample *t*-test can be used to test between group differences.

3.6 Two-sample *t*-test

A two-sample *t*-test is basically a test of how different two group means are in terms of their variance. Clearly, if there was no difference between the groups, the difference to variance ratio would be close to zero. The *t* value becomes larger as the difference between the groups increases in respect to their variances. An approximate formula for calculating a *t* value, when variances are equal is

$$t = \frac{(x_1 - x_2)}{\sqrt{(s_p^2/n_1 + s_p^2/n_2)}}$$

where x is the mean, s_p^2 is the pooled variance and n is the sample size of each group. Thus, *t* is the difference between the mean values for the two groups divided by the standard error of the difference. When variances of the two groups are not equal, that is when Levene's test for equality of variances is significant, individual group variances, and not the pooled variance, are used in calculating the *t* value. Box 3.3 shows the SPSS commands to obtain a two-sample *t*-test in which the numbered coding for each group has to be entered.

The first Group Statistics table shows summary statistics, which are identical to the statistics obtained in *Analyze → Descriptive Statistics → Explore*. However, there is no information in this table that would allow the normality of the distributions in each group or the presence of influential outliers to be assessed. Thus, it is important to always obtain full descriptive statistics using the *Explore* command to check for normality prior to conducting a two-sample *t*-test.

Box 3.3 SPSS commands to obtain a two-sample *t*-test

SPSS Commands

babies.sav – IBM SPSS Statistics Data Editor
    Analyze → Compare Means → Independent Samples T Test
Independent-Samples T-Test
        Highlight Birth weight, Birth length and Head circumference and click
            into Test Variable(s)
        Highlight Gender and click into Group Variable
        Click on Define Groups
Define Groups
        Use specified values: Enter coding: 1 for Group 1 and 2 for Group 2
        Click Continue
Independent-Samples T-Test
        Click OK

T-Test

Group Statistics

	Gender	*N*	Mean	Std. deviation	Std. error mean
Birth weight (kg)	Male	119	3.4414	0.32525	0.02982
	Female	137	3.5316	0.42849	0.03661
Birth length (cm)	Male	119	50.333	0.7833	0.0718
	Female	137	50.277	0.8534	0.0729
Head circumference (cm)	Male	119	34.942	1.3061	0.1197
	Female	137	34.253	1.3834	0.1182

In the Independent Samples Test table, the first test is Levene's test of equal variances. A *P* value for this test that is less than 0.05 indicates that the variances of the two groups are significantly different and therefore that the *t* statistics calculated assuming variances are not equal should be used. The variable birth weight does not pass the test for equal variances with a *P* value of 0.007 but this was expected because the statistics in the Descriptives table showed a 1:1.7, or almost twofold, difference in variance (Table 3.3). For this variable, the statistics calculated assuming variances are not equal is appropriate. However, both birth length and head circumference pass the test of equal variances and the differences between genders can be reported using the *t* statistics that have been calculated assuming equal variances.

For birth weight, the appropriate *t* statistic can be read from the line *Equal variances not assumed*. The *t* statistic for birth length and head circumference can be read from the line *Equal variances assumed*. The *t*-test *P* value indicates the likelihood that the differences in mean values occurred by chance. If the likelihood is small, that is, the *P* value is less than 0.05, the null hypothesis can be rejected. For birth weight, the *P* value for the difference between the genders does not reach statistical significance with a *P* value of 0.057. This *P* value indicates that there is a 5.7%, or 57 in 1000, chance of finding this difference if the two groups in the population have equal means.

Independent Samples Test

		Levene's test for equality of variances		t-Test for equality of means					95% confidence interval of the difference	
		F	Sig.	t	df	Sig. (two-tailed)	Mean diff-erence	Std. error diff-erence	Lower	Upper
Birth weight (kg)	Equal variances assumed	7.377	0.007	−1.875	254	0.062	−0.09021	0.04812	−0.18498	0.00455
	Equal variances not assumed			−1.911	249.659	0.057	−0.09021	0.04721	−0.18320	0.00277
Birth length (cm)	Equal variances assumed	2.266	0.133	0.538	254	0.591	0.0554	0.1030	−0.1473	0.2581
	Equal variances not assumed			0.541	253.212	0.589	0.0554	0.1023	−0.1461	0.2569
Head circum-ference (cm)	Equal variances assumed	0.257	0.613	4.082	254	0.000	0.6895	0.1689	0.3568	1.0221
	Equal variances not assumed			4.098	252.221	0.000	0.6895	0.1682	0.3581	1.0208

For birth length, there is clearly no difference between the genders with a P value of 0.591. For head circumference, there is a highly significant difference between the genders with a P value of <0.0001. The head circumference of female babies is significantly different from the head circumference of male babies. This P value indicates that there is less than a 1 in 1000 chance of this difference being found by chance if the null hypothesis is true.

3.7 Confidence intervals

Confidence intervals are invaluable statistics for estimating the precision around a summary statistic such as a mean value and for estimating the magnitude of the difference between two groups. For mean values, the 95% confidence interval is calculated as follows:

$$\text{Confidence interval (CI)} = \text{mean} \pm (1.96 \times SE)$$

where SE = standard error.

Thus, using the data from the Group Statistics table provided in the SPSS output for a t-test, the confidence interval for birth weight for males would be calculated as follows:

$$95\% \text{confidence interval} = 3.441 \pm (1.96 \times 0.0298) = 3.383, 3.499$$

Table 3.5 Interpretation of 95% confidence intervals

Relative position of the 95% confidence intervals in two group	Statistical significance between groups
Do not overlap	Highly significant difference
Just touch	Significant at approximately $P < 0.01$
Overlap by less than 25% of the average length of the two intervals	Significant at approximately $P < 0.05$
Overlap, but one summary statistic is not within the confidence interval for the other group	Possibly significant, but not highly
Overlap so that one confidence interval crosses the summary statistics of the other group	Definitely not significant

These values correspond approximately to the 95% confidence interval lower and upper bounds shown in the Descriptives table. To calculate the 99% confidence interval, the critical value of 2.57 instead of 1.96 would be used in the calculation. This would give a wider confidence interval that would indicate the range in which the true population mean lies with more certainty.

The confidence intervals of two groups can be used to assess whether there is a significant difference between the two groups. If the 95% confidence interval of one group does not overlap with the confidence interval of another, there will be a statistically significant difference between the two groups. The interpretation of the overlapping of confidence intervals when two groups are compared is shown in Table 3.5.

3.7.1 Interpreting the overlap of 95% confidence intervals

Figure 3.6 shows the mean values of an outcome measurement, say per cent change from baseline, in three independent groups. The degree of overlap of the confidence intervals reflects the P values. For the comparison of group I versus III the confidence intervals do not overlap and the group means are significantly different at $P < 0.0001$. For the comparison of group I versus II, the confidence intervals overlap to a large extent and the group means are not significantly different at $P = 0.52$. For the comparison of group II versus III, where one summary statistic is not within the confidence interval of the other group, the difference between group means is marginally significant at $P = 0.049$.

In the data set, **babies.sav** the means and confidence intervals of the outcome variable for each group can be summarized as shown in Table 3.6. The degree of overlap of the 95% confidence intervals confirms the between group P values.

Finally, in the Independent Samples Test table, the mean difference and its 95% confidence interval were also reported. The mean difference is the difference between the mean values for males and females. The direction of the mean difference is determined by the coding used for gender. With males coded as 1 and females as 2, the differences are represented as males − females. Therefore, this section of the table indicates that males have a mean birth weight, that is, 0.09021 kg lower than females but a mean birth length, that is, 0.0554 cm longer and a mean head circumference, that is, 0.6895 cm larger than females. For reporting, these figures would be rounded to no more than two decimal places.

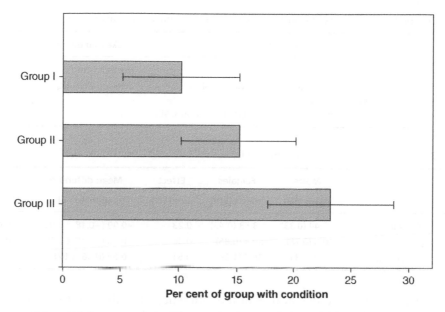

Figure 3.6 Interpretation of the overlap between 95% confidence intervals.

Table 3.6 Summary of mean values and interpretation of 95% confidence intervals

	M (95% CI) Males	*M* (95% CI) Females	Overlap of CI	Significance
Birth weight	3.44 (3.38, 3.50)	3.53 (3.46, 3.60)	Slight	$P = 0.06$
Birth length	50.3 (50.1, 50.5)	50.3 (50.1, 50.4)	Large	$P = 0.59$
Head circumference	34.9 (34.7, 35.2)	34.3 (34.0, 34.5)	None	$P < 0.0001$

Obviously, a zero value for a mean difference would indicate no difference between groups. Thus, a 95% confidence interval around the mean difference that contains the value of zero, as it does for birth length, suggests that the two groups are not significantly different. A confidence interval that is shifted away from the value of zero, as it is for head circumference, indicates with 95% certainty that the two groups are different. The slight overlap with zero for the 95% confidence interval of the difference for birth weight reflects the marginal *P* value.

3.8   Reporting the results from two-sample *t*-tests

A summary of the types of statistics that is used to describe centre, spread and precision is shown in Table 3.7.

The results from two-sample *t*-tests can be reported as shown in Table 3.8. In addition to reporting the *P* value for the difference between genders, it is important to report the characteristics of the groups in terms of their mean values and standard deviations, the effect size and the mean between group difference and 95% confidence interval. Except for effect size, these statistics are all provided on the SPSS *t*-test output.

Table 3.7 Summary statistics to describe normal and skewed distributions

Statistic	Normal distribution	Skewed distribution
Centre	Mean (*M*)	Median (Mdn)
Spread	Standard deviation (SD) Variance (SD²)	Inter-quartile (IQR) range
Precision	Standard error (SE) = SD/$\sqrt{n}$ 95% confidence interval (95% CI) = 1.96 × SE	

Table 3.8 Summary of birth details by gender

	Males mean (SD)	Females mean (SD)	Effect size (SD)	Mean difference and 95% CI	P value
Birth weight (kg)	3.44 (0.33)	3.53 (0.43)	0.23	−0.09 (−0.18, −0.003)	0.06
Birth length (cm)	50.3 (0.78)	50.3 (0.85)	0.06	0.06 (−0.15, 0.26)	0.59
Head circumference (cm)	34.9 (1.31)	34.3 (1.38)	0.51	0.69 (0.36, 1.02)	<0.0001

The *P* values show the significance of the differences, but the effect size and mean difference give an indication of the magnitude of the differences between the groups. As such, these statistics give a meaningful interpretation to the *P* values.

3.8.1   Reporting results in a graph

Graphs are important tools for conveying the results of research studies. The most informative figures are clear and self-explanatory. For mean values from continuous data, dot plots are the most appropriate graph to use. In summarizing data from continuous variables, it is important that bar charts are used only when the distance from zero has a meaning and therefore when the zero value is shown on the axis.

Box 3.4 SPSS commands to draw a dot plot

SPSS Commands

babies.sav –IBM SPSS Statistics Data Editor
    Graphs → Legacy Dialogs → Error Bar
Error Bar
        Click Simple, tick Summaries for groups of cases (default)
        Click Define
Define Simple Error Bar: Summaries for Groups of Cases
        Highlight Birth weight and click into Variable
        Highlight Gender and click into Category Axis
        Click OK

Box 3.4 shows how to create a dot plot with error bars in SPSS. The commands in Box 3.4 can then be repeated for birth length and head circumference to produce the graphs shown in Figure 3.7. Note that the scales on the *y*-axis of the three graphs shown

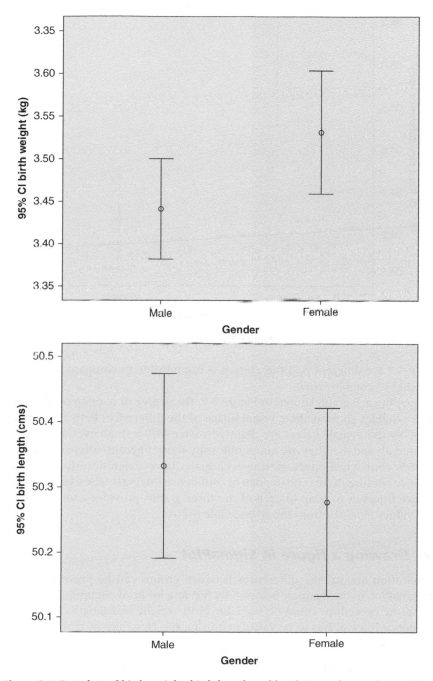

Figure 3.7 Dot plots of birth weight, birth length and head circumference by gender.

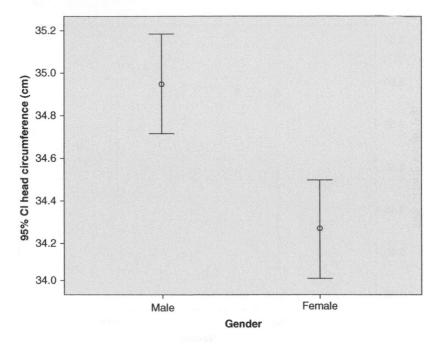

Figure 3.7 (*continued*)

in Figure 3.7 are different and therefore it is not possible to compare the graphs with one another or combine them.

However, in each graph shown in Figure 3.7, the degree of overlap of the confidence intervals provides an immediate visual image of the differences between genders. The graphs show that female babies are slightly heavier with a small overlap of 95% confidence intervals and that they are not significantly shorter because there is a large overlap of the 95% confidence intervals. However, males have a significantly larger head circumference because there is no overlap of confidence intervals. The extent to which the confidence intervals overlap in each of the three graphs provides a visual explanation of the P values obtained from the two-sample t-tests.

3.8.2   Drawing a figure in SigmaPlot

For publication quality, the differences between groups can be presented in a graph using SigmaPlot. In the example below, only the data for head circumference are plotted but the same procedure could be used for birth weight and length. First, the width of confidence interval has to be calculated using the Descriptives table obtained from *Analyze → Descriptive Statistics → Explore*.

$$\text{Width of 95\%CI} = \text{mean} - \text{lower bound of 95\%CI}$$

Thus, the width of the confidence interval for head circumference is as follows:

$$\text{Width of 95\%CI} = 34.94 - 34.71 = 0.23 (\text{males})$$

$$= 34.25 - 34.02 = 0.23 (\text{females})$$

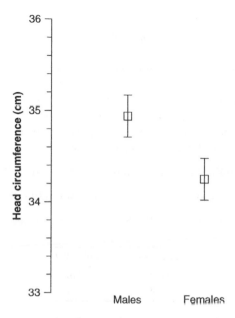

Figure 3.8 Mean head circumference at 1 month by gender.

The numerical values of the mean and the width of the 95% confidence interval are then entered into the SigmaPlot spreadsheet as follows and the commands in Box 3.5 can be used to draw a dot plot as shown in Figure 3.8.

Column 1	Column 2
34.94	0.23
34.25	0.23

Box 3.5 SigmaPlot commands for drawing a dot plot

SigmaPlot Commands

Data 1*

   At top of the screen Click on Graph → Create Graph
   Click on Scatter Plot in sub-menu
   Click on Simple Scatter – Error Bars in Scatter Group
Create Graph – Error Bars
   Symbol Values = Worksheet Columns (default), click Next
Create Graph – Data Format
   Highlight Single Y, click Next
Create Graph – Select Data
   Data for Y = use drop box and select Column 1
   Data for Error = use drop box and select Column 2,
   Click Finish

Once the plot is obtained, the graph can be customized by changing the axes, axis labels, graph colours and so on using options under the menu *Graph Page* – the fourth tab at the top of the screen.

Alternatively, the absolute mean differences between males and females could be presented in a graph. Birth length and head circumference were measured in the same scale (cm) and therefore can be plotted on the same figure. Birth weight is in different units (kg) and would need to be presented in a different figure.

The width of the confidence intervals is calculated from the mean difference and lower 95% confidence interval of the difference, as follows:

$$\text{Width of 95\%CI for birth length} = 0.055 - (-0.147) = 0.202$$

$$\text{Width of 95\%CI for head circumference} = 0.689 - 0.357 = 0.332$$

These values are then entered into the SigmaPlot spreadsheet as follows:

Column 1	Column 2
0.055	0.202
0.689	0.332

Box 3.6 shows how a horizontal scatter plot can be drawn in SigmaPlot to produce Figure 3.9. The decision whether to draw horizontal or vertical dot plots is one of personal choice; however, horizontal plots have the advantage that longer descriptive labels can be included in a way that they can be easily read.

Box 3.6 SigmaPlot commands for horizontal dot plot

SigmaPlot Commands

Data 1*

    Click on Create Graph tab at top of the screen
    Click on Scatter in sub-menu
    Click on Simple Scatter – Error Bars in Scatter group
Create Graph – Error Bars
    Symbol Values = Worksheet Columns (default), click Next
Create Graph – Data Format
    Highlight Many X, click Next
Create Graph – Select Data
    Data for X1 = use drop box and select Column 1
    Data for Error 1 = use drop box and select Column 2
Click Finish

3.9 Rank-based non-parametric tests

Rank-based non-parametric tests are used when the data do not conform to a normal distribution. If the data are clearly skewed, if outliers have an important effect on the mean value or if the sample size in one or more of the groups is small, say between 20

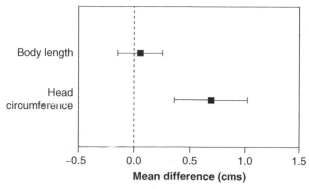

Figure 3.9 Mean difference in body length and head circumference between males and females at 1 month of age.

and 30 cases, then a rank-based non-parametric test should probably be used. These tests rely on ranking and summing the scores in each group and may lack sufficient power to detect a significant difference between two groups when the sample size is very small.

The non-parametric test that is equivalent to a two-sample t test is the Mann–Whitney U test. The Mann–Whitney U test is based on the ranking of measurements from two samples to estimate whether the samples are from the same population. In this test, no assumptions are made about the distribution of the measurements in either group.

The assumptions for the Mann–Whitney U test are shown in Box 3.7.

Box 3.7 Assumptions for Mann–Whitney U test to compare two independent samples

The assumptions for the Mann–Whitney U test are:
- the data are randomly sampled from the population
- the groups are independent, that is, each participant is in one group only

---

Research question

The spreadsheet **surgery.sav**, which was used in Chapter 2, contains the data for 141 babies who attended hospital for surgery, their length of stay and whether they had an infection during their stay.

Question: Do babies who have an infection have a longer stay in hospital?

Null hypothesis: That there is no difference in length of stay between babies who have an infection and babies who do not have an infection.

Variables: Outcome variable = length of stay (continuous)
                 Explanatory variable = infection (categorical, binary)

Descriptive statistics and the distribution of the outcome variable length of stay in each group can be inspected using the commands shown in Box 3.2 with length of stay as the dependent variable and infection as the factor.

The Descriptives table shows that the mean and median values for length of stay for babies with no infection are 33.20 and 22.50, respectively, 10.70 units apart and for babies with an infection, the values are 45.52 and 37.00, or 8.52 units apart. The variances are unequal at 1098.694 for no infection and 1492.804 for infection, that is, a ratio of 1:1.4. The skewness statistics are all above 2 and the kurtosis statistics are also high, indicating that the data are peaked and are not normally distributed.

Case Processing Summary

	Infection	Cases					
		Valid		Missing		Total	
		N	Per cent	N	Per cent	N	Per cent
Length of stay	No	80	94.1	5	5.9	85	100.0%
	Yes	52	92.9	4	7.1	56	100.0%

Descriptives

		Infection		Statistic	Std. error
Length of stay	No	Mean		33.20	3.706
		95% Confidence interval for mean	Lower bound	25.82	
			Upper bound	40.58	
		5% trimmed mean		28.25	
		Median		22.50	
		Variance		1098.694	
		Std. deviation		33.147	
		Minimum		0	
		Maximum		244	
		Range		244	
		Inter-quartile range		20	
		Skewness		4.082	0.269
		Kurtosis		21.457	0.532
	Yes	Mean		45.52	5.358
		95% confidence interval for mean	Lower bound	34.76	
			Upper bound	56.28	
		5% trimmed mean		40.36	
		Median		37.00	
		Variance		1492.804	
		Std. deviation		38.637	
		Minimum		11	
		Maximum		211	
		Range		200	
		Inter-quartile range		29	
		Skewness		2.502	0.330
		Kurtosis		7.012	0.650

The *P* values for the Kolmogorov–Smirnov and the Shapiro–Wilk tests are shown in the column labelled Sig. and are less than 0.05 for both groups, indicating that the data do not pass these tests of normality in either group.

Tests of Normality

	Infection	Kolmogorov–Smirnov[a]			Shapiro–Wilk		
		Statistic	df	Sig.	Statistic	df	Sig.
Length of stay	No	0.252	80	0.000	0.576	80	0.000
	Yes	0.262	52	0.000	0.707	52	0.000

[a]Lilliefors significance correction.

The histograms and plots shown in Figure 3.10 confirm the results of the tests of normality. The histograms show that both distributions are positively skewed with tails to the right. The Q–Q plot for each group does not follow the line of normality and is significantly curved. The box plots show a number of extreme and outlying values. The maximum value for length of stay of babies with no infection is 6.36 z scores above the mean, while for babies with an infection the maximum value is 4.28 z scores above the mean.

The normality statistics for babies with an infection and babies without an infection are summarized in Table 3.9, with 'No' indicating that the distribution is outside the normal range.

For both groups, the data are positively skewed and could possibly be transformed to normality using a logarithmic transformation. Without transformation, the most appropriate test for analysing length of stay is a rank-based non-parametric test, which can be obtained using the commands shown in Box 3.8.

Box 3.8 SPSS commands to obtain a non-parametric test for two independent groups

SPSS Commands

surgery.sav – IBM SPSS Statistics Data Editor
  Analyze → Nonparametric Tests → Independent Samples
Nonparametric Tests: Two or More Independent Samples
  Click on the Objective tab, tick Automatically compare distributions
   across groups (default)
  Click on the Fields tab, tick Use custom field assignments (default)
  Under Fields – highlight length of stay and click into Test Fields,
   highlight Infection and click into Groups
  Click on the Settings tab, select Choose tests, tick Customize tests,
   tick Mann–Whitney U (2 samples)
  Click Run

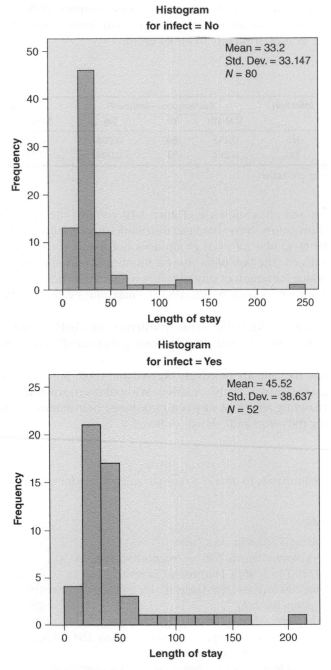

Figure 3.10 Histograms and plots of length of stay by infection.

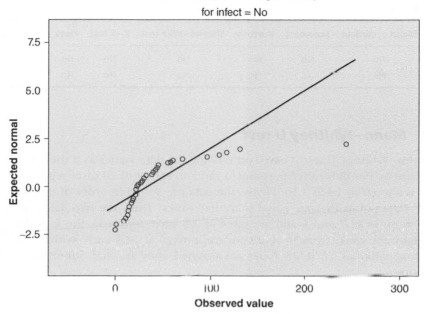

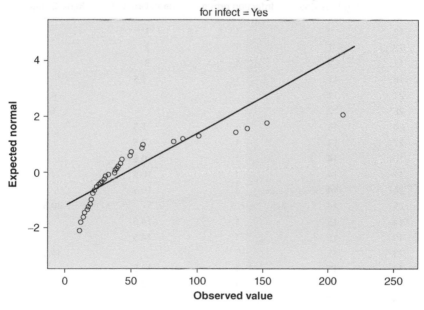

Figure 3.10 (*continued*)

Table 3.9   Summary of statistics to assess whether data are within normal limits or outside normal range

Group	Mean − median	Skewness	Kurtosis	Shapiro–Wilk test	K–S test	Plots	Overall decision
No	No	No	No	No	No	No	No
Yes	No	No	No	No	No	No	No

3.9.1   Mann–Whitney U test

The Mann–Whitney U test is based on ranking the data values as if they were from a single sample. For illustrative purposes, a random subset of 20 cases with valid length of stay is shown in Table 3.10. Firstly, the data are sorted in order of magnitude and ranked. Data points that are equal share tied ranks. Thus, the two data points of 13 share the ranks of 7 and 8 and are rated at 7.5 each. Similarly, the four data points of 17 share the ranks from 17 to 20 and are ranked at 18.5 each, which is the mean of the four rankings. Once the ranks are assigned, they are then summed for each of the groups.

Table 3.10   Ranking data to compute non-parametric statistics

ID	Length of stay	Infection group	Rank Group 1	Rank Group 2
32	0	1	1	
33	1	1	2	
12	9	1	3	
16	11	1	4.5	
22	11			4.5
28	12			6
20	13	1	7.5	
27	13	1	7.5	
10	14	1	10.5	
11	14	1	10.5	
24	14	1	10.5	
25	14			10.5
14	15	1	14.5	
19	15	1	14.5	
23	15			14.5
30	15	1	14.5	
13	17	1	18.5	
15	17	1	18.5	
17	17	1	18.5	
21	17	2		18.5
		Sum of ranks	156	54
		N	15	5
		Mean	10.5	10.8

The Hypothesis Test Summary table shows that the $P = 0.004$ and provides evidence that there is a significant difference in the distributions of the two groups.

Hypothesis Test Summary

	Null Hypothesis	Test	Sig.	Decision
1	The distribution of Length of stay is the same across categories of Infection.	Independent-Samples Mann-Whitney U Test	.004	Reject the null hypothesis.

Asymptotic significances are displayed. The significance level is .05.

Non-parametric tests

By double clicking on the Hypothesis Test Summary table, the Model Viewer screen will open. The Model View has a two panel views, with the Hypothesis Test Summary table shown on the left hand side, referred to as the Main View. On the right side, the linked Auxiliary View is displayed which shows the following population pyramid chart and test table. The chart displays back-to-back histograms for each category of the group, that is, 'No' infection and 'Yes' infection. The number of cases in each group and the mean rank of each group are also reported. The mean rank are for each group is reported. The mean ranks provide an indication of the direction of effect but because the data are ranked, the dimension is different from the original measurement and is therefore difficult to communicate.

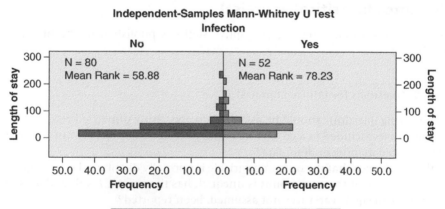

Total N	132
Mann-Whitney U	2,690.000
Wilcoxon W	4,068.000
Test Statistic	2,690.000
Standard Error	214.535
Standardized Test Statistic	2.843
Asymptotic Sig. (2-sided test)	.004

Table 3.11 Length of stay for babies with infection and without infection

	Infection absent ($n = 80$) Mdn (IQR)	Infection present ($n = 52$) Mdn (IQR)	P value
Length of stay (days)	22.5 (20)	37.0 (29)	0.004

The Mann–Whitney U and the Wilcoxon W that are obtained from SPSS are two derivations of the same test and are best reported as the Mann–Whitney U test. The asymptotic significance value is reported when the sample size is large, say more than 30 cases. The difference between the groups could be reported in a table as shown in Table 3.11.

Another approach to non-normal data is to divide the outcome variable into categorical centile groups as discussed in Chapter 8. Decision about whether to use non-parametric tests, to transform the variable or to categorize the values requires careful consideration. The decision should be based on the size of the sample, the effectiveness of the transformation in normalizing the data and the ways in which the relationship between the explanatory and outcome variables is best presented.

3.10   Notes for critical appraisal

Questions to ask when assessing descriptive statistics published in the literature are shown in Box 3.9.

Box 3.9 Questions for critical appraisal

The following questions should be asked when appraising published results:
- are any cases included in a group more than once, for example, are any follow-up data treated as independent data?
- is there evidence that the outcome variable is normally distributed in each group?
- if the variance of the two groups is unequal, has the correct P value, that is, the P value with equal variances not assumed, been reported?
- are the summary statistics appropriate for the distributions?
- are there any influential outliers that could have increased the difference in mean values between the groups?
- are mean values presented appropriately in figures as dot plots or are histograms used inappropriately?
- are mean values and the differences between groups presented with 95% confidence intervals?

References

1. Altman DG, Bland JM. Standard deviations and standard errors. *BMJ* 2005; **331**: 903.
2. Cohen J. *Statistical power analysis for the behavioural sciences*, 2nd edn. Lawrence Erlbaum Associates: Hillsdale, NJ, 1988.
3. Cohen J. A power primer. *Psychol Bull* 1992; **1**: 155–159.
4. Hattie, JA, Marsh, HW, Neill, JT, Richards, GE. Adventure education and outward bound: out-of-class experiences that make a lasting difference. *Rev Educ Res* 1977; **67**: 43–87.
5. Hedges, LV. Distribution theory for Glass's estimator of effect size and related estimators. *J Educ Stat* 1981; **6**: 107–128.
6. Peat JK, Mellis CM, Williams K, Xuan W. *Health science research: a handbook of quantitative methods*. Allen and Unwin: Crows Nest, Australia, 2002.
7. Stevens J. *Applied multivariate statistics for the social sciences*, 3rd edn. Lawrence Erlbaum Associates: Mahwah, NJ, 1996.
8. Tabachnick BG, Fidell LS. *Using multivariate statistics*, 4th edn. Allyn and Bacon: Boston, USA, 2001.

CHAPTER 4

Paired and one-sample *t*-tests

A statistician is a person who likes to prove you wrong, 5% of the time.
TAKEN FROM AN INTERNET BULLETIN BOARD

Objectives

The objectives of this chapter are to explain how to:

- analyse paired or matched data
- use paired *t*-tests and one-sample *t*-tests
- interpret results from non-parametric paired tests
- calculate an effect size
- report changes or differences in paired data in appropriate units

In addition to two-sample (independent) *t*-tests, there are also two other parametric *t*-tests that can be used to analyse continuous data, that is, paired *t*-tests and one-sample (single sample) *t*-tests. All three types of *t*-test can be one-tailed or two-tailed tests. However, one-tailed *t*-tests are rarely used in health sciences research.

4.1 Paired *t*-tests

A paired *t*-test is used to estimate whether the means of two related measurements are significantly different from one another. This test is used when two continuous variables are related because they are collected from the same participant at different times, from different sites on the same person at the same time or from cases and their matched controls.[1] Examples of paired study designs are

- data from a longitudinal study;
- measurements collected before and after an intervention in an experimental study;
- differences between related sites in the same person, for example limbs, eyes or kidneys;
- matched cases and controls.

For a paired *t*-test, there is no explanatory (group) variable. The outcome of interest is the difference in the outcome measurements between each pair or between each case

---

Medical Statistics: A Guide to SPSS, Data Analysis and Critical Appraisal, Second Edition.
Belinda Barton and Jennifer Peat.
© 2014 John Wiley & Sons, Ltd. Published 2014 by John Wiley & Sons, Ltd.
Companion website: www.wiley.com/go/barton/medicalstatistics2e

and its matched control, that is, the within-pair differences. When using a paired *t*-test, the variation between the pairs of measurements is the most important statistic and the variation between the participants, as when using a two-sample *t*-test, is of little interest. The null hypothesis for a paired *t*-test is that the mean of the differences between the two related measurements is equal to zero, that is, no difference.

4.1.1 Data sheet layout

For related measurements, the data for each pair of values must be entered on the same row of the spreadsheet. Thus, the number of rows in the data sheet is the same as the number of participants when the outcome variable is measured more than once for each participant or is the number of participant-pairs when cases and controls are matched. When each participant is measured on two or more occasions, the sample size is the number of participants. In a matched case–control study, the number of case–control pairs is the sample size and not the total number of participants. For this reason, withdrawals, loss of follow-up data and inability to recruit matched controls reduce both power and the generalizability of the paired *t*-test because participants with missing paired values or cases who are not matched with controls are excluded from the analyses.

4.1.2 Assumptions for a paired t-test

Independent two-sample *t*-tests cannot be used for analysing paired or matched data because the assumption that the two groups are independent, that is, data are collected from different or non-matched participants, would be violated. Treating paired or matched measurements as independent samples will artificially inflate the sample size and lead to inaccurate analyses.

The assumptions for using paired *t*-tests are shown in Box 4.1.

Box 4.1 Assumptions for a paired *t*-test

For a paired *t*-test, the following assumptions must be met:
- the outcome variable must be on a continuous scale
- the differences between the pairs of measurements are normally distributed

---

The data file **growth.sav** contains the body measurements of 277 babies measured at 1 month and at 3 months of age.

The decision of whether to use a one- or two-tailed test must be made when the study is designed. If a one-tailed *t*-test is used, the null hypothesis is more likely to be rejected than if a two-tailed test is used (Chapter 3). In general, two-tailed tests should always be used unless there is a good reason for not doing so and a one-tailed test should only be used when the direction of effect is specified in advance.[2] In this example, it makes sense to test for a significant increase in body measurements because there is certainty that a decrease will not occur and there is only one biologically plausible direction of effect. Therefore, a one-tailed test is appropriate for the alternate hypothesis.

Questions:	Does the weight of babies increase significantly in a 2-month growth period?
	Does the length of babies increase significantly in a 2-month growth period?
	Does the head circumference of babies increase significantly in a 2-month growth period?
Null	The weight of babies is not different between the two time periods.
hypotheses:	The length of babies is not different between the two time periods.
	The head circumference of babies is not different between the two time periods.
Variables:	Outcome variables = weight, length and head circumference measured at 1 month of age and 3 months of age (continuous)

4.1.3   Testing the assumptions of a paired t-test

To test the assumption that the differences between the two outcome variables are normally distributed, the differences between measurements taken at 1 month and at 3 months must first be computed as shown in Box 4.2.

Box 4.2 SPSS commands to transform variables

SPSS Commands

growth.sav – IBM SPSS Statistics Data Editor
> *Transform → Compute Variable*

Compute Variable
> *Target Variable = diffwt*
> *Numeric Expression = Weight at 3mo – Weight at 1mo*
> *Click Type & Label*

Compute Variable: Type and Label
> *Tick Label and enter Weight 3mo-1mo*
> *Click Continue*

Compute Variable
> *Click OK*

By clicking on the *Reset* button in *Compute Variable*, all fields will be reset to empty and the command sequence shown in Box 4.2 can be used to compute the following variables:

diffleng = Length at 3mo – Length at 1mo, and
diffhead = Head circumference at 3mo – Head circumference at 1mo

In Data View, once the new variables are created, they should be labelled, have the number of decimal places adjusted to be appropriate, and the measurement level option correctly entered as Scale. The distribution of these differences between the paired measurements can then be examined using the commands shown in Box 4.3 to obtain histograms. Alternatively, the SPSS Chart Builder can be used to create and edit histograms. The SPSS Chart Builder can be used to create a number of different charts include bar, line pie and scatter/dot.

Box 4.3 SPSS commands to obtain frequency histograms

SPSS Commands

growth.sav – IBM SPSS Statistics Data Editor
   Graphs → Legacy Dialogs → Histogram
Histogram
   Variable = Weight 3mo-1mo
   Tick Display normal curve
   Click OK

While only histograms have been obtained in this example, in practice a thorough investigation of all tests of normality should be undertaken using *Analyze → Descriptive Statistics → Explore* and other options discussed in Chapter 2.

The command sequence in Box 4.3 can then be repeated with the difference variables Length 3m-1mo and Head 3mo-1mo to produce the histograms shown in Figure 4.1. The histograms indicate that the difference variables for weight and length are fairly normally distributed. The distribution of scores for the difference variable for head circumference is quite skewed. The checks of normality as discussed in Chapter 2 indicate that this variable is not normally distributed. Therefore, a non-parametric test is more appropriate to analyse this variable, which is discussed later in this chapter.

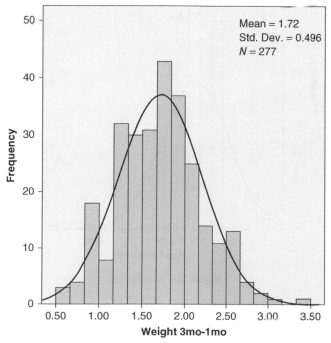

Figure 4.1 Histograms of differences between babies at 1 month and 3 months for weight, length and head circumference.

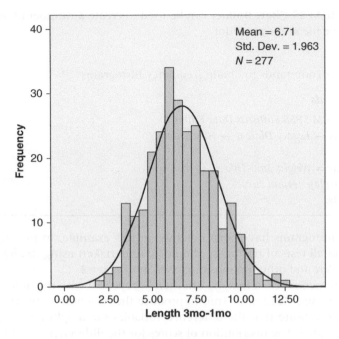

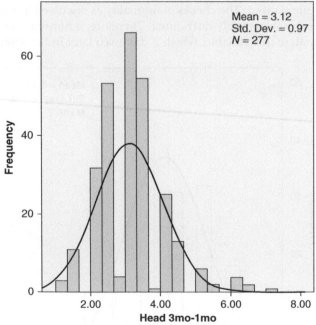

Figure 4.1 (*continued*)

Research example

The SPSS commands to conduct a paired samples *t*-test to examine whether there has been a significant increase in weight and length are shown in Box 4.4. By entering the data variables at 3 months before the data variables at 1 month, the direction of the summary statistics will be in the appropriate direction and have the correct signs.

Box 4.4 SPSS commands to obtain a paired samples *t*-test

SPSS Commands

growth.sav – IBM SPSS Statistics Data Editor
       Analyze → Compare Means → Paired-Samples T Test
Paired-Samples T-Test
       Highlight Weight at 3mo and click into Variable 1 then highlight Weight at 1mo and
          click into Variable 2 in the Paired Variables box
       Highlight Length at 3mo and click into Variable 1 then highlight Length at 1mo and
          click into Variable 2 in the Paired Variables box
       Highlight Head circumference at 3m and click into Variable 1 and highlight Head
          circumference at 1mo and click into Variable 2 in the Paired Variables box
       Click OK

T-Test

Paired Samples Statistics

		Mean	N	Std. deviation	Std. error mean
Pair 1	Weight at 3 months (kg)	6.131	277	0.7741	0.0465
	Weight at 1 month (kg)	4.415	277	0.6145	0.0369
Pair 2	Length at 3 months (cm)	61.510	277	2.7005	0.1623
	Length at 1 month (cm)	54.799	277	2.3081	0.1387

The Paired Samples Statistics table provides summary statistics for each variable but does not give any information that is relevant to the paired *t*-test. The Paired Samples Correlations table shows the correlations between each of the paired measurements. This table is not relevant because it does not make sense to test the hypothesis that two related measurements are associated with one another.

Paired Samples Correlations

		N	Correlation	Sig.
Pair 1	Weight at 3 months (kg) and weight at 1 month (kg)	277	0.768	0.000
Pair 2	Length at 3 months (cm) and Length at 1 month (cm)	277	0.703	0.000

Paired Samples Test

		Paired differences						
		Mean	Std devia- tion	Std error mean	95% confidence interval of the Difference		t	df	Sig. (two- tailed)
					Lower	Upper			
Pair 1	Weight at 3 months (kg)– Weight at 1 months (kg)	1.7167	0.4961	0.0298	1.6580	1.7754	57.591	276	0.000
Pair 2	Length at 3 months (cm)– Length at 1 month (cm)	6.7105	1.9635	0.1180	6.4782	6.9427	56.881	276	0.000

The Paired Samples Test table provides important information about the *t*-test results. The second column, which is labelled Mean, gives the main outcome measurement that is the mean within-pair difference. When conducting a paired *t*-test, the means of the differences between the pairs of measurements are computed as part of the test.

4.1.4   Interpretation of the results

The mean paired differences column in the Paired Samples table indicates that at 3 months, babies were on an average 1.717 kg heavier in weight and 6.71 cm longer in length than at 1 month of age. These mean values provide an indication that babies increased in measurements over a 2-month period. However, they do not provide information as to whether this increase was statistically significant.

The 95% confidence intervals of the differences are calculated as the mean paired differences ± (1.96 * SE of mean paired differences). These are shown in the Paired Samples Test table and do not contain the value of zero for any variable, which also provides evidence that the difference in body size between 1 and 3 months is statistically significant. The *t* value is calculated as the mean differences divided by their standard error. Because the standard error becomes smaller as the sample size becomes larger, the *t* value increases as the sample size increases for the same mean difference. Thus, in this example with a large sample size of 277 babies, relatively small mean differences are highly statistically significant.

In the last column in the Paired Samples Test table, labelled Sig. (two-tailed), the *P* values for a two-tailed test are reported and highly statistically significant with $P < 0.0001$. However, the alternative hypothesis for this study was one-tailed; therefore, the *P* values have to be adjusted by halving them. The *P* values are <0.0001 so that halving them will also render a highly significant *P* value. The *P* values (one-tailed) from the paired *t*-tests for all three variables indicate that each null hypothesis should be rejected and that there is a significant increase in body measurements between the two time periods. As with any statistical test, it is important to decide whether the size of mean difference

Table 4.1   Growth in weight and length from 1 month to 3 months in 277 term babies

	1 month Mean (SD)	3 months Mean (SD)	Mean difference (95% CI)	P value	Effect size
Weight	4.42 (0.61)	6.13 (0.77)	1.72 (1.66, 1.78)	<0.0001	3.46
Length	54.80 (2.31)	61.51 (2.70)	6.71 (6.48, 6.94)	<0.0001	3.42

between measurements would be considered clinically important in addition to being statistically significant.

4.1.5   Calculating the effect size

For paired data, the effect size Cohen's d is calculated as the mean difference divided by the standard deviation. For weight, the effect size is $1.717/0.496 = 3.46$ and for length, the effect size is $6.710/1.964 = 3.42$. These effect sizes are very large but are expected in babies studied in a critical growth period. The results from this study could be reported as shown in Table 4.1. The means and standard deviations are reported to two decimal places, which is one more decimal place above the number that the original measurements were taken in.

4.2   Non-parametric test for paired data

A non-parametric equivalent of the paired *t*-test is the Wilcoxon signed rank test, which is also called the Wilcoxon matched pairs test. This test is used when lack of normality in the differences of the scores is a concern, that is when the differences did not come from a normally distributed population, or when the sample size is small. The Wilcoxon signed rank test is used to test the null hypothesis that the median of the differences between pairs of observations is equal to zero.

The assumptions of the Wilcoxon signed rank test are (i) that the paired differences are independent and (ii) the differences come from a distribution in which the differences between paired measurements are symmetrically distributed around the median value. For this test, the number of outliers should not be large relative to the sample size. When the sample size is small, symmetry may be difficult to assess.

In this test, the absolute differences (i.e. sign of the difference is ignored) between paired scores are ranked. Then the ranks where there is a positive difference between the two observations are summed. Similarly, the ranks where there is a negative difference between the two observations are summed. Difference scores that are equal to zero, indicating no difference between pairs, are excluded from the analysis. The smaller of the two summed totals is the test statistic, which is used to determine whether the null hypothesis should be rejected. This test is not suitable when a large proportion of paired differences are equal to zero because this effectively reduces the sample size.

The difference variable for head circumference (*diffhead*) in the **growth.sav** data set did not have a normal distribution and can be analysed using the Wilcoxon signed rank test, which can obtained using the SPSS commands in Box 4.5.

Box 4.5 SPSS commands to conduct a non-parametric paired test

SPSS Commands

growth.sav – IBM SPSS Statistics Data Editor
    Analyze → Nonparametric Tests → Related Samples
Nonparametric Tests: Two or More Related Samples
    Click on the Objective tab, tick Automatically compare observed data to hypothesized
        (default)
    Click on the Fields tab, tick Use custom field assignments (default)
    Under Fields – highlight Head circumference at 1 mo and click into Test Fields,
        highlight Head circumference at 3 mo and click into Test Fields
    Click on the Settings tab, Select Choose Tests (default), tick Customize tests
        and tick Wilcoxon matched-pair signed-rank (2 samples)
    Click Run

Hypothesis Test Summary

	Null Hypothesis	Test	Sig.	Decision
1	The median of differences between Head circumference at 1 mo (cm) and Head circumference at 3 mo (cm) equals 0.	Related-Samples Wilcoxon Signed Rank Test	.000	Reject the null hypothesis.

Asymptotic significances are displayed. The significance level is .05.

Non-parametric tests

The P value that is displayed in the Hypothesis Test Summary table is computed based on the ranks of the absolute values of the differences between 1 month and 3 months. The test statistics with a P value of <0.0001 shows that the alternative hypothesis should be accepted and that the median of the paired differences does not equal zero and that observations increased or decreased over time (two-tailed test).

By double clicking on the Hypothesis Test Summary table, the Model Viewer window is opened and the following information is obtained (see page 99).

The histogram displays the size of the rank difference between pairs of observation and the frequency of the difference. The difference is calculated as the head circumference scores at 3 months minus the head circumference scores at 1 month, as shown underneath the histogram. The number of negative ranks where the head circumference at 3 months is lower than that at 1 month is reported as negative differences in the histogram. The number of positive ranks where head circumference at 3 months is higher than that at 1 month of age is reported as positive differences. The zero ranks, that is, no difference between observations is not reported in the histogram. As the legend next to the bar chart indicates no babies have a negative rank, that is, a lower head circumference at 3 months than at 1 month of age, as expected. The legend also shows that there are no ties, that is, no babies with the same difference scores. Although this legend does not provide any useful information for communicating the size of effect, it does indicate the direction of the effect, with the head circumference of babies increasing from 1 month to 3 months of age.

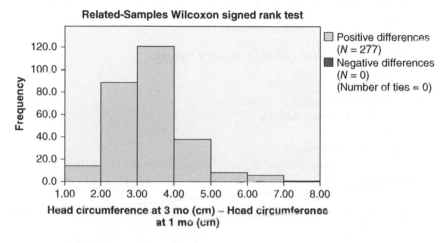

Related-Samples Wilcoxon signed rank test

Positive differences (*N* = 277)
Negative differences (*N* = 0)
(Number of ties = 0)

Head circumference at 3 mo (cm) – Head circumference at 1 mo (cm)

Total *N*	277
Test statistic	38,503.000
Standard error	1,330.486
Standardized test statistic	14.470
Asymptotic sig. (two-sided test)	.000

In reporting the results of this non-parametric test, the median and interquartile range rather than the mean and standard deviation would be reported since the mean difference may be a biased measure of central tendency when the data are not normally distributed. In addition to reporting the total sample size and the *P* value, the *Z* statistic of 14.47, which is the standardized *W* value obtained from the Wilcoxon signed-ranks test should be reported.

4.3   Standardizing for differences in baseline measurements

With paired data, the absolute differences between the pairs may not be of interest. It is often important that the differences are standardized for between-subject differences in baseline values. One method is to compute a per cent change from baseline. Another method is to calculate the ratio between the follow-up and baseline measurements. It is important to choose a method that is appropriate for the type of data collected and that is easily communicated.

For babies' growth, per cent change is a simple method to standardize for differences in body size at baseline, that is, at 1 month of age. The commands shown in Box 4.6 can be used to compute per cent growth in weight, and similarly for length and head circumference.

Box 4.6 SPSS commands to compute per cent changes

SPSS Commands

growth.sav – IBM SPSS Statistics Data Editor
     Transform → Compute Variable
Compute Variable
     Target Variable = perwt
     *Numeric Expression = (Weight at 3mo – Weight at 1mo) * 100/Weight at 1mo*
     Click Type & Label
Compute Variable: Type and Label
     Tick Label and enter Percent change in weight
     Click Continue
Compute Variable
     Click Paste
*Syntax1 – IBM SPSS Syntax Editor
     Select Run → All

The paste and run commands list the calculations in the syntax window as shown below. This information can then be printed and stored for documentation. Once the computations are complete, the new variables need to be labelled in the Variable View window.

COMPUTE perwt=(weight3m - weight1m)*100/weight1m.
VARIABLE LABELS perwt 'Percent change in weight'.
EXECUTE.

COMPUTE perleng=(length3m - length1m)*100/length1m.
VARIABLE LABELS perleng 'Percent change in length'.
EXECUTE.

COMPUTE perhead=(head3m - head1m)*100/head1m.
VARIABLE LABELS perhead 'Percent change in head'.
EXECUTE.

An assumption of paired *t*-tests is that the differences between the pairs of measurements are normally distributed; therefore, the distributions of the per cent changes need to be examined. The histograms shown in Figure 4.2 can be obtained using the commands shown in Box 4.3. The histograms for per cent change in weight and head circumference have a small tail to the right, but the sample size is large and the tails are not so marked that the assumptions for using a paired *t*-test would be violated. However, the distributions should be fully checked for normality using *Analyze → Descriptive Statistics → Explore* as discussed in Chapter 2.

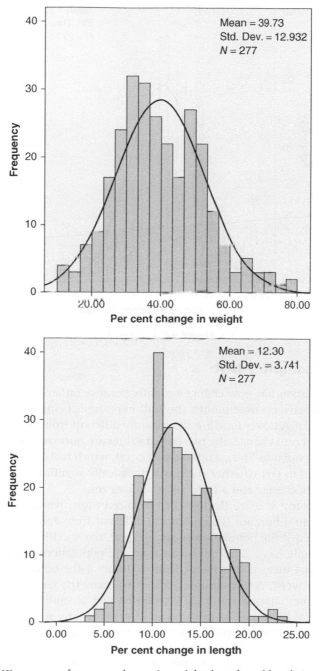

Figure 4.2 Histograms of per cent change in weight, length and head circumference.

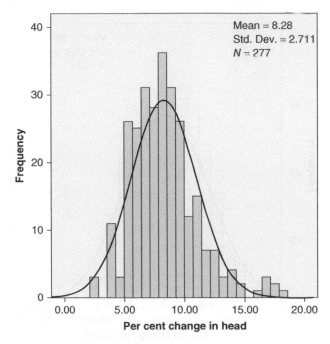

Figure 4.2 (*continued*)

4.4 Single-sample *t*-test

The research question has now changed slightly because rather than considering absolute differences between time points, the null hypothesis being tested is whether the mean per cent changes over time are significantly different from zero. With differences converted to a per cent change, the two paired values are now converted to a single continuous outcome variable. Thus, a one-sample *t*-test, which is also called a single-sample *t*-test, can be used to test whether there is a statistically significant difference between the mean per cent change and a fixed value such as zero.

A one-sample *t*-test is more flexible than a paired *t*-test, which is limited to testing whether the mean difference is significantly different from zero. A one-sample *t*-test can be used to test if the population mean is equal to a specified value. For example, to test if the sample has a different mean from the population mean of 100 points if the outcome being measured is IQ, or from 40 hours if the outcome measured is the average working week. A one-sample *t*-test is a parametric test and the assumptions are that firstly, the data are normally distributed and secondly, the observations are independent. Also, the outcome must be an interval or ratio scale of measurement. If the assumptions of a one sample *t*-test are not satisfied, a non-parametric equivalent test, that is, a Wilcoxon signed rank test may be conducted. This rank test is available in SPSS using the following commands *Analyze → Nonparametric Tests → One Sample*.

Computing per cent changes provides control over the units that the changes are expressed in and their direction of effect. However, if the differences computed in Box 4.2 were used as the outcome and a one-sample *t*-test was used to test for a difference from zero, the one-sample *t*-test would give exactly the same summary statistics and *P* values as the paired *t*-test simply because the paired *t*-test automatically computes mean differences and tests for a difference from zero.

For the research question, the command sequence shown in Box 4.7 can be used to compute a one-sample *t*-test to test whether the per cent changes in weight, length and head circumference are significantly different from zero.

Box 4.7 SPSS commands to conduct a one-sample *t*-test

SPSS Commands

growth.sav – IBM SPSS Statistics Data Editor
   Analyze → Compare Means → One-Sample T Test
One-Sample T Test
   Highlight the variables Per cent change in weight, Per cent change in length and
       Per cent change in head circumference and click into the Test Variable(s) box
   Test Value = 0 (default setting)
   Click OK

T-Test

One-Sample Statistics

	N	Mean	Std. deviation	Std. error mean
Per cent change in weight	277	39.726	12.9322	0.7770
Per cent change in length	277	12.298	3.7413	0.2248
Per cent change in head	277	8.277	2.7115	0.1629

The One-Sample Statistics table gives more relevant statistics with which to answer the research question because the mean within-participant per cent changes and their standard deviations are provided. The means in this table show that the per cent increase in weight over 2 months is larger than the per cent increase in length and head circumference.

One-Sample Test

	t	df	Sig. (two-tailed)	Mean difference	95% confidence interval of the difference	
					Test value = 0	
					Lower	Upper
Per cent change in weight	51.126	276	0.000	39.7264	38.197	41.256
Per cent change in length	54.708	276	0.000	12.2980	11.856	12.741
Per cent change in head	50.803	276	0.000	8.2767	7.956	8.597

In the One-Sample Test table, the *t* values are again computed as mean difference divided by the standard error and, in this table, are highly significant for all measurements. The highly significant *P* values are reflected in the 95% confidence intervals, none of which contain the zero value. The outcomes are now all in the same units, that is per cent change, and therefore growth rates between the three variables can be directly compared. This was not possible before when the variables were in their original units of measurement. As before, Cohen's *d* can be calculated as the mean divided by the standard deviation using the values reported in the One-Sample Statistics table.

Table 4.2 Mean body measurements and per cent change between 1 and 3 months in 277 babies

	1 month Mean (SD)	3 months Mean (SD)	Per cent increase and 95% CI	P value
Weight (kg)	4.42 (0.62)	6.13 (0.77)	39.7 (38.2, 41.3)	<0.0001
Length (cm)	54.8 (2.3)	61.5 (2.7)	12.3 (11.9, 12.7)	<0.0001
Head circumference (cm)	37.9 (1.4)	41.0 (1.4)	8.3 (7.9, 8.6)	<0.0001

These effect sizes of d for percentage change are 3.07 for weight, 3.29 for length and 3.06 for head circumference. These differ slightly from the effect sizes computed for a paired t-test because the variables are now in different standardized units and the mean difference and per cent increase have different standard deviations. The effect sizes rank length as having the largest effect size, whereas weight has the largest per cent increase.

This summary information can be reported as shown in Table 4.2. In some disciplines such as psychology, the t value is also reported with its degrees of freedom, for example as $t(276) = 51.13$ with the effect size of $d = 3.07$. However, since the only interpretation of the t value and its degrees of freedom is the P value, it is often excluded from summary tables.

Research question

The research question can now be extended to ask if certain groups, such as males and females, have different patterns or rates of growth.

Questions:	Over a 2-month period:
	Do males increase in weight significantly more than females?
	Do males increase in length significantly more than females?
	Do males increase in head circumference significantly more than females?
Null hypothesis:	Over a 2-month period:
	There is no difference between males and females in weight growth.
	There is no difference between males and females in length growth.
	There is no difference between males and females in head circumference growth.
Variables:	Outcome variables = per cent increase in length, weight and head circumference (continuous)
	Explanatory variable = gender (categorical, binary)

The research question then becomes a two-sample *t*-test again because there is a continuously distributed variable (per cent change) and a binary group variable with two levels that are independent (male, female). Once again, the distributions of per cent change should be fully checked for normality using *Analyze → Descriptive Statistics → Explore* as discussed in Chapter 2 and that test assumptions have been satisfied before conducting a two-sample or independent *t*-test. The SPSS commands shown in Box 3.3 can be used to obtain the following output.

T-Test

Group Statistics

	Gender	*N*	Mean	Std. deviation	Std. error mean
Per cent change in weight	Male	148	42.0051	13.26558	1.09042
	Female	129	37.1121	12.06764	1.06250
Per cent change in length	Male	148	12.6818	3.30790	0.27191
	Female	129	11.8577	4.15334	0.36568
Per cent change in head	Male	148	8.2435	2.50656	0.20604
	Female	129	8.3147	2.93850	0.25872

The means in the Group Statistics table show that males have a higher increase in weight and length, but a slightly lower increase in head circumference than females. These statistics are useful for summarizing the magnitude of the differences in each gender.

In the Independent Samples Test table, the Levene's test of equality of variances shows that the variances are not significantly different between genders for weight ($P = 0.374$) and head circumference ($P = 0.111$). For these two variables, the *Equal variances assumed* rows in the table are used. However, the variance in per cent change for length is significantly different between the genders ($P = 0.034$) and therefore the appropriate *t* value, degrees of freedom and *P* value for this variable are shown in the *Equal variances not assumed* row. An indication that the variances are unequal could be seen in the previous Group Statistics table, which shows that the standard deviation for per cent change in length is 3.3079 for males and 4.1533 for females. An estimate of the variances can be obtained by squaring the standard deviations to give 10.94 for males and 17.25 for females, which is a variance ratio of 1:1.6.

Thus, the Independent Samples Test table shows that per cent increase in weight is significantly different between the genders at $P = 0.002$, per cent increase in length does not reach significance between the genders at $P = 0.072$ and per cent increase in head circumference is not clearly not different between the genders at $P = 0.828$. This is reflected in the 95% confidence intervals, which do not cross zero for weight, cross zero marginally for length and encompass zero for head circumference.

Independent Samples Test

		Levene's test for equality of variances		t-Test for equality of means						
									95% confidence interval of the difference	
		F	Sig.	t	df	Sig. (two-tailed)	Mean difference	Std. error difference	Lower	Upper
Per cent change in weight	Equal variances assumed	0.792	0.374	3.193	275	0.002	4.89304	1.53240	1.87633	7.90976
	Equal variances not assumed			3.214	274.486	0.001	4.89304	1.52247	1.89583	7.89025
Per cent change in length	Equal variances assumed	4.518	0.034	1.837	275	0.067	0.82410	0.44873	−0.05928	1.70748
	Equal variances not assumed			1.808	243.779	0.072	0.82410	0.45569	−0.07350	1.72170
Per cent change in head	Equal variances assumed	2.561	0.111	−0.217	275	0.828	−0.07114	0.32717	−0.71521	0.57294
	Equal variances not assumed			−0.215	253.173	0.830	−0.07114	0.33074	−0.72248	0.58021

4.5 Testing for a between-group difference

If no between-gender differences were found, the summary statistics for the entire sample could be presented. However, the growth patterns for weight are different between males and females. One-sample *t*-tests can be used to test whether the mean per cent increase is significantly different from zero for each gender. This can be achieved using the *Split File* option shown in Box 4.8. After the commands have been completed, the message *Split File On* will appear in the bottom right hand side of the Data Editor screen. The advantage of using *Split File* rather than *Select Cases* is that the SPSS output will be automatically documented by group status.

Box 4.8 SPSS commands to split data into separate groups for analysis

SPSS Commands

growth.sav – IBM SPSS Statistics Data Editor
      Data → Split File
Split File
      Click Compare groups
      Highlight Gender and click over into Groups Based on
      Click OK

The one-sample *t*-test for each gender can then be obtained using the commands shown in Box 4.7 to produce the following output.

T-Test

One-Sample Statistics

Gender		N	Mean	Std. deviation	Std. error mean
Male	Per cent change in weight	148	42.0051	13.26558	1.09042
	Per cent change in length	148	12.6818	3.30790	0.27191
	Per cent change in head	148	8.2435	2.50656	0.20604
Female	Per cent change in weight	129	37.1121	12.06764	1.06250
	Per cent change in length	129	11.8577	4.15334	0.36568
	Per cent change in head	129	8.3147	2.93850	0.25872

One-Sample Test

Gender		Test value = 0					
						95% confidence interval of the difference	
		t	*df*	Sig. (two-tailed)	Mean difference	Lower	Upper
Male	Per cent change in weight	38.522	147	0.000	42.00513	39.8502	44.1601
	Per cent change in length	46.640	147	0.000	12.68183	12.1445	13.2192
	Per cent change in head	40.010	147	0.000	8.24352	7.8363	8.6507
Female	Per cent change in weight	34.929	128	0.000	37.11209	35.0098	39.2144
	Per cent change in length	32.426	128	0.000	11.85773	11.1342	12.5813
	Per cent change in head	32.138	128	0.000	8.31466	7.8027	8.8266

The One-Sample Statistics table gives the same summary statistics as obtained in the two-sample *t*-test. The One-Sample Test table provides a *P* value for the significance of the per cent change from baseline for each gender and also gives the 95% confidence intervals around the mean changes. Another alternative to obtaining summary means for each gender is to use the commands shown in Box 4.9, but with the *Split File* option removed.

Box 4.9 SPSS commands to obtain summary mean values

SPSS Commands

growth.sav – IBM SPSS Statistics Data Editor
   Data → Split File
Split File
   Click Analyze all cases, do not create groups
   Click OK
growth – SPSS Data Editor
   Analyze → Compare Means → Means
Means
   Click variables for weight, length, head circumference at 1 month (weight1m,
      length1m, head1m) and at 3 months (weight3m, length3m, head3m) and all three
      percent changes (perwt, perlen, perhead) into the Dependent List box
   Click Gender over into the Independent List box
   Click OK

Means

Report

Gender		Weight at 1 month (kg)	Length at 1 month (cm)	Head circumference at 1 month (cm)	Weight at 3 months (kg)	Length at 3 months (cm)	Head circumference at 3 months (cm)	Per cent change in weight	Per cent change in length	Per cent change in head circumference
Male	Mean	4.534	55.249	38.259	6.389	62.218	41.393	42.0051	12.6818	8.2435
	N	148	148	148	148	148	148	148	148	148
	Std. deviation	0.6608	2.5636	1.325	0.7829	2.6185	1.1411	13.26558	3.30790	2.50656
Female	Mean	4.278	54.283	37.526	5.836	60.698	40.632	37.1121	11.8577	8.3147
	N	129	129	129	129	129	129	129	129	129
	Std. deviation	0.5269	1.8539	1.3160	0.6507	2.5704	1.4575	12.06764	4.15334	2.93850
Total	Mean	4.415	54.799	37.918	6.131	61.510	41.039	39.7264	12.2980	8.2767
	N	277	277	277	277	277	277	277	277	277
	Std. deviation	0.6145	2.3081	1.3685	0.7741	2.7005	1.3504	12.93223	3.74134	2.71147

Table 4.3   Mean body measurements and per cent change between 1 and 3 months in 148 male and 129 female babies

		1 month Mean (SD)	3 months Mean (SD)	Per cent change and 95% CI	P value for change from baseline	P value for difference between genders
Weight (kg)	Male	4.53 (0.66)	6.39 (0.78)	42.0 (39.9, 44.2)	<0.0001	0.002
	Female	4.28 (0.53)	5.84 (0.65)	37.1 (35.0, 39.2)	<0.0001	
Length (cm)	Male	55.2 (2.6)	62.2 (2.6)	12.7 (12.1, 13.2)	<0.0001	0.072
	Female	54.3 (1.9)	60.7 (2.6)	11.9 (11.1, 12.6)	<0.0001	
Head	Male	38.3 (1.3)	41.4 (1.1)	8.2 (7.8, 8.7)	<0.0001	0.828
Circumference (cm)	Female	37.5 (1.3)	40.6 (1.5)	8.3 (7.8, 8.8)	<0.0001	

The results could be reported as shown in Table 4.3. Although a one-tailed *P* value is used for the significance of increases in body size because we only expect babies to increase in body size, a two-tailed *P* value is used for between-gender comparisons because the direction of effect between genders is not certain.

4.5.1   *Plotting the results*

When plotting summary statistics of continuous variables, the choice of whether to use bar charts or dot points is critical. Bar charts should always begin at zero so that their lengths can be meaningfully compared. When the distance from zero has no meaning, mean values are best plotted as dot points. For example, mean length would not be plotted using a bar chart because no baby has a zero length. However, bar charts are ideal for plotting per cent changes where a zero value is plausible. The results can be plotted as bar charts in SigmaPlot (Figure 4.3) by entering the data as follows and using the commands shown in Box 4.10. The means for males are entered in column 1 and the 95% confidence interval width in column 2. The values for females are entered in columns 3 and 4. The column titles should not be entered in the spreadsheet cells.

Column 1	Column 2	Column 3	Column 4
42.0	2.1	37.1	2.1
12.7	0.6	11.9	0.6
8.2	0.4	8.3	0.4

Box 4.10 SigmaPlot commands for graphing per cent change results

SigmaPlot Commands

Data 1*
    Click on Create Graph tab at top of the screen
    Click on Bar in sub-menu
    Click on Grouped Horizontal Bar – Error Bars in Bar Group
Create Graph – Error Bars
    Symbol Values = Worksheet Columns (default), click Next
Create Graph – Data Format
    Highlight Many X, click Next
Create Graph – Select Data
    Data for Set 1 = use drop box and select Column 1
    Data for Error 1 = use drop box and select Column 2
    Data for Set 2 = use drop box and select Column 3
    Data for Error 2 = use drop box and select Column 4
    Click Finish

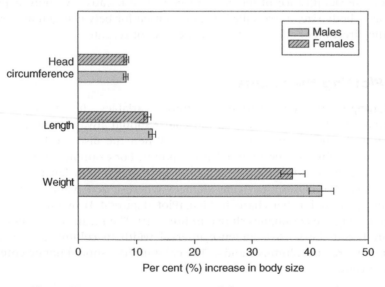

Figure 4.3 Per cent increase in growth from age 1 to 3 months.

The graph can then be customized by changing the axes, fills, labels etc in *Graph →
Graph Properties* menus.

4.6 Notes for critical appraisal

Questions to ask when assessing statistics from paired or matched data are shown in
Box 4.11.

Box 4.11 Questions for critical appraisal

The following questions should be asked when appraising published results from paired or matched data:
- Has an appropriate paired *t*-test or single sample test been used?
- Do the within-pair differences need to be standardized for baseline differences, that is, presented as per cent changes or ratios?
- Are the within-pair differences normally distributed?
- If summary statistics are reported, are they in the same units of change so that they can be directly compared if necessary?
- Have rank-based non-parametric tests been used for non-normally distributed differences?
- Have descriptive data been reported for each of the pair of variables in addition to information of mean changes?

References

1. Bland JM, Altman DG. Matching. *BMJ* 1994; **309**: 1128.
2. Bland JM, Altman DG. One and two sided tests of significance. *BMJ* 1994; **309**: 248.

CHAPTER 5

Analysis of variance

I discovered, though unconsciously and insensibly, that the pleasure of observing and reasoning was a much higher one that that of skill and sports.
CHARLES DARWIN

Objectives

The objectives of this chapter are to explain how to:
- decide when to use an analysis of variance (ANOVA) test
- conduct and interpret the output from a one-way or a factorial ANOVA using SPSS
- understand between-group and within-group differences
- classify factors into fixed, interactive or random effects
- test for a trend across the groups within a factor
- understand sample size requirements
- calculate effect size
- perform post-hoc tests
- build a multivariate analysis of covariance (ANCOVA) model
- report the findings from an ANOVA model
- check the assumptions of ANOVA and ANCOVA

When data are normally distributed, a two-sample *t*-test can only be used to assess the significance of the difference between the mean values of two independent groups. To compare differences in the mean values of three or more independent groups simultaneously, an analysis of variance (ANOVA), which is a parametric test, can be used. Thus, ANOVA is suitable when the outcome measurement is a continuous normally distributed variable and when the explanatory variable is categorical with three or more groups. An ANOVA model can also be used for comparing the effects of several categorical explanatory variables at one time or for comparing differences in the mean values of one or more groups after adjusting for a continuous variable, that is, a covariate. This is referred to as an analysis of covariance (ANCOVA). A covariate is any variable that correlates with the outcome variable. For example, ANCOVA would be used to test for the effects of gender and socioeconomic status on weight after adjusting for height.

Both ANCOVA and ANCOVA are applications of the general linear model (GLM). In general, GLM is used to build a model to predict an outcome variable from one or more explanatory variables which may be categorical or continuous variables. The GLM may

---

Medical Statistics: A Guide to SPSS, Data Analysis and Critical Appraisal, Second Edition.
Belinda Barton and Jennifer Peat.
Companion website: www.wiley.com/go/barton/medicalstatistics2e

be univariate with only one explanatory variable or multivariate with a number of explanatory variables. Therefore, in GLM, the outcome is expressed as a function of the model and prediction error. In the univariate case, where there is only one outcome variable, the linear model consists of weights or coefficients, an intercept and a prediction error.

5.1 Building ANOVA and ANCOVA models

For both ANOVA and ANCOVA, the theory behind the model must be reliable in that there must be biological plausibility or scientific reason for the effects of the factors being tested. In this, it is important that the factors are independent and not closely related to one another. For example, it would not make sense to test for differences in mean values of an outcome between groups defined according to education and socioeconomic status when these two variables are related to each other. Once the results of an ANOVA are obtained, they can only be generalized to the population if the data were collected from a random sample, and a significant P value can only be used to indicate association and cannot be taken as evidence of causality.

When building an ANOVA or ANCOVA model, it is important to build the model in a logical and considered way. The process of model building is as much an art as a science. Descriptive and summary statistics should always be obtained first to provide a good working knowledge of the data before beginning the bivariate analyses or multivariate modelling. In this way, the model can be built up in a systematic way, which is preferable to including all variables in the model and then deciding which variables to remove, that is, using a backward elimination process. Table 5.1 shows the steps that can be used in the model building process.

Table 5.1   Steps in building an ANOVA model

Type of analysis	SPSS procedure	Purpose
Univariate analyses	Explore	Examine cell sizes Obtain univariate means Test for normality
Bivariate analyses	Crosstabulations One-way ANOVA	Ensure adequate cell sizes Estimate differences in means and homogeneity of variances Examine trends across groups within a factor
Multivariate analyses	Factorial ANOVA ANCOVA	Test several explanatory factors or adjust for covariates Test normality of residuals Test influence of multivariate outliers

5.2 ANOVA models

5.2.1 Assumptions for ANOVA models

The assumptions for ANOVA, which must be met in all types of ANOVA models, are shown in Box 5.1.

Box 5.1 Assumptions for using ANOVA

The assumptions that must be met when using one-way or factorial ANOVA are as follows:

- the participants must be independent, that is each participant appears only once in their group
- the groups must be independent, that is each participant must be in one group only
- the outcome variable is normally distributed
- all cells have an adequate sample size
- the cell size ratio is no larger than 1:4
- the variances are similar between groups (homogeneity of variance)
- the residuals are normally distributed
- there are no influential outliers

The first two assumptions are similar to the assumptions for two-sample t-tests (see Section 3.1) and any violation will invalidate the analysis. In practice, this means that each participant should appear on one data row of the spreadsheet only and thus will be included in the analysis only once. When cases appear in the spreadsheet on more than one occasion then repeated measures ANOVA or a linear mixed model should be used as described in Chapter 6.

When an ANOVA is conducted, the data are divided into cells according to the number of groups in the explanatory variable. Small cell sizes, that is, cell sizes less than 10, are always problematic because of the lack of precision in calculating the mean value for the cell. The minimum cell size in theory is 10 but in practice 30 is preferred. In addition to creating imprecision, low cell counts lead to a loss of statistical power. The assumption of a low cell size ratio is also important for example if one cell has 10 cases and another cell has 60 cases then the ratio would be 1:6. A cell size imbalance of more than 1:4 across the model would be a concern.

It may be difficult to avoid small cell sizes in non-experimental studies because it is not possible to predict the number of cases in each cell prior to data collection. Even in experimental studies in which equal numbers can be achieved in some groups, drop-outs and missing data can lead to unequal cell sizes. If small cells are present, they can be re-coded or combined into larger cells but only if it is possible to meaningfully interpret the re-coding. Alternatively, the group with small cells can be omitted from the analysis although this will lead to a loss of generalizability.

Both the assumptions of a normal distribution and equality of the variance of the outcome variable between cells should be tested before ANOVA is conducted. However, as with a t-test, ANOVA is robust to some deviations from normality of distributions and some imbalance of variances. The assumption that the outcome variable is normally distributed is of most importance when the sample size is small and/or when univariate outliers increase or decrease mean values between cells by an important amount and therefore influence perceived differences between groups. The main effects of non-normality and unequal variances, especially if there are outliers, are to bias the P values. However, the direction of the bias may not be clear.

When variances are not significantly different between cells, the model is said to be homoscedastic (also referred to as homogeneity of variance). The assumption of equal variances is of most importance when there are small cells, say cells with less than 30 cases, when the cell size ratio is larger than 1:4 or when there are large differences in variance between cells, say larger than 1:10. The main effect of unequal variance is to reduce statistical power and thus lead to type II errors (i.e. failure to reject the null hypothesis). Equality of variances should be tested in bivariate analyses before running an ANOVA model and then reaffirmed in the final model.

5.2.2   Within- and between-group variance

To interpret the output from an ANOVA model, it is important to have a concept of the mathematics used in conducting the test. In one-way ANOVA, the data are divided into their groups as shown in Figure 5.1 and a mean for each group is computed. Each mean value is considered to be the predicted value for that particular group of participants. In addition, a grand mean is computed as shown in Table 5.2. The grand mean which is also shown in Figure 5.1, is the mean for all of the data and will only be the average of the three group means when the sample size in each group is equal.

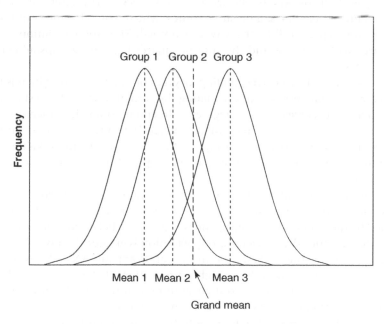

Figure 5.1 Concept of an ANOVA model.

Table 5.2   Means computed in one-way ANOVA

Group₁	Group₂	Group₃	Total sample
Group mean₁	Group mean₂	Group mean₃	Grand mean

The ANOVA analysis is then based on calculating the difference of each participant's observed value from their group mean, which is regarded as their predicted value, and also the difference from the grand mean. Thus, the following calculations are made for each participant:

Within-group difference = group mean − observed measurement

Between-group difference = grand mean − observed measurement

The within-group difference is the variation of each participant's measurement from their own group mean and is thought of as the explained variation. The between-group difference is the variation of each participant's measurement from the grand mean and is thought of as the unexplained variation. An important assumption in ANOVA is that the within-group differences, which are also called residual or error values, are normally distributed.

In calculating ANOVA statistics, the within-group differences for the participants are squared and then the squared differences are summed to compute the within-group variance, which is denoted as the 'Sum of Squares within Groups' (SS_W). The between-group difference for each participant is also squared and these squared differences are then summed to compute the between-group variance, which is denoted as the 'Sum of Squares between Groups' (SS_B). The effect of squaring the values is to remove the effects of negative values, which would balance out the positive values if the non-squared differences were summed. The 'Total Variation' is the sum of the squares within groups and the sum of squares between groups added together ($SS_T = SS_W + SS_B$).

Each sum of squares has a corresponding 'degrees of freedom' (df), which is the number of observations that are used in calculating the sum of squares. Each sum of squares is then divided by its corresponding degrees of freedom, to obtain a mean square. This gives a 'mean square within groups' (MS_W), which is also referred to as mean square error and a 'mean square between groups' (MS_B). The mean square values represent the variation among participants in the same group and the variation between group means, respectively.

The F value that is calculated for an ANOVA is the mean between-group variance divided by the mean within-group variance (MS_B/MS_W), that is, the unexplained variance divided by the explained variance, and is thus a ratio between mean squares. The F value indicates whether the between-group variation is greater than would be expected by chance. The higher the F value, the more significant the ANOVA test because the groups (factors) are accounting for a higher proportion of the variance. Obviously, if more of the participants are closer to their group mean than to the grand mean, then the within-group variance will be lower than the between-group variance and F will be large. If the within-group variance is equal to the between-group variance, then F will be equal to approximately 1 indicating that there is no significant difference in means between the groups of the factor (i.e. null hypothesis is true).

If there are only two groups in a factor and only one factor, then a one-way ANOVA is equivalent to a two-sample t-test and F is equal to t^2. This relationship holds because t is calculated from the mean divided by the standard error (SE) in the same units as the original measurements whereas F is calculated from the variance, which is in squared units.

5.3   One-way analysis of variance

A one-way ANOVA is used when the effect of only one categorical variable with more than two nominal or ordinal levels (explanatory variable) on a single continuous variable (outcome) is explored. For example, when the effect of socioeconomic status, which has three groups (low, medium and high), on weight is examined. The concept of ANOVA can be thought of as an extension of a two-sample t-test applied to more than two groups with similar assumptions. However, the terminology used for ANOVA is quite different. In ANOVA, the explanatory variable, which is called a factor, has more than two groups.

The null hypothesis for a one-way ANOVA is that the population means for all groups are equal. The alternative hypothesis is that at least one mean is significantly different from one of the others. A factorial ANOVA is used when the effects of two or more categorical variables (explanatory variables) on a single continuous variable (outcome) are explored, for example when the effects of gender and socioeconomic status on weight are examined.

The ANOVA test is called an analysis of variance and not an analysis of means because this test is used to assess whether the mean values of different groups are far enough apart in terms of their spread (variance) to be considered significantly different. Figure 5.1 shows how a one-way ANOVA model in which the factor has three groups can be conceptualized.

If a factor has four groups, it is possible to compare the groups by conducting three independent two-sample t-tests, that is, to test the mean values of group 1 versus 2, group 2 versus 3 and group 3 versus 4. However, this approach of conducting multiple two-sample t-tests increases the probability of obtaining a significant result merely by chance (a type I error). The probability of a type I error not occurring for each t-test is 0.95 (i.e. $1 - 0.05$). The three tests are independent; therefore, the probability of a type I error not occurring over all three tests is $0.95 \times 0.95 \times 0.95$, or 0.86. Therefore, the probability of at least one type I error occurring over the three two-sample t-tests is $1 - 0.86$, or 0.14, which is higher than the P level set at 0.05.[1] A one-way ANOVA is used to examine the differences between several groups within a factor in one model, thereby reducing the number of pairwise comparisons and the chance of a type I error occurring.

5.3.1   Sample size for a one-way ANOVA

In general, when using a one-way ANOVA with three groups, the required sample size can be estimated on the basis of the effect size Cohen's d calculated between the largest and smallest mean values. A sample size of approximately 600 per group is required to show that a small effect size of 0.15 is statistically significant, 160 per group to show that a medium effect size of 0.3 is statistically significant and 90 per group to show that a moderate effect size of 0.4 is statistically significant. If the effect size is large at 0.8, only 25 per group are required for significance. This assumes a power of 80%, a significance level equal to 0.05 and that the groups have equal variance and equal sample sizes. Deviation from these assumptions will require larger numbers. However, the larger the number of groups, the smaller the number of participants is required in each group to maintain statistical power. For example, for a Cohen's d effect size of

0.30 to be significant 160 per group is needed if there are three groups, 120 per group if there are four groups and 96 per group if there are six groups (power = 80%, $P <$ 0.05, two-tailed). Detailed sample size calculation tables for ANOVA are shown on the StatsToDo website provided in the section of this book, Useful Websites.

Research question

The spreadsheet **weights.sav** contains the data from a population sample of 550 term babies who had their weight recorded at 1 month of age. The babies also had their parity recorded, that is, their birth order in their family.

Question:	Are the weights of babies related to their parity?
Null hypothesis:	That there is no difference in mean weight between groups defined by parity.
Variables:	Outcome variable = weight (continuous)
	Explanatory variable = parity (categorical, four groups)

The first statistics to obtain are the cell means and cell sizes. The number of children in each parity group can be obtained using the *Analyze → Descriptive Statistics → Frequencies* command sequences shown in Box 1.7 with parity entered as the variable.

The Frequency table shows that the sample size of each group is large and all cells have more than 30 participants. The cell size ratio is 62:192 or 1:3 and does not violate the ANOVA assumptions. Thus, the ANOVA model will be robust to some degrees of non-normality, outliers and unequal variances. However, it is still important to validate the ANOVA assumptions of normality and equal variances between groups. An aware-ness of any violations of these assumptions before running the model may influence how the results are interpreted, especially if any P values are of marginal significance. On the one hand, a small cell with a small variance compared to the other groups has the effect of inflating the F value, that is, of increasing the chance of a type I error. On the other hand, a small cell with large variance compared to the other groups reduces the F value and increases the chance of a type II error.

Frequency table

Parity

		Frequency	Per cent	Valid per cent	Cumulative per cent
Valid	Singleton	180	32.7	32.7	32.7
	One sibling	192	34.9	34.9	67.6
	Two siblings	116	21.1	21.1	88.7
	Three or more siblings	62	11.3	11.3	100.0
	Total	550	100.0	100.0	

Summary statistics and checks for normality can be obtained using the *Analyze → Descriptive Statistics → Explore* command sequence shown in Box 2.2. In this example, the dependent variable is weight and the factor is parity. The plots that are most useful to request are the box plots, histograms and normality plots.

The Descriptives table shows that means and medians for weight in each group are approximately equal and the values for skewness and kurtosis are all between −1 and +1, suggesting that the data are close to normally distributed. The variances in each group are 0.384, 0.351, 0.366 and 0.287, respectively. The variance ratio between the lowest and highest values is 0.287:0.384, which is 1:1.3.

Descriptives

	Parity			Statistic	Std. error
Weight (kg)	Singleton	Mean		4.2589	0.04617
		95% confidence	Lower bound	4.1678	
		Interval for mean	Upper bound	4.3501	
		5% trimmed mean		4.2588	
		Median		4.2500	
		Variance		0.384	
		Std. deviation		0.61950	
		Minimum		2.92	
		Maximum		5.75	
		Range		2.83	
		Interquartile range		0.95	
		Skewness		0.046	0.181
		Kurtosis		−0.542	0.360
	One sibling	Mean		4.3887	0.04277
		95% confidence	Lower bound	4.3043	
		Interval for mean	Upper bound	4.4731	
		5% trimmed mean		4.3709	
		Median		4.3250	
		Variance		0.351	
		Std. deviation		0.59258	
		Minimum		3.17	
		Maximum		6.33	
		Range		3.16	
		Interquartile range		0.84	
		Skewness		0.467	0.175
		Kurtosis		0.039	0.349
	Two siblings	Mean		4.4601	0.05619
		95% confidence	Lower bound	4.3488	
		Interval for mean	Upper bound	4.5714	
		5% trimmed mean		4.4525	
		Median		4.4700	
		Variance		0.366	
		Std. deviation		0.60520	
		Minimum		3.09	
		Maximum		6.49	
		Range		3.40	
		Interquartile range		0.82	
		Skewness		0.251	0.225
		Kurtosis		0.139	0.446

	Parity			Statistic	Std. error
Weight (kg)	Three or more siblings	Mean		4.4342	0.06798
		95% confidence	Lower bound	4.2983	
		Interval for mean	Upper bound	4.5701	
		5% trimmed mean		4.4389	
		Median		4.4450	
		Variance		0.287	
		Std. deviation		0.53526	
		Minimum		3.20	
		Maximum		5.48	
		Range		2.28	
		Interquartile range		0.71	
		Skewness		−0.029	0.304
		Kurtosis		−0.478	0.599

The Kolmogorov–Smirnov and the Shapiro–Wilk statistics in the Tests of Normality table suggest that the data for singletons, babies with two siblings, and babies with three or more siblings conform to normality with P values above 0.05. However, the data for babies with one sibling do not appear to conform to a normal distribution based on these tests because the P values of 0.049 and 0.018 are less than 0.05. However, since these are conservative tests, failure to pass these statistical tests of normality does not always mean that ANOVA cannot be used unless other tests also indicate non-normality.

Tests of Normality

		Kolmogorov–Smirnov[a]			Shapiro–Wilk		
	Parity	Statistic	df	Sig.	Statistic	df	Sig.
Weight (kg)	Singleton	0.038	180	0.200*	0.992	180	0.381
	One sibling	0.065	192	0.049	0.983	192	0.018
	Two siblings	0.059	116	0.200*	0.990	116	0.579
	Three or more siblings	0.070	62	0.200*	0.985	62	0.672

*This is a lower bound of the true significance.
[a]Lilliefors significance correction.

The histograms shown in Figure 5.2 confirm the tests of normality and show that the distribution for babies with one sibling has slightly spread tails so that it does not conform absolutely to a bell-shaped curve. The normal Q–Q plots shown in Figure 5.2 have small deviations at the extremities. The normal Q–Q plot for babies with one sibling deviates slightly from normality at both extremities. Although the histogram for babies with three or more siblings is not classically bell shaped, the normal Q–Q plot suggests that this distribution conforms to an approximately normal bell curve.

The box plots in Figure 5.2 indicate that there are two outlying values, one in the group of babies with one sibling and one in the group of babies with two siblings. It is unlikely that these outlying values, which are also univariate outliers, will have a large influence on the summary statistics and ANOVA results because the sample size of each group is large. However, the outliers should be confirmed as correct values and not data

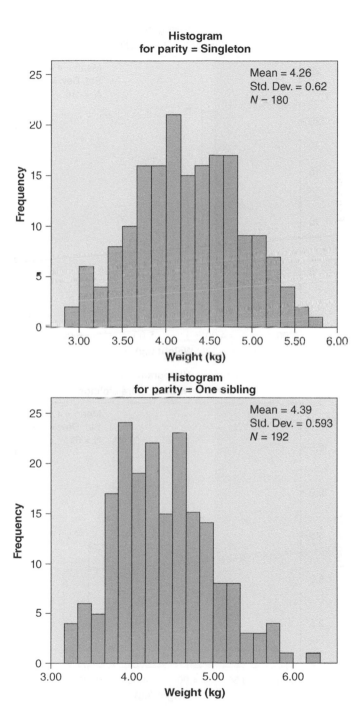

Figure 5.2 Histograms and plots of weight by parity.

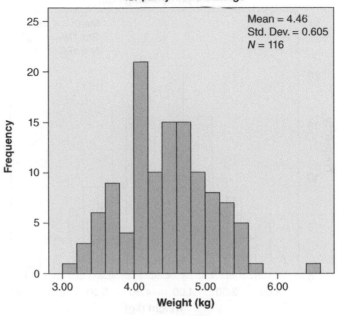

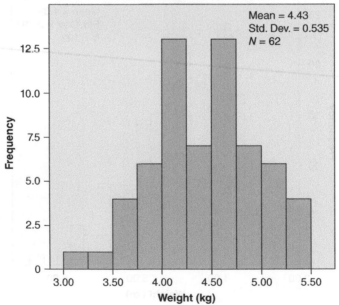

Figure 5.2 (*continued*)

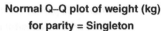
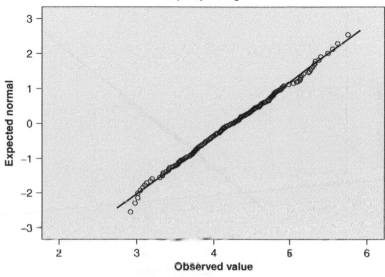

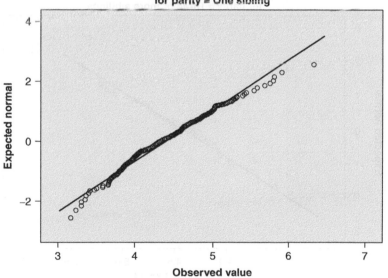

Figure 5.2 (*continued*)

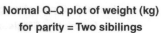

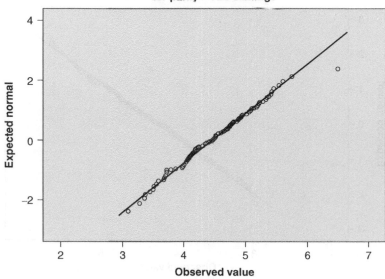

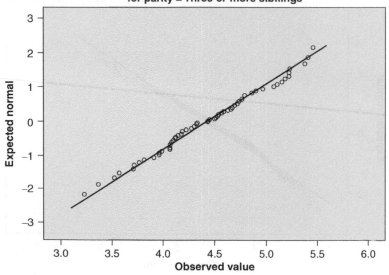

Figure 5.2 (*continued*)

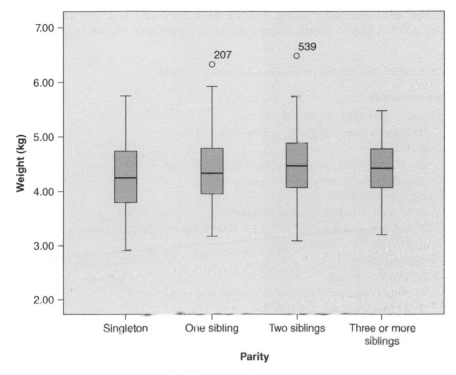

Figure 5.2 (*continued*)

Table 5.3   Characteristics of the data set

Characteristic	
Independence of observations	Yes
Smallest cell size	62
Cell ratio	1:3
Variance ratio	1:1.3
Approximately normal distribution in each group	Yes
Number of outlying values	2
Number of univariate outliers	2

entry or data recording errors. Once they are verified as correctly recorded data points, the decision to include or omit outliers from the analyses is the same as for any other statistical tests. In a study with a large sample size, it is expected that there will be a few outliers (see Chapter 2). In this data set, the outliers will be retained in the analyses and the residuals will be examined for the presence of extreme values (discussed later in this chapter) to ensure that these outliers do not have an undue influence on the results. The characteristics of the sample that need to be considered before conducting an ANOVA test and the features of the data set are summarized in Table 5.3.

After the assumptions for using ANOVA have been checked and are validated, a one-way ANOVA can be obtained using the SPSS commands shown in Box 5.2.

Box 5.2 SPSS commands to obtain a one-way ANOVA

SPSS Commands

weights.sav – IBM SPSS Statistics Data Editor
     Analyze → Compare Means → One-Way ANOVA
One-Way ANOVA
     Highlight Weight and click over into Dependent List
     Highlight Parity and click over into Factor
     Click on Post-hoc
One-Way ANOVA: Post Hoc Multiple Comparisons
     Equal Variances Assumed: Tick LSD, Bonferroni and Duncan, click Continue
One-Way ANOVA
     Click on Options
One-Way ANOVA: Options
     Statistics: Tick Descriptive and Homogeneity of variance test
     Tick Means Plot and click Continue
     Missing Values: Excludes cases analysis by analysis (default)
One-Way ANOVA
     Click OK

The summary statistics in the Descriptives table produced in a one-way ANOVA are identical to the statistics obtained using the command sequence *Analyze → Descriptive Statistics → Explore*. The descriptive statistics provided by the ANOVA commands show useful summary information but do not give enough details to check the normality of the distribution of weight in each group.

One way

Descriptives

Weight (kg)

	N	Mean	Std. deviation	Std. error	95% confidence interval for mean Lower bound	95% confidence interval for mean Upper bound	Minimum	Maximum
Singleton	180	4.2589	0.61950	0.04617	4.1678	4.3501	2.92	5.75
One sibling	192	4.3887	0.59258	0.04277	4.3043	4.4731	3.17	6.33
Two siblings	116	4.4601	0.60520	0.05619	4.3488	4.5714	3.09	6.49
Three or more siblings	62	4.4342	0.53526	0.06798	4.2983	4.5701	3.20	5.48
Total	550	4.3664	0.60182	0.02566	4.3160	4.4168	2.92	6.49

Homogeneity of variances is a term that is used to indicate that groups have the same or similar variances (see Chapter 3). In the Test of Homogeneity of Variances table, the P value of 0.590 in the significance column, which is larger than the critical value of

0.05, indicates that the variances of the groups are not significantly different from one another.

Test of Homogeneity of Variances

Weight (kg)

Levene statistic	df1	df2	Sig.
0.639	3	546	0.590

The ANOVA table shows how the sum of squares is partitioned into between-group (SS_B) and within-group effects (SS_W). The average of each sum of squares is needed to calculate the F value. Therefore, each sum of squares is divided by its respective degree of freedom (df) to compute the mean variance, that is, the mean square. The degrees of freedom for the between-group sum of squares is the number of groups minus 1, that is, $4 - 1 = 3$, and for the within-group sum of squares is the number of cases in the total sample minus the number of groups, that is, $550 - 4 = 546$.

ANOVA

Weight (kg)

	Sum of squares	df	Mean square	F	Sig.
Between groups	3.477	3	1.159	3.239	0.022
Within groups	195.365	546	0.358		
Total	198.842	549			

In this model, the F value, which is the between-group mean square divided by the within-group mean square, is large at 3.239 and is significant at $P = 0.022$. Therefore, the null hypothesis is rejected and we conclude that there is a significant difference in the mean population values of the four parity groups.

5.4   Effect size for ANOVA

One of the most commonly reported measures of effect size for ANOVA is eta squared (η^2), which is an index of the strength of association between a factor and a dependent variable. Eta squared is the proportion of total variation attributable to the factor. Eta squared is calculated as the ratio of the factor variance to the total variance and values range from 0 to 1.

In the example above, the amount of variation in weight that is explained by parity can be calculated as the between-group sum of squares for weight divided by the total sum of squares as follows:

$$\eta^2 = SS_B/SS_T$$

$$= 3.477/198.842$$

$$= 0.017$$

This statistic indicates that only 1.7% of the variation in weight is explained by parity. Alternatively, eta squared can be obtained using the SPSS commands *Analyze → Compare*

Means → Means, clicking on Options and requesting *ANOVA table and eta*. This will produce the same ANOVA table as above and include eta squared but does not include a test of homogeneity or allow for post-hoc testing.

Eta squared can be converted to Cohen's *f* which gives an average standardized difference between the mean values of the groups. This statistic is most accurate when the group sizes are approximately equal. The formula is as follows:

$$\text{Cohen's } f = \frac{\sqrt{\eta^2}}{(1 - \eta^2)}$$

Thus for the model above, Cohen's $f = \sqrt{0.017/(1 - 0.017)} = 0.13$. For Cohen's f, a value of 0.1 is considered a small effect size, 0.25 is considered a medium effect size and 0.4 is considered a large effect size.[2] From this, we can conclude that parity only has a small association with weight at 1 month.

However, eta squared is a biased estimate of the strength of association, in that it overestimates the effects, especially for small sample sizes.[3] Another measure of effect size that is less biased is omega squared (ω^2). While SPSS does not calculate omega squared for ANOVA, it can be calculated as follows when there are equal sample sizes in all cells:

$$\omega^2 = SS_B - (k - 1) \times MS_W/(SS_T + MS_W), \text{ where } k \text{ is the number of groups.}$$

Thus for this example, if the sample size in all cells had been equal,

$$\omega^2 = 3.477 - (3 - 1) \times \frac{0.358}{(198.842 + 0.358)} = 0.014$$

The omega squared value obtained is slightly lower than the eta squared value.

5.5 Post-hoc tests for ANOVA

Although the ANOVA statistics show that there is a significant difference in mean weights between parity groups, they do not indicate which group means are significantly different from one another. Specific group mean differences can be assessed using planned contrasts, which are decided before the ANOVA is conducted and which strictly limit the number of comparisons made.[4] The planned comparisons should have a theoretical and/or empirical basis so that the comparisons to be made can be decided upon. Alternatively, post-hoc tests, which may involve all possible comparisons between group means can be used. Post-hoc tests are often considered to be data dredging and therefore inferior to the thoughtfulness of planned or *a priori* comparisons.[5] Some post-hoc tests preserve the overall type I error rate, but for other post-hoc tests the chance of a type I error increases with the number of comparisons made.

It is always better to conduct a small number of planned comparisons rather than a large number of unplanned post-hoc tests. Strictly speaking, the between-group differences that are of interest and the specific between-group comparisons that are made should be decided prior to conducting the ANOVA. In addition, planned and post-hoc tests should only be requested after the main ANOVA has shown that there is a statistically significant difference between group means. When the *F* test is not significant, it is unwise to explore whether there are any between-group differences.[4]

A post-hoc test may consist of pairwise comparisons, group-wise comparisons or a combination of both. Pairwise comparisons are used to determine which groups are statistically significantly different from each other. Group-wise comparisons are used to identify subsets of means that differ significantly from each other. Post-hoc tests also vary from being conservative, such as Scheffe's to being more liberal such as Fisher's least significance difference (LSD) where no adjustment is made for multiple comparisons. A conservative test is one in which the actual P value is larger than the true P level, and the probability of a type I error occurring will be less than the level of significance specified (α). Thus, conservative tests may incorrectly fail to reject the null hypothesis because a larger effect size between means is required for significance. A liberal test is one in which the actual P value is smaller than the true P value and the probability of a type I error occurring will be greater than the level of significance specified. Thus, liberal tests may result in the incorrect acceptance of the null hypothesis. Table 5.4 shows some commonly used post-hoc tests, their assumptions and the type of comparisons made.

The choice of post-hoc test should be determined by equality of the variances, equality of group sizes and by the acceptability of the test in a particular research discipline. For example, Scheffe and Tukey's honestly significant difference tests are often used in psychological research, Bonferroni in clinical applications and Duncan in epidemiological studies. The advantages of using a conservative post-hoc test have to be balanced against the probability of type II errors, that is, missing real differences.[6] Conservative post-hoc tests have been criticized because they increase the type II error rate.[7] One suggestion which is becoming more widely accepted is that liberal tests such as Fisher's LSD are used for exploratory studies and more conservative tests such as Bonferroni are used for large, clinical confirmatory studies.[8] Exploratory studies are those in which data is collected with one or more objectives but the study may also be used to test hypotheses

Table 5.4 Types of comparisons produced by post-hoc tests

Post-hoc test	Requires equal group sizes	Group-wise subsets	Pairwise comparisons with a 95% CI
Equal variance assumed			
Conservative tests			
Scheffe	No	Yes	Yes
Tukey's honestly significant difference (HSD)	Yes	Yes	Yes
Bonferroni	No	No	Yes
Liberal tests			
Student–Newman–Keuls (SNK)	Yes	Yes	No
Duncan	Yes	Yes	No
Fisher's least significance difference (LSD)	Yes	No	Yes
Equal variance not assumed			
Games Howell	No	No	Yes
Dunnett's C	No	No	Yes

that are generated by the data. For such studies, a flexible approach to data analyses is required. On the other hand, confirmatory studies are those which are designed to collect definitive proof of a predefined hypothesis that will be used in final decision making in clinical settings. Between the two extremes of exploratory studies and confirmatory studies, there is a wide range of different types of investigations – in all studies it is important to make a considered decision about what method, if any, is used to control the type I error rate.

In the ANOVA test for the **weights.sav** data, the following post-hoc pairwise comparisons, Fisher's LSD and Bonferroni post-hoc tests were requested:

Post-hoc tests

Multiple Comparisons

Dependent variable: weight (kg)

(I) Parity		(J) Parity	Mean difference (I–J)	Std. error	Sig.	Lower bound	Upper bound
LSD	Singleton	One sibling	−0.12975*	0.06206	0.037	−0.2517	−0.0078
		Two siblings	−0.20114*	0.07122	0.005	−0.3410	−0.0612
		Three or more siblings	−0.17525*	0.08809	0.047	−0.3483	−0.0022
	One sibling	Singleton	0.12975*	0.06206	0.037	0.0078	0.2517
		Two siblings	−0.07139	0.07034	0.311	−0.2096	0.0668
		Three or more siblings	−0.04550	0.08738	0.603	−0.2171	0.1261
	Two siblings	Singleton	0.20114*	0.07122	0.005	0.0612	0.3410
		One sibling	0.07139	0.07034	0.311	−0.0668	0.2096
		Three or more siblings	0.02589	0.09410	0.783	−0.1590	0.2107
	Three or more siblings	Singleton	0.17525*	0.08809	0.047	0.0022	0.3483
		One sibling	0.04550	0.08738	0.603	−0.1261	0.2171
		Two siblings	−0.02589	0.09410	0.783	−0.2107	0.1590
Bonferroni	Singleton	One sibling	−0.12975	0.06206	0.222	−0.2941	0.0346
		Two siblings	−0.20114*	0.07122	0.029	−0.3897	−0.0126
		Three or more siblings	−0.17525	0.08809	0.283	−0.4085	0.0580
	One sibling	Singleton	0.12975	0.06206	0.222	−0.0346	0.2941
		Two siblings	−0.07139	0.07034	1.000	−0.2577	0.1149
		Three or more siblings	−0.04550	0.08738	1.000	−0.2769	0.1859
	Two siblings	Singleton	0.20114*	0.07122	0.029	0.0126	0.3897
		One sibling	0.07139	0.07034	1.000	−0.1149	0.2577
		Three or more siblings	0.02589	0.09410	1.000	−0.2233	0.2751
	Three or more siblings	Singleton	0.17525	0.08809	0.283	−0.0580	0.4085
		One sibling	0.04550	0.08738	1.000	−0.1859	0.2769
		Two siblings	−0.02589	0.09410	1.000	−0.2751	0.2233

*The mean difference is significant at the 0.05 level.

5.5.1   *Fisher's least significant difference (LSD) post-hoc test*

The Fisher's LSD test is the most liberal post-hoc test because it performs all possible tests between means. With no adjustments made for multiple comparisons, the results of the Fisher's LSD test amount to multiple *t*-testing. A requirement of this test is that the overall ANOVA has to be significant.

The Multiple Comparisons table shows the mean difference between each pair of groups, the significance and the confidence intervals around the difference in means between groups. SigmaPlot can be used to plot the mean differences and 95% confidence intervals as a scatter plot with horizontal error bars using the commands shown in Box 3.6 to obtain Figure 5.3. This figure shows that three of the comparisons have error bars that cross the zero line of no difference. The differences are not statistically significant using the Fisher's LSD test. The remaining three comparisons do not cross the zero line of no difference and are statistically significant as indicated by the *P* values in the Multiple Comparisons table.

5.5.2 *Bonferroni post-hoc test*

The Bonferroni post-hoc comparison is a conservative test in which the critical *P* value of 0.05 is divided by the number of comparisons made. Thus, if five comparisons are made, the critical value of 0.05 is divided by 5 and the adjusted new critical value is $P = 0.01$. In SPSS the *P* levels in the Multiple Comparisons table have already been adjusted for the number of multiple comparisons. Therefore, each *P* level obtained from a Bonferroni test in the Multiple Comparisons table should be evaluated at the critical level of 0.05.

By using the Bonferroni test, which is a conservative test, the significant differences between some groups identified by the Fisher's LSD test are not significant. The mean values are identical but the confidence intervals are adjusted so that they are wider as shown in Figure 5.4. The 95% error bars show that only one comparison does not cross the zero line of difference compared to three comparisons using the LSD test.

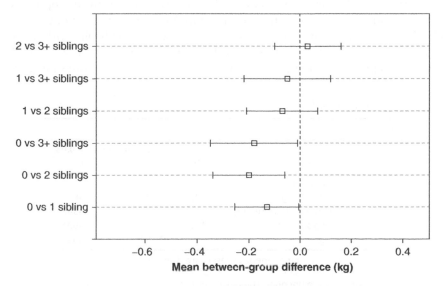

Figure 5.3 Between-group comparisons with no adjustment for multiple testing.

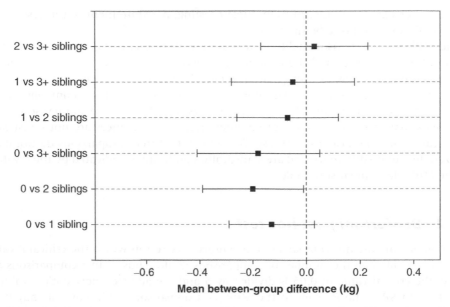

Figure 5.4 Between-group comparisons using Bonferroni corrected confidence intervals.

5.5.3 Duncan post-hoc test

The Duncan test shown in the Homogeneous Subsets table is one of the more liberal post-hoc tests. Under this test, there is a progressive comparison between the largest and smallest mean values until a difference that is not significant at the $P < 0.05$ level is found and the comparisons are stopped. In this way, the number of comparisons is limited. The output from this test is presented as subsets of groups that are not significantly different from one another. The between-group P value (0.05) is shown in the top row of the Homogenous Subtests table and the within-group P values at the foot of the columns. Thus in the table, the mean values for groups of singletons and babies with one sibling are not significantly different from one another with a P value of 0.104. Similarly, the mean values of groups with one sibling, two siblings, or three or more siblings are not

Homogeneous Subsets

Weight (kg)

| | Parity | N | Subset for alpha = 0.05 | |
			1	2
Duncan[a,b]	Singleton	180	4.2589	
	One sibling	192	4.3887	4.3887
	Three or more siblings	62		4.4342
	Two siblings	116		4.4601
	Sig.		0.104	0.403

Means for groups in homogeneous subsets are displayed.
[a]Uses harmonic mean sample size = 112.633.
[b]The group sizes are unequal. The harmonic mean of the group sizes is used. Type I error levels are not guaranteed.

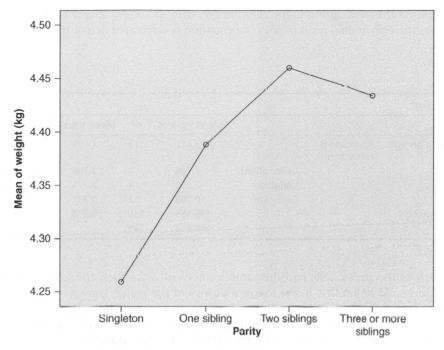

Figure 5.5 Means plot of weight by parity.

significantly different from one another with a *P* value of 0.403. Singletons do not appear in the same subset as babies with two siblings or with three or more siblings which indicates that the mean weight of singletons is significantly different from these two groups at the $P < 0.05$ level.

Means plot

A means plot provides a visual presentation of the mean value for each group. The means plot obtained by the commands in Box 5.2 and shown in Figure 5.5 indicates that there is a trend for weight to increase with increasing parity and helps in the interpretation of the post-hoc tests. It also provides visual evidence as to why the group with one sibling is not significantly different from singletons or babies with two siblings or with three or more siblings, and why singletons are significantly different from the groups with two siblings or with three or more siblings.

   If the means plot shown in Figure 5.5 was to be published, it would be best plotted in SigmaPlot with 95% confidence intervals around each mean value included to help interpret the between-group differences. Also, the line connecting the mean value of each group should be removed because the four groups are independent of one another.

5.6   Testing for a trend

The increase in weight with increasing parity suggests that it is appropriate to test whether there is a significant linear trend for weight to increase across the groups within this factor. A trend test can be performed by rerunning the one-way ANOVA and ticking the *Polynomial* option in the *Contrasts* box with the *Degree: Linear* (default) option used. As the polynomial term implies, an equation is calculated across the model.

One way

ANOVA

Weight (kg)

			Sum of squares	df	Mean square	F	Sig.
Between groups	(Combined)		3.477	3	1.159	3.239	0.022
	Linear term						
		Unweighted	1.706	1	1.706	4.768	0.029
		Weighted	2.774	1	2.774	7.754	0.006
		Deviation	0.703	2	0.351	0.982	0.375
Within groups			195.365	546	0.358		
Total			198.842	549			

   If each of the parity cells had the same number of cases then the unweighted linear term would be used to assess the significance of the trend. However, the cell sizes are unequal and therefore the weighted linear term is used. The table shows that the weighted linear term sum of squares is significant at the $P = 0.006$ level. The P value for the linear term-weighted indicates that the slope of the line through the plot is significantly different from zero. That is, there is a significant linear trend in the group means. The descriptive statistics show that the mean weight increases as parity increases.

5.7   Reporting the results of a one-way ANOVA

In addition to presenting the between-group comparisons shown in Figure 5.3, the results from the one-way ANOVA can be summarized as shown in Table 5.5. When reporting the table, it is important to include details stating that weight was approximately normally distributed in each group and that the group sizes were all large (minimum 62) with a cell size ratio of 1:3 and a variance ratio of 1:1.3. The significant difference in weight at 1 month between children with different parities can be described as $F = 3.24$, $df = 3,546$, $P = 0.022$ with a significant linear trend for weight to increase with increasing parity ($P = 0.006$). The degrees of freedom are conventionally shown as the between-group and within-group degrees of freedom separated with a comma.

Table 5.5   Reporting results from a one-way ANOVA

Parity	N	Mean (SD)	F (df)	P value	P value trend
Singletons	180	4.26 (0.62)	3.24 (3,546)	0.022	0.006
One sibling	192	4.39 (0.59)			
Two siblings	116	4.46 (0.61)			
Three or more siblings	62	4.43 (0.54)			

Although the inclusion of the *F* value and degrees of freedom is optional since their only interpretation is the *P* value, some journals request that they are reported.

When designing the study, only one post-hoc test should be planned and conducted if the ANOVA was significant. If the Bonferroni post-hoc test had been conducted, it could be reported that the only significant difference in mean weights was between singletons and babies with two siblings ($P = 0.029$) with no significant differences between any other groups.

If Duncan's post-hoc test had been conducted, it could be reported that babies with two siblings and babies with three or more siblings were significantly different from singletons ($P < 0.05$). However, babies with one sibling did not have a mean weight that was significantly different from either singletons ($P = 0.104$) or from babies with two siblings, or with three or more siblings ($P = 0.403$).

5.8 Factorial ANOVA models

A factorial ANOVA is used to test for differences in mean values between groups when there are two or more factors, or explanatory variables, with two or more groups each included in a single multivariate analysis. In SPSS, factorial ANOVA is accessed through the *Analyze → General Linear Models → Univariate* command sequence. The term 'univariate' may seem confusing in this context but in this case refers to the fact that there is only one outcome variable rather than only one explanatory variable.

In a factorial ANOVA, the data are divided into cells according to the number of participants in each group of each factor stratified by the other factors. The more explanatory variables that are included in a model, the greater the likelihood of creating small or empty cells. The cells can be conceptualized as shown in Table 5.6. The number of cells in a model is calculated by multiplying the number of groups in each factor. For a model with three factors that have three, two and four groups, respectively, as shown in Table 5.6, the number of cells is $3 \times 2 \times 4$, or 24 cells in total.

In factorial ANOVA, the within-group differences are calculated as the distance of each participant from its cell mean rather than from the group mean as in one-way ANOVA. However, the between-group differences are again calculated as the difference of each participant from the grand mean, that is, the mean of the entire data set. As with one-way ANOVA, all of the differences are squared and summed, and then the mean square is calculated.

Table 5.6   Cells in the analysis of a model with three factors (three-way ANOVA)

FACTOR 1						
FACTOR 2	Group 1		Group 2		Group 3	
FACTOR 3	Group 1	Group 2	Group 1	Group 2	Group 1	Group 2
Group 1	$m_{1,1,1}$	$m_{2,1,1}$	$m_{1,2,1}$	$m_{2,2,1}$	$m_{1,3,1}$	$m_{2,3,1}$
2	$m_{1,1,2}$	$m_{2,1,2}$	$m_{1,2,2}$	$m_{2,2,2}$	$m_{1,3,2}$	$m_{2,3,2}$
3	$m_{1,1,3}$	$m_{2,1,3}$	$m_{1,2,3}$	$m_{2,2,3}$	$m_{1,3,3}$	$m_{2,3,3}$
4	$m_{1,1,4}$	$m_{2,1,4}$	$m_{1,2,4}$	$m_{2,2,4}$	$m_{1,3,4}$	$m_{2,3,4}$

5.8.1   *Fixed factors, random factors and interactions*

Fixed or random effect factors can be incorporated in factorial ANOVA models. When both random and fixed effect factors are included, this is referred to as a mixed model. Factorial ANOVA is mostly used to examine the effects of fixed factors. A fixed factor is a factor in which all possible groups or all levels of the factor are included, for example, males and females or number of siblings. Usually, treatment effects such as a treatment group and a control group are fixed. With fixed factors, inferences can be made only to the levels of the factor used in the study. When using fixed factors, the differences between the specified groups are the statistics of interest.

Factors are considered to be random when only a sample of a wider range of groups or all possible levels is included. For example, factors may be classified as having random effects when only three or four ethnic groups are represented in the sample but the results will be generalized to all ethnic groups in the community. In this case, only general differences between the groups are of interest because the results will be used to make inferences to all possible ethnic groups rather than to only the groups in the sample. That is, inferences from the data are for all levels of the factor in the population from which the levels were selected.

It is important to classify groups as random factors if the study sample was selected by recruiting, for example, specific sports teams, schools or doctors' practices and the results will be generalized to all sports teams, schools or doctors' practices or if different sports teams, schools or doctors' practices would be selected in the future. In these types of study designs, there is a cluster sampling effect and the group is entered into the model as a random factor.

The classification of factors as fixed or random effects has implications for interpreting the results of the ANOVA model. In random effect models, any unequal variance between cells is less important when the numbers in each cell are equal. However, when there is increasing inequality between the numbers in each cell, then differences in variance become more problematic. The use of fixed or random effects can give very different P values because the F statistic is computed differently. For fixed effects, the F value is calculated as the between-group mean square divided by the error mean square whereas for random effects, the F value is calculated as the between-group mean square divided by the interaction mean square.

Sometimes the effect of one fixed factor is modified by another fixed factor. That is, there is an interaction between factors since the effects of one factor depend on the level of another factor. The presence of a significant interaction between two or more factors, or between a factor and a covariate can be tested in a factorial ANOVA model. The interaction term is computed as a new variable by multiplying the factors and then included in the model or can be requested in an SPSS option. Thus, with a factorial ANOVA it is possible to examine the effect of the explanatory variable (also referred to as the 'main effect'), as well as the presence of any interaction effects on the outcome variable. When there is a significant interaction, the main effects are not interpreted in isolation since this may lead to erroneous conclusions and the interaction is the most important effect. To interpret the results in more detail, the interaction can be explored further by examining the effect of one explanatory variable at a fixed level of the other explanatory variable, referred to as simple main effects. However, depending on the number of levels of a factor, it is recommended that not all possible simple effects conducted as this will increase the probability of a Type I error occurring.

Research question

Differences in weights between genders can be tested using a two-sample t-test and differences between different parities were tested in the previous example using a one-way ANOVA. However, maternal education status (Year 10 school, Year 12 school or university), in addition to gender and parity can be tested together as explanatory factors in a three-way ANOVA model. These factors are all fixed factors.

Question:	Are the weights of babies related to their gender, parity or maternal level of education?
Null hypothesis:	That there is no difference in mean weight between groups defined according to gender, parity and level of education
Variables:	Outcome variable = weight (continuous)
	Explanatory variables = gender (categorical, two groups), parity (categorical, four groups) and maternal education (categorical, three groups)

The number of cells in the ANOVA model will be 2 (gender) × 3 (maternal education) × 4 (parity), or 24 cells. First, the summary statistics need to be obtained to verify that there are an adequate number of babies in each cell. This can be achieved by splitting the file by gender which has the smallest number of groups and then generating two tables of parity by maternal education as shown in Box 5.3.

Box 5.3 SPSS commands to obtain cell sizes

SPSS Commands

weights.sav – IBM SPSS Statistics Data Editor
    Data → Split File
Split File
        Tick Organise output by groups
        Highlight Gender and click into Groups Based on
        Click OK
weights – SPSS Data Editor
        Analyze → Descriptive Statistics → Crosstabs
Crosstabs
        Highlight Maternal education and click into Row(s)
        Highlight Parity and click into Column(s)
        Click OK

The Crosstabulations tables show that even with a large sample size of 550 babies, including three factors in the model will create some small cells with less than 10 cases and that there is a large cell imbalance. For males, the cell size ratio is 4:55, or 1:14, and for females the cell size ratio is 2:45, or 1:23. Without maternal education included, all cell sizes as indicated by the Total row and Total column totals are quite large. To increase the small cell sizes, it would make sense to combine the groups of two siblings and three or more siblings. This combining of cells is possible because the theory is valid and because the post-hoc tests indicated that the means of these two groups are not significantly different from one another. By combining these groups, the smallest cells will be larger at 8 + 4 or 12 for males and 13 + 2 or 15 for females. The cell ratios will then be 12:55, or 1:4.6 for males and 15:45, or 1:3 for females. The ratio for males is close to the assumption of 1:4 and within this assumption for females.

Gender = 1 male

Maternal education * parity crosstabulation[a]

Count

			Parity			
		Singleton	One sibling	Two siblings	Three or more siblings	Total
Maternal education	Year 10	15	40	26	17	98
	Year 12	22	16	8	4	50
	Tertiary	55	42	22	8	127
Total		92	98	56	29	275

[a]Gender = male.

Gender = 2 female

Maternal education * parity crosstabulation[a]

Count

			Parity			
		Singleton	One sibling	Two siblings	Three or more siblings	Total
Maternal education	Year 10	24	36	21	19	100
	Year 12	19	15	13	2	49
	Tertiary	45	43	26	12	126
Total		88	94	60	33	275

[a]Gender = female.

To combine the parity groups, the recode commands shown in Box 1.9 can be used after removing the Split file option as shown in Box 5.4.

Box 5.4 SPSS commands to remove split file

SPSS Commands

weights.sav – IBM SPSS Statistics Data Editor
   Data → Split File
   Tick Analyse all cases, do not create groups
   Click OK

The SPSS commands to obtain summary means for parity and maternal education in males and females separately are shown in Box 5.5.

Box 5.5 SPSS commands to obtain summary means

SPSS Commands

weights.sav   IBM SPSS Statistics Data Editor
    Analyze → Compare Means → Means
Means
    Highlight Weight and click into Dependent List
    Highlight Gender, Maternal education and Parity recoded (3 levels), click into
       Independent List
    Click OK

The Means tables show mean values in each group for each factor. There is a difference of 4.59 − 4.14, that is, 0.45 kg between genders, a difference of 4.41 − 4.35, that is, 0.06 kg between the highest and lowest maternal education groups and a difference of 4.45 − 4.26, that is, 0.19 kg between the highest and lowest parity groups. These values are not effect sizes in units of the standard deviations, so the differences cannot be directly compared. In ANOVA, effect sizes can be calculated, but the number of groups and the pattern of dispersion of the mean values across the groups need to be taken into account.[5] However, the absolute differences show that the largest difference is for gender followed by parity and that there is an almost negligible difference for maternal education. The effect of maternal education is so small that it is unlikely to be a significant predictor in a multivariate model.

Means

Weight (kg) * gender

Weight (kg)

Gender	Mean	N	Std. deviation
Male	4.5923	275	0.62593
Female	4.1405	275	0.48111
Total	4.3664	550	0.60182

Weight (kg) * maternal education

Weight (kg)

Maternal education	Mean	N	Std. deviation
Year 10	4.3529	198	0.55993
Year 12	4.4109	99	0.69464
Tertiary	4.3596	253	0.59611
Total	4.3664	550	0.60182

Weight (kg) * parity recoded (three levels)

Weight (kg)			
Parity re-coded (three levels)	Mean	*N*	Std. deviation
Singleton	4.2589	180	0.61950
One sibling	4.3887	192	0.59258
Two or more siblings	4.4511	178	0.58040
Total	4.3664	550	0.60182

The summary statistics can also be used to verify the cell size and variance ratios. A summary of this information validates the model and helps to interpret the output from the three-way ANOVA. The cell size ratio when parity is recoded into three cells has been found to be adequate. The variance ratio for each factor, for example for parity, can be calculated by squaring the standard deviations from the Means table. For parity, the variance ratio is $(0.58)^2:(0.62)^2$ or 1:1.14.

Next, the distributions of the variables should be checked for normality using the methods described in Chapter 2 and for one-way ANOVA. The largest difference between mean values is between genders; therefore, it is important to examine the distribution for each gender to identify any outlying values or outliers. In fact, the distribution of each group for each factor should be checked for the presence of any outlying values or univariate outliers. The SPSS output is not included here but the analyses should proceed in the knowledge that there are no influential outliers and no significant deviations from normality for any variable in the model.

5.9   An example of a three-way ANOVA

A three-way ANOVA is defined by three factors; in this example, the factors are gender, parity and maternal education. The commands for running a three-way ANOVA to test for the effects of gender (two groups), parity (three groups) and maternal education (three groups) on weight and to test for a linear trend between weight and levels of parity are shown in Box 5.6.

Box 5.6 SPSS commands to obtain a three-way ANOVA

SPSS Commands

weights.sav – IBM SPSS Statistics Data Editor
> *Analyze → General Linear Model → Univariate*

Univariate
> *Highlight Weight and click into Dependent Variable*
> *Highlight Gender, Maternal education and Parity recoded (3 levels) and click into*
> > *Fixed Factor(s)*
> *Click on Model*

Univariate: Model
    Click on Custom
    Under Build Term(s): Type, pull down menu and click on Main effects
    Highlight gender, education and parity1 and click over into Model
    Sum of squares: Type III on pull down menu (default)
    Tick Include intercept in model (default), click Continue
Univariate
    Click on Contrasts
Univariate Contrasts
    Factors: Highlight parity1
    Change Contrasts: pull down menu, select Polynomial, click Change, click Continue
Univariate
    Click on Plots
Univariate: Profile Plots
    Highlight gender, click into Horizontal Axis
    Highlight parity1, click in Separate Lines, click Add, click Continue
Univariate
    Click on Options
Univariate: Options
    Highlight gender, education and parity1 and click into Display
    Means for
    Tick Compare main effects
    Confidence interval adjustment: LSD (none)(default)
    Click Continue
Univariate
    Click OK

The results from the three-way ANOVA are shown in the Tests of Between-Subject Effects table. In the table, the corrected model type III sum of squares is the sum of squares for the main effects. The first two rows show tests for the corrected model and intercept which usually are not of interest and can be ignored. The corrected model sum of squares divided by the corrected total sum of squares, that is, 32.613/198.842 or 0.164, is the variation that can be explained by the model and is the R squared value shown in the table footnote. This value indicates that gender, maternal education and parity together explain 0.164 or 16.4% of the variation in weight. This is considerably higher than the 1.7% explained by parity only in a previous model.

The F values are the within-group mean square divided by the error mean square. The F values for the three factors show that both gender and parity are significant predictors of weight at 1 month with $P < 0.0001$ and $P = 0.001$, respectively, but that maternal educational status is not a significant predictor with $P = 0.373$. After combining two of the parity groups and adjusting for gender differences in the parity groups, the significance of parity in predicting weight has increased to $P = 0.001$ compared with $P = 0.022$ obtained from the one-way ANOVA previously conducted.

Univariate analysis of variance

Tests of Between-Subject Effects

Dependent variable: weight (kg)

Source	Type III sum of squares	df	Mean square	F	Sig.
Corrected model	32.613[a]	5	6.523	21.346	0.000
Intercept	9012.463	1	9012.463	29,494.120	0.000
GENDER	28.528	1	28.528	93.361	0.000
EDUCATION	0.604	2	0.302	0.989	0.373
PARITY1	4.327	2	2.164	7.080	0.001
Error	166.229	544	0.306		
Total	10,684.926	550			
Corrected total	198.842	549			

[a]R squared $= 0.164$ (adjusted R squared $= 0.156$).

The sums of squares for the model, intercept, factors and the error term when added up manually equal 9244.764. This is less than the total sum of squares of 10,684.926 shown in the table, which also includes the sum of squares for all possible interactions between factors in the model, even though the inclusion of interactions was not requested.

The polynomial linear contrast in the Contrast Results table again shows that there is a significant linear trend for weight to change with parity at the $P < 0.0001$ level. Examination of mean weight by parity indicates that there is an increasing linear trend, with weight increasing as parity increases. The subscript to this Custom Hypothesis Tests table indicates that the outcome is being assessed over the three parity groups, that is, the groups labelled 1, 2 and 3. The quadratic term is not relevant because there is no evidence to suggest that the relationship between weight and parity is curved rather than linear, and consistent with this, the quadratic contrast is not significant.

Custom Hypothesis Tests

Contrast results (K matrix)

Parity recoded (three levels) polynomial contrast[a]		Dependent variable Weight (kg)
Linear	Contrast estimate	0.157
	Hypothesized value	0
	Difference (estimate − hypothesized)	0.157
	Std. error	0.042
	Sig.	0.000
	95% confidence interval for difference Lower bound	0.074
	Upper bound	0.240
Quadratic	Contrast estimate	−0.025
	Hypothesized value	0
	Difference (estimate − hypothesized)	−0.025
	Std. error	0.040
	Sig.	0.542
	95% confidence interval for difference Lower bound	−0.104
	Upper bound	0.055

[a]Metric $= 1.000, 2.000, 3.000.$

Marginal means

The Estimated Marginal Means table shows mean values adjusted for the other factors in the model, that is, the predicted mean values. Marginal means that are similar to the unadjusted mean values provide evidence that the model is robust. If the marginal means change by a considerable amount after adding an additional factor to the model, then the added factor is an important confounder or covariate. The significance of the comparisons in the Pairwise Comparisons table is based on a t value, that is, the mean difference/SE, for the difference in marginal means without any adjustment for multiple comparisons.

Estimated Marginal Means

Estimates

Dependent variable: weight (kg)

Gender	Mean	Std. error	95% confidence interval	
			Lower bound	Upper bound
Male	4.603	0.035	4.535	4.672
Female	4.148	0.035	4.079	4.216

Pairwise Comparisons

Dependent variable: weight (kg)

(I) gender	(J) gender	Mean difference (I − J)	Std. error	Sig.[a]	95% confidence interval for difference[a]	
					Lower bound	Upper bound
Male	Female	0.456*	0.047	0.000	0.363	0.548
Female	Male	−0.456*	0.047	0.000	−0.548	−0.363

Based on estimated marginal means.
*The mean difference is significant at the 0.05 level.
[a]Adjustment for multiple comparisons: least significant difference (equivalent to no adjustments).

Univariate Tests

Dependent variable: weight (kg)

	Sum of squares	df	Mean square	F	Sig.
Contrast	28.528	1	28.528	93.361	0.000
Error	166.229	544	0.306		

The F tests the effect of gender. This test is based on the linearly independent pairwise comparisons among the estimated marginal means.

The estimated marginal mean is the mean value of a factor averaged across other levels of the factors, that is, averaged over all cell means. In this model, the marginal means are averaged over parity and maternal education. The standard errors are identical in the two groups because the pooled data for all cases are used to compute a single estimate of the standard error. For this reason, it is important that the assumptions of equal variance and similar cell sizes in all groups are met. The marginal mean for males is 4.603 kg compared to a mean of 4.592 kg in the unadjusted analysis, and for females is 4.148 kg compared to 4.141 kg in the unadjusted analysis. Thus, the difference between genders in the adjusted ANOVA analysis is 0.455 kg compared with a difference of 0.452 kg that can be calculated from the previous Means table.

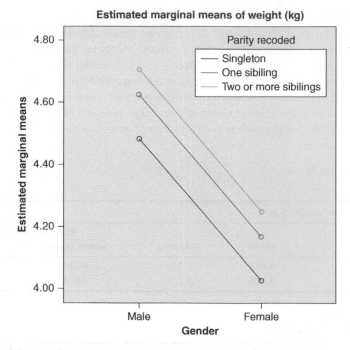

Figure 5.6 Profile plot of marginal means of weight by gender and parity.

Pairwise comparisons for maternal education and parity were also requested although they have not been included here.

The Profile plot shown in Figure 5.6 indicates that the relative values in mean weights between groups defined according to parity are the same for both genders. In the plot, if the lines cross one another this would indicate an interaction between factors. However, in Figure 5.6, the lines are parallel which indicates that there is no interaction between gender and parity. Interactions are discussed in more detail in Chapter 7.

5.9.1   Reporting the results of a three-way ANOVA

The results from the three-way ANOVA can be presented as shown in Table 5.7.

The results could be described as follows: 'Table 5.7 shows the unadjusted mean weights of babies at 1 month of age by group. The F and P values were derived from a three-way ANOVA. The cell size was within the assumption of 1:4 for females and close to this assumption for males and the variance ratio was less than 1:2. There was a significant difference in weight between males and females and between groups defined according to parity, but not between groups defined according to maternal education status. A polynomial contrast indicated that there was a significant linear trend between weight and levels of parity ($P < 0.0001$). Pairwise contrasts showed that the difference in marginal means between males and females was 0.46 kg (95% CI 0.36, 0.55, $P < 0.0001$). In addition, the difference in marginal means between singletons and babies with one sibling was statistically significant at −0.14 kg (95% CI −0.25, −0.03, $P = 0.015$) and the difference between singletons and babies with two or more siblings

Table 5.7   Mean weights of babies at 1 month of age by gender, parity and maternal education

	N	Weight (kg) Mean (SD)	F (df)	P value	P value trend
Gender					
Males	275	4.59 (0.63)	93.36 (1, 544)	<0.0001	–
Females	275	4.14 (0.48)			
Parity					
Singletons	180	4.26 (0.62)	7.08 (2, 544)	0.001	<0.0001
One sibling	192	4.39 (0.59)			
Two or more siblings	178	4.45 (0.58)			
Maternal education					
Year 10 school	198	4.35 (0.56)	0.99 (2, 544)	0.373	–
Year 12 school	99	4.41 (0.69)			
Tertiary education	253	4.36 (0.60)			

was statistically significant at -0.22 kg (95% CI -0.34, -0.11, $P < 0.0001$). Profile plots indicated that there was no interaction between gender and parity'.

5.10   Analysis of covariance (ANCOVA)

An ANCOVA is used when the effects of one or more categorical factors (explanatory variables) on a single continuous variable (outcome or dependent variable) are explored after adjusting for the effects of one or more continuous variables (covariates). The ANCOVA analysis first produces a regression of the outcome on the covariate and then adjusts the cell means for the effect of the covariate. Regression which provides a line of best fit through the data is discussed in detail in Chapter 7. Adjusting for a covariate has the effect of reducing the residual (error) term by reducing the amount of noise in the model. As in regression, it is important that the association between the outcome and the covariate is linear. In ANCOVA, the residual terms are the distances of each individual from the regression line and not from the cell mean, thus the residual distances are smaller than in ANOVA.

The assumptions for ANCOVA are identical to the assumptions for ANOVA but the additional assumptions shown in Box 5.7 must also be met.

Box 5.7 Additional assumptions for ANCOVA

The following assumptions for ANCOVA must be met in addition to the assumptions shown in Box 5.1 for ANOVA:
- the measurement of the covariate is reliable
- if there is more than one covariate, there is low collinearity between covariates

- the association between the covariate and the outcome is linear
- there is homogeneity of the regression, that is, the slopes across the data in each cell are the same as the slope in the total sample
- there is no interaction between the covariate and the factors
- there are no multivariate outliers

In building the ANCOVA model, the choice of covariates must be made carefully and should be limited to those that can be measured reliably. Few covariates are measured without any error but unreliable covariates lead to a loss of statistical power. Covariates such as age and height can be measured reliably but other covariates such as reported hours of sleep or time spent exercising may be subject to significant reporting bias.

It is also important to limit the number of covariates to variables that are not significantly related to one another. As in all multivariate models, multicollinearity, that is a significant association or correlation between explanatory variables, can result in an unstable model and unreliable estimates of effect, which can be difficult to interpret. Ideally, the correlation between covariates (which is discussed in Chapter 7) should be low with an r value of less than 0.7.

5.10.1   Effect size for ANCOVA

Partial eta squared, which is an estimate of effect size, is the ratio of variance accounted by a factor to the variance accounted by a factor and its associated error variance. Partial eta squared is calculated as the sum of squares for the factor divided by the sum of squares for the factor plus the sum of squares for the error as follows:

Partial $\eta^2 = SS_B/SS_B + SS_E$, where SS_E is the sum of the squares for the error term.

Partial eta squared differs from eta squared (described in Section 5.4), in that, the latter's denominator is the sum of the squares total (i.e. total variance). For partial eta squared, the variances for other factors are partialled out, that is, removed from the total non-error variation.[3]

Partial eta squared values for each factor can be directly compared but cannot be added to indicate how much of the variance of the outcome variable is accounted for by the explanatory variables. Eta squared values sometimes over-estimate effect because the values add to over 1.0 when summed and for this reason they are considered a biased estimate of the true effect size in the population although they are widely used. As for one-way ANOVA, partial eta squared can be converted to Cohen's f. In SPSS, partial eta squared values can be obtained for ANCOVA, factorial ANOVA and repeated measures ANOVA (see Chapter 6).

Research question

Weight is related to the length of a baby and therefore it makes sense to use ANCOVA to test whether the significant differences in weight between gender and parity groups are maintained after adjusting for length. In testing this, length is added into the model as a covariate. The SPSS commands for running an ANCOVA model are shown in Box 5.8. Maternal education has been omitted from this model because the previous three-way ANOVA showed that this variable does not have a significant relationship with babies' weights.

Box 5.8 SPSS commands for obtaining an ANCOVA model

SPSS Commands

weights.sav – IBM SPSS Statistics Data Editor
    Analyze → General Linear Model → Univariate
    Univariate
    Click on Reset
    Highlight Weight and click into Dependent Variable
    Highlight Gender and Parity recoded (3 levels) and click into Fixed Factor(s)
    Highlight Length, click into Covariate(s)
    Click on Model
Univariate: Model
    Click on Custom
    Under Build Term(s): Type pull down menu and click on Main effects
    Highlight gender, parity1 and length and click over into Model
    Sum of squares: Type III on pull down menu (default)
    Tick Include intercept in model (default), click Continue
Univariate
    Click on Contrasts
Univariate Contrasts
    Factors: Highlight parity1
    Change Contrast: pull down menu, select Polynomial, click Change, click Continue
Univariate
    Click on Options
Univariate: Options
    Highlight gender and Parity1, click into Display Means for
    Tick Compare main effects
    Confidence interval adjustment: using LSD (none)(default)
    Tick Estimates of effect size
    Click Continue
Univariate
    Click OK

The Tests of Between-Subject Effects table shows that by adding a covariate that is a significant predictor of weight, the explained variation has increased from 16.4% to 55.9% as indicated by the R square value. All three factors in the model are statistically significant but parity is now less significant at $P = 0.003$ compared to $P = 0.001$ in the former three-way ANOVA model. These P values, which are adjusted for the covariate, are more accurate than the P values from the previous one-way and three-way ANOVA models. The partial eta squared values are also displayed in the Tests of Between-Subject Effects table. Length has the largest partial eta squared value and can be calculated using the figures shown as follows: $79.155 / (79.155 + 87.678) = 0.474$.

Tests of Between-Subjects Effects

Dependent variable: weight (kg)

Source	Type III sum of squares	df	Mean square	F	Sig.	Partial eta squared
Corrected model	111.164[a]	4	27.791	172.747	0.000	0.559
Intercept	20.805	1	20.805	129.322	0.000	0.192
Gender	8.378	1	8.378	52.074	0.000	0.087
Parity1	1.929	2	0.965	5.996	0.003	0.022
Length	79.155	1	79.155	492.024	0.000	0.474
Error	87.678	545	0.161			
Total	10,684.926	550				
Corrected total	198.842	549				

[a]R squared = 0.559 (Adjusted R squared = 0.556).

The Contrast Results table shows that the linear trend between weight and parity remains significant, but slightly less so at $P = 0.001$.

Custom Hypothesis Tests

Contrast results (K matrix)

Parity re-coded (three levels) Polynomial contrast[a]		Dependent variable Weight (kg)
Linear	Contrast estimate	0.098
	Hypothesized value	0
	Difference (estimate − hypothesized)	0.098
	Std. error	0.030
	Sig.	0.001
	95% confidence interval for difference — Lower bound	0.039
	Upper bound	0.157
Quadratic	Contrast estimate	−0.035
	Hypothesized value	0
	Difference (estimate − hypothesized)	−0.035
	Std. error	0.029
	Sig.	0.238
	95% confidence interval for difference — Lower bound	−0.092
	Upper bound	0.023

[a]Metric = 1.000, 2.000, 3.000.

When there is a significant covariate in the model, the marginal means are calculated with the covariate held at its mean value. Again, the marginal means are predicted means and not observed means. In this model, the marginal means are calculated at the mean value of the covariate length, that is, 54.841 as shown in the footnote of the estimates table. In this situation, the marginal means need to be treated with caution because they may not correspond with any situation in real life where the covariate is held at its mean value and is balanced between groups. In observational studies, the marginal means from such analyses often have no interpretation apart from group comparisons.

Estimated Marginal Means

Estimates

Dependent variable: weight (kg)

Gender	Mean	Std. error	95% confidence interval	
			Lower bound	Upper bound
Male	4.494[a]	0.025	4.445	4.542
Female	4.238[a]	0.025	4.190	4.287

[a] Covariates appearing in the model are evaluated at the following values: Length (cm) − 54.841.

Pairwise Comparisons

Dependent variable: weight (kg)

(I) gender	(J) gender	Mean difference (I − J)	Std. error	Sig.[a]	95% confidence interval for difference[a]	
					Lower bound	Upper bound
Male	Female	0.255*	0.035	0.000	0.186	0.325
Female	Male	−0.255*	0.035	0.000	−0.325	−0.186

Based on estimated marginal means.
*The mean difference is significant at the 0.05 level.
[a] Adjustment for multiple comparisons: least significant difference (equivalent to no adjustments).

Univariate Tests

Dependent variable: weight (kg)

	Sum of squares	df	Mean square	F	Sig.
Contrast	8.378	1	8.378	52.074	0.000
Error	87.678	545	0.161		

The *F* tests the effect of gender. This test is based on the linearly independent pairwise comparisons among the estimated marginal means.

5.11   Testing the model assumptions of ANOVA/ANCOVA

It is important to conduct tests to check that the assumptions of an ANOVA or ANCOVA model have been met. By rerunning the model with different options, statistics can be obtained to test that the residuals are normally distributed, that there are no influential multivariate outliers, that the variance is homogeneous and that there are no interactions between the covariate and the factors. Here, the assumptions are being tested only when the final model is obtained but in practice the assumptions would be tested at each stage in the model building process. The SPSS commands shown in Box 5.9 can be used to test the model assumptions.

Box 5.9 SPSS commands for testing the assumptions of ANOVA/ANCOVA model

SPSS Commands

weights.sav – IBM SPSS Statistics Data Editor
    Analyze → General Linear Model → Univariate
Univariate
    Click on Reset
    Highlight Weight and click into Dependent Variable
    Highlight Gender and Parity recoded (3 levels) and click into Fixed Factor(s)
    Highlight Length, click into Covariate(s)
    Click on Model
Univariate: Model
    Click on Custom
    Under Build Term(s): Type pull down menu and click on Main effects
    Highlight gender, parity1 and length and click over into Model
    Pull down menu, click on All 2-way
    Highlight gender, parity1 and length, click over into Model
    Sum of squares: Type III on pull down menu (default)
    Tick Include intercept in model (default), click Continue
Univariate
    Click on Save
Univariate: Save
    Under Predicted Values tick Unstandardized
    Under Residuals tick Standardized
    Under Diagnostics tick Cook's distances and Leverage values
    Click Continue
Univariate
    Click on Options
Univariate Options
    Tick on Estimates of effect size, Homogeneity tests, Spread vs level plot
    Residual plot, and Lack of fit, click Continue
Univariate
    Click OK

5.11.1 Homogeneity of variance

In the Levene's Test of Equality of Error Variances table, the Levene's test indicates that the differences in variances are not significantly different with a P value of 0.085. If the P value had been significant at < 0.05, the variance ratio (largest variance divided by the smallest variance) should also be checked to confirm that it is greater than 2. If the variances are not equal, an option would be to halve the critical P values for any between-group differences say to $P = 0.025$ instead of $P = 0.05$. This is an arbitrary decision but would reduce the type I error rate. A less rigorous option would be to select a post-hoc test that adjusts for unequal variances. Alternatively, regression would be the preferred method of analysing the data.

Univariate Analysis of Variance

Levene's test of equality of error variances[a]

Dependent variable: weight (kg)			
F	df1	df2	Sig.
1.947	5	544	0.085

Tests the null hypothesis that the error variance of the dependent variable is equal across groups.
[a]Design:Intercept + GENDER + PARITY1 + LENGTH + GENDER ∗ PARITY1 + GENDER ∗ LENGTH + PARITY1 ∗ LENGTH

The Sig. column in the Tests of Between-Subject Effects table shows that gender and length are significant predictors of weight with $P < 0.0001$ and that parity is a marginal predictor with $P = 0.057$. However, there is a significant interaction between gender and length at $P < 0.0001$ although there are no significant interactions between gender and parity ($P = 0.478$) or parity and length ($P = 0.079$).

Tests of Between-Subject Effects

Dependent variable: weight (kg)					
Source	Type III sum of squares	df	Mean square	F	Sig.	Partial eta squared
Corrected model	114.742[a]	9	12.749	81.862	0.000	0.577
Intercept	18.697	1	18.697	120.056	0.000	0.182
GENDER	2.062	1	2.062	13.237	0.000	0.024
PARITY1	0.898	2	0.449	2.884	0.057	0.011
LENGTH	73.731	1	73.731	473.425	0.000	0.467
GENDER * PARITY1	0.230	2	0.115	0.739	0.478	0.003
GENDER * LENGTH	2.434	1	2.434	15.631	0.000	0.028
PARITY1 * LENGTH	0.793	2	0.397	2.547	0.079	0.009
Error	84.099	540	0.156			
Total	10,684.926	550				
Corrected total	198.842	549				

[a]R squared = 0.577 (adjusted R squared = 0.570).

5.11.2 *Interactions*

When interactions are present in any multivariate model, the main effects of the variables involved in the interaction are no longer of interest because it is the interaction that describes the relationship between the variables and the outcome. However, the main effects must always be included in the model even though they are no longer of interest. Inclusion of the interaction between gender and length violates the ANCOVA model assumption that there is no association between the interaction, the covariate (length) and the factor (gender). In this case, regression with centred variables would be the preferred analysis. Alternatively, the ANCOVA could be conducted for males and females separately although this will reduce the precision around the estimates of effect simply because the sample size in each model is approximately halved.

5.11.3   Lack of fit

The lack of fit test divides the total variance into the variance due to the interaction terms not included in the model (lack of fit) and the variance in the model (pure error). An F value that is not significant as in this table at $P = 0.070$ indicates that the model cannot be improved by adding further interaction terms, which in this case would have been the three-way interaction term between gender, parity and length. However, any significant interaction that includes the covariate would violate the assumption of the model.

Lack of Fit Tests

Dependent variable: weight (kg)

Source	Sum of squares	df	Mean square	F	Sig.	Partial eta squared
Lack of fit	20.907	114	0.183	1.236	0.070	0.249
Pure error	63.192	426	0.148			

It is important to examine the variance across the model using a spread-vs-level plot because the cell sizes in the model are unequal. The spread-vs-level plot shows one point for each cell. If the variance is not related to the cell means then unequal variances will not be a problem. However, if there is a relation such as the variance increasing with the mean of the cell, then unequal variances will bias the F value.

The first spread-vs-level plot shown in Figure 5.7 (see p.153) indicates that the standard deviation on the y-axis increases with the mean weight of each gender and parity cell as shown on the x-axis. However, the range in standard deviations is relatively small, that is, from approximately 0.45–0.65. This ratio of less than 1:2 for standard deviation, or 1:4 for variance, will not violate the ANOVA assumptions. The second Spread-vs-Level plot shown in Figure 5.7 shows the same pattern as the first Spread-vs-Level plot and the spread values of variance on the y axis are the square of the standard deviation values shown in the first plot (variance = square of standard deviation).

If the variances are widely unequal, it is sometimes possible to reduce the differences by transforming the measurement. If there is a linear relation between the variance and the means of the cells and all the data values are positive, taking the square root or logarithm of the measurements may be helpful. Transforming variables into units that are not easy to communicate are last resort methods to avoid violating the assumptions of ANOVA or ANCOVA. In practice, the use of a different statistical test such as multiple regression analysis may be preferable because the assumptions are not as restrictive.

5.11.4   Testing residuals: Unbiased and normality

One assumption of ANOVA and ANCOVA is that the residuals are unbiased. This means that the differences between the observed and predicted values for each participant are not systematically different from one another. Using the commands in Box 5.9 the matrix plot shown in Figure 5.8 (see p.154) can be obtained. This plot shows that the observed and predicted values have a linear relationship with no systematic differences

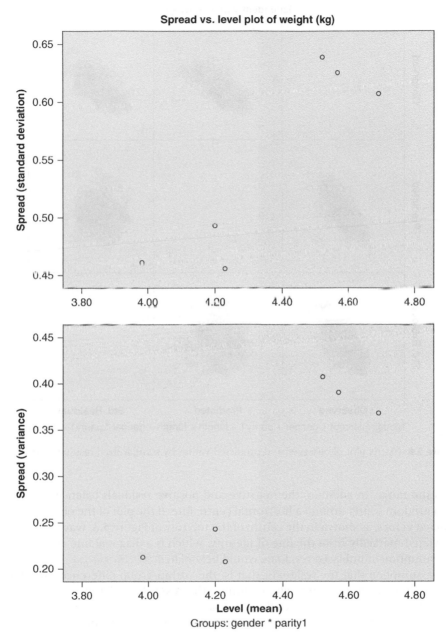

Figure 5.7 Spread by standard deviation and variance by level (mean) plot of weight for each gender and parity group.

Dependent variable: weight (kg)

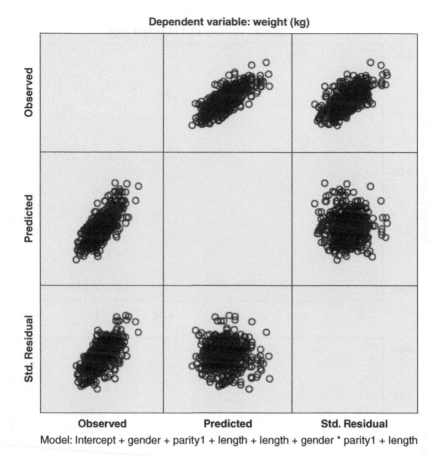

Model: Intercept + gender + parity1 + length + length + gender * parity1 + length

Figure 5.8 Matrix plot of observed and predicted values by standardized residuals for weight.

across the range. In addition, the negative and positive residuals balance one another with a random scatter around a horizontal centre line. If the plot of the observed against predicted values, as shown in the centre of the top row of Figure 5.8, was funnel shaped or deviated markedly from the line of identity, which is a diagonal line across the plot, the assumption of unbiased residuals would be violated.

The assumption that the residuals, that is, the within-group differences, have a normal distribution can be tested when running the ANOVA model. It is important that this assumption is satisfied especially if the sample size is relatively small because the effect of non-normally distributed residuals or of multivariate outliers is to bias the P values.

When residuals are requested in *Save* as shown in Box 5.9, the residual for each case is created as a new variable at the end of the SPSS Data View spreadsheet, with the variable name of ZRE_1 and variable label of 'Standardized Residual for weight'. The distribution of the residuals can be explored in more detail using standard tests of normality in *Analyze* → *Descriptive Statistics* → *Explore* as shown in Box 2.2, with the new variable Standardized Residual for weight as the dependent variable.

Descriptives

			Statistic	Std. error
Standardized residual for	Mean		0.0000	0.04229
	95% confidence	Lower bound	−0.0831	
WEIGHT	Interval for mean	Upper bound	0.0831	
	5% trimmed mean		0.0014	
	Median		−0.0295	
	Variance		0.984	
	Std. deviation		0.99177	
	Minimum		−2.69	
	Maximum		3.16	
	Range		5.85	
	Inter-quartile range		1.32	
	Skewness		0.069	0.104
	Kurtosis		0.178	0.208

Extreme values

			Case number	Value
Standardized residual for WEIGHT	Highest	1	256	3.16
		2	101	3.08
		3	404	3.03
		4	32	2.80
		5	447	2.73
	Lowest	1	252	−2.69
		2	437	−2.48
		3	311	−2.37
		4	35	−2.37
		5	546	−2.34

Tests of Normality

	Kolmogorov–Smirnov[a]			Shapiro–Wilk		
	Statistic	df	Sig.	Statistic	df	Sig.
Standardized residual for WEIGHT	0.020	550	0.200*	0.995	550	0.069

*This is a lower bound of the true significance.
[a]Lilliefors significance correction.

The descriptive statistics and the tests of normality show that the standardized residuals are normally distributed with a mean residual of zero and a standard deviation very close to unity at 0.992, as expected. The histogram and normal Q–Q plot shown in Figure 5.9 indicate only small deviations from normality in the tails of the distribution.

For an approximately normal distribution, 99% of standardized residuals will by definition fall within three standard deviations of the mean. Therefore, 1% of the sample is expected to be outside this range. In this sample size of 550 children, it would be expected that 1% of the sample, that is five children, would have a standardized residual outside the area that lies between −3 and +3 standard deviations from the mean. The Extreme Values table shows that residual scores for three children are more than three standard deviations from the mean and the largest standardized residual is 3.16.

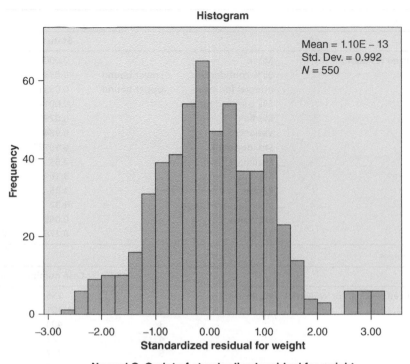

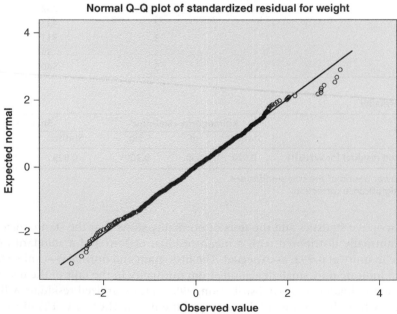

Figure 5.9 Histogram and plot of standardized residuals by weight.

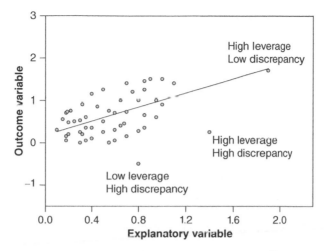

Figure 5.10 Distribution of data points and outliers.

The number of outliers is less than would be expected by chance. In addition, all three outliers have values that are just outside the cut-off range and therefore are not of concern.

5.11.5 *Identifying multivariate outliers: leverage and discrepancy*

To identify multivariate outliers, statistics such as leverage and discrepancy for each data point can be calculated. Leverage measures how far or remote a data point is from the remaining data but does not indicate whether the remote data point is on the same line as other cases or far away from the line. Thus, leverage does not provide information about the direction of the distance from the other data points.[9] Discrepancy indicates whether the remote data point is in line with other data points. Figure 5.10 shows how remote points or outliers can have a high leverage and/or a high discrepancy.

Cook's distances are a measure of influence, that is, a product of leverage and discrepancy. Influence measures the change in regression coefficients (see Chapter 7) if the data point is removed.[9] A recommended cut-off for detecting influential cases is a Cook's distance greater than $4 / (n - k - 1)$, where n is the sample size and k is the number of explanatory variables in the model. In this example, any distance that is greater than $4 / (550 - 3 - 1)$, or 0.007, should be investigated. Obviously the larger the sample size the smaller the Cook's distance becomes. Therefore in practice, Cook's distances above 1 should be investigated because these cases are regarded as influential cases or outliers.

A leverage value that is greater than $2(k + 1)/n$, where k is the number of explanatory variables in the model and n is the sample size, is of concern. In the working example, this value would be $2 \times (3 + 1)/550$, or 0.015. As with Cook's distance, this leverage calculation is also influenced by sample size and the number of explanatory variables in the model. In practice, leverage values less than 0.2 are acceptable and leverage values greater than 0.5 need to be investigated. Leverage is also related to Mahalanobis distance, which is another technique to identify multivariate outliers when regression is used (see Chapter 7).[9]

Cook's distances and the leverage values obtained from the SPSS commands in Box 5.9 are added to the SPSS Data View spreadsheet with COO_1 and LEV_1 as the variable names. Cook's distances can be plotted in a histogram using the SPSS commands shown in Box 5.10. These commands can be repeated for leverage values.

Box 5.10 SPSS commands to examine potential multivariate outliers

SPSS Commands

Weights.sav – IBM SPSS Statistics Data Editor
    Graphs → Legacy Dialogs → Histogram
Histogram
    Highlight Cook's distance for weight, click into Variable
    Click OK

The plots shown in Figure 5.11 (see p.159) indicate that there are no multivariate outliers because there are no Cook's distances greater than 1 or leverage points greater than 0.2.

Deciding whether points are problematic will always be context specific and several factors need to be taken into account including sample size and diagnostic indicators. If problematic points are detected, it is reasonable to remove them, rerun the model and decide on an action depending on their influence on the results. Possible solutions are to recode values to remove their undue influence, to recruit a study sample with a larger sample size if the sample being tested is small or to limit the generalizability of the model.

5.12   Reporting the results of an ANCOVA

If the model assumptions had all been met, the results of the final ANCOVA model could be reported in a similar way to reporting the three-way ANOVA. In addition, it is important to report how any univariate or multivariate outliers were treated in the analysis and which interactions were tested. The statistics reported should include information to assure readers that all ANCOVA assumptions had been met and should include values of partial eta squared or omega squared values to convey the relative contribution of each factor to the model. Other statistics to report are the total amount of variation explained and the significance of each factor in the model.

In the present ANCOVA model, because there was a significant interaction between factors, it is better to analyse the data using regression as described in Chapter 7.

5.13   Notes for critical appraisal

There are many assumptions for ANOVA and ANCOVA and it is important that all assumptions are tested and met to avoid inaccurate P values. Some of the most important questions to ask when critically appraising a journal article in which ANOVA or ANCOVA is used to analyse the data are shown in Box 5.11.

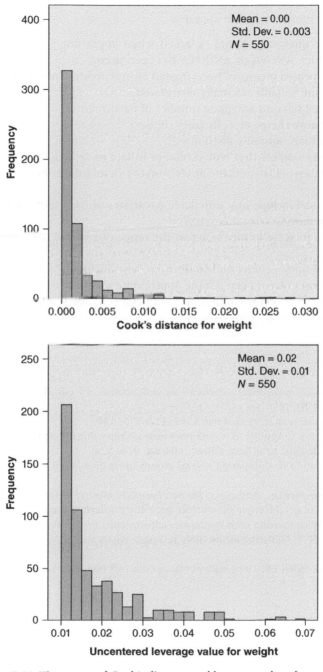

Figure 5.11 Histograms of Cook's distance and leverage values for weight.

Box 5.11 Questions for critical appraisal

The following questions should be asked when appraising published results from analyses in which ANOVA or ANCOVA has been used:
- Have any repeated measures been treated as independent observations?
- Is the outcome variable normally distributed?
- Does each cell have an adequate number of participants?
- Are the variances between cells fairly similar?
- Are the residuals normally distributed?
- Are there any outliers that would tend to inflate or reduce differences between groups or that would distort the model and the standard errors, and therefore the P values?
- Does the model include any unreliable covariates or covariates that do not have a linear relationship with the outcome?
- If there is an increase in means across the range of a factor, has a trend test been used?
- Have tests of homogeneity and collinearity been included?
- Would regression have been a more appropriate statistical test to use?
- Do the P values reflect the differences between cell means and the group sizes?

References

1. Stevens, J. *Applied multivariate statistics for the social sciences*, 3rd edn. Lawrence Erlbaum Associates: Mahwah, NJ, 1996.
2. Cohen J. A power primer. *Psychol Bull* 1992; **112**: 155–159.
3. Pierce CA, Block RA, Aguinis, H. Cautionary note on reporting eta-squared values from multifactor ANOVA designs. *Educ Psychol Meas* 2004; **64**: 916–924.
4. Altman DG, Bland JM. Comparing several groups using analysis of variance. *BMJ* 1996; **312**: 1472–1473.
5. Norman GR, Streiner DL. *Biostatistics. The bare essentials*. Mosby: Missouri, USA, 1994.
6. Bland JM, Alman DG. Multiple significance tests: the Bonferroni method. *BMJ* 1995; **310**: 170.
7. Perneger TV. What's wrong with Bonferroni adjustments. *BMJ* 1998; **316**: 1236–1238.
8. Bender R, Lange S, Adjusting for multiple testing – when and how? *J Clin Epidemol* 2001; **54**: 343–349.
9. Tabachnick BG, Fidell LS. *Using multivariate statistics*, 4th edn. Allyn and Bacon: Boston, USA, 2001.

CHAPTER 6

Analyses of longitudinal data

All that really belongs to us is time; even he who has nothing else has that.
BALTASAR GRACIAN (1601–1658)

Objectives

The objectives of the chapter are to explain how to:
- decide which type of model to use to analyze data collected in a longitudinal study where repeated or multiple measurements on participants are obtained
- obtain and interpret the results of repeated measures ANOVA and linear mixed models
- check that the assumptions for repeated measures ANOVA and linear mixed models are met
- report results in a graph or a table
- critically appraise analyses of longitudinal data reported in the literature

---

In longitudinal studies, the outcome is measured repeatedly over time for each participant. Time is commonly measured as weeks, months or years but may be represented by other estimates such as age or school grade. For example, to assess the efficacy of a treatment for the relief of asthma, a participant's forced expiratory volume (FEV) is measured at weekly intervals for 1 month. When the outcome variable is continuous, two of the statistical methods that can be used to investigate changes in outcome and trends over time, both within and between study groups are:

i. a general linear model using the repeated measures option in SPSS which provides both a multivariate analysis of variance (MANOVA) and a univariate repeated measures analysis of variance (ANOVA); or
ii. a linear mixed model

The choice of method that is most suited for modelling a particular longitudinal data set requires careful consideration because different models may produce different estimates, standard errors and associated P values for the same data set.

6.1 Study design

Repeated measures ANOVA and linear mixed models are ideal for analyzing data from cohort or experimental studies which have a prospective or longitudinal design.

Medical Statistics: A Guide to SPSS, Data Analysis and Critical Appraisal, Second Edition.
Belinda Barton and Jennifer Peat.
© 2014 John Wiley & Sons, Ltd. Published 2014 by John Wiley & Sons, Ltd.
Companion website: www.wiley.com/go/barton/medicalstatistics2e

Cohort studies are often used to compare the health outcomes of groups of people whose exposures are different and as such have the advantage that they can be used to demonstrate possible causation in that the exposure can be measured before the outcome develops. For analyzing data from cohort studies, models which offer the ability to compare differences at time points and/or between-exposure groups are ideal. Repeated measures ANOVA and linear mixed models can also be used to analyze data from randomized controlled trials and other experimental and non-experimental studies in which data of outcomes in different treatment groups is collected at baseline and at ongoing time points typically following a treatment intervention.

6.2   Sample size and power

To obtain accurate estimates of effect and unbiased P values in a model, it is important that the sample size, cell size and accuracy of the measurements are adequate to support the model. Estimates of the sample size required to support longitudinal data analyses vary. In general, the sample size should be calculated on the basis of the number of variables to be tested in the model including the outcome (dependent) variable. A rough rule of thumb for the multivariate approach (i.e. MANOVA) is that the sample size should be greater than $a + 10$ participants, where a is the number of levels for repeated measures.[1] However, larger numbers are preferable in order to increase precision by reducing the size of the standard errors. The number of participants needs to be much larger than the number of repeat measures because when the number of measurements exceeds the number of participants, the model used to analyze the data will have low statistical power. Calculation of the sample size required for repeated measures and linear mixed models can be complex and there are a few computing packages available (see Useful Websites). However, the calculation of power and sample size is not available for all types of mixed models. Generally the information that is required to calculate sample size for repeated measures or longitudinal analysis is an estimated effect size, the number of repeated measures and an estimate of the correlations among pairs of the repeated measures.

   Cell size, that is the number of participants in each group of a fixed factor or in each sub-group if there are two or more factors, is an important consideration. If the cell size ratio between the smallest and largest cells is larger than 1:4, the ANOVA assumptions will not be met. Bias in estimates of effect from ANOVA models will increase as the cell imbalance increases but this not an important consideration in linear mixed models. In ANOVA, small cells are problematic because the mean and variance cannot be estimated accurately for the cell. Groups with small numbers may need to be combined with other groups if the theory is logical. If combining cells is not logical, groups with small cell sizes can be omitted from the model, although this may reduce the generalizability of the results. When the sample size is small, alternative outcome measurements such as area under the curve or average values should be considered rather than using a repeated measures or longitudinal analysis.[2]

   The method used to develop a multivariate model can have an important influence on the results. Including all potentially predictive variables into a single model may introduce multicollinearity and may result in a number of small or empty cells and therefore reduce the statistical power. A sequential approach in which variables are added into the model one at a time in order of clinical importance or univariate evidence of effect conserves power because variables can be removed from the model if they are not significant predictors. At each step, the model can be examined for fit and signs of mulitcollinearity which can provide important insights into relationships between explanatory variables and developmental pathways.

Any degree of error in measuring a variable is likely to increase variance and reduce statistical power. On the other hand, variables that explain a significant proportion of the variance and improve the fit of a model increase statistical power. There is obviously a trade-off between including all variables that improve the fit of a model and reducing the number of variables in order to maximize cell sizes and the precision that can be gained from the sample size.

6.3 Covariates

Covariates included in repeated measures or linear mixed models may be fixed covariates or time varying covariates. For example, when weight increase of infants is modelled, body length is an important covariate. In longitudinal data sets in which the covariate is measured at each time point the measurements may be highly correlated, and a time varying covariate such as age will also increase with time. In repeated measures ANOVA, time varying covariates can be included or the covariate measured at a single time point, usually the first time point, may be included. In linear mixed models, if a covariate such as body length is included for each time point, the default option is that the mean value of the covariate across the model will be used. Repeated measures ANOVA and mixed models will give different results when a covariate is included because the covariate for a single time point is used in repeated measures ANOVA, whereas the mean covariate value across the time points for each participant is used in a linear mixed model.

6.4 Assumptions of repeated measures ANOVA and mixed models

The assumptions that must be met to use both repeated measures ANOVA and a linear mixed model are shown in Box 6.1.

Box 6.1 Assumptions for using repeated measures ANOVA and linear mixed models

- the participants must be independent, that is, each participant is in only one level of each group and does not influence another participant's score;
- the factors must be independent, that is, fixed factors and covariates must not be highly related to one another;
- the outcome variable is normally distributed within each cell at each time point;
- the residuals across the model are normally distributed;
- there are no influential univariate or multivariate outliers

Additional assumptions for univariate repeated measures ANOVA
- there is sphericity across the model, that is, the variance of pairs of measures is constant
- there is homogeneity, that is, the variances in the groups are equal.

The assumptions of normality should always be tested although both repeated measures ANOVA and mixed models are fairly robust to some degree of non-normality as long as there are no influential outliers. If the assumption of normality of residuals is not met, the direction of bias is not always clear. This may not be too important if the P value is large and clearly non-significant or if the P value is small and clearly significant. However, bias is a major problem if the P value is close to the margin of significance or the sample size is small.

Outliers can have an important effect on the perceived differences between groups by making the groups seem more different or more alike. In both repeated measures ANOVA and linear mixed models, the residuals can be saved to the spreadsheet to test for normality of distribution and to identify outliers with a high residual value. The direction of bias caused by outliers is usually to artificially skew the mean value of a group in the direction of the outlier. Influential outliers can be recoded with a nominal value to remove their influence – a value that is commonly used is one that is marginally outside the range of the remainder of the data.[3] Alternatively, outliers can be omitted from the model although this may have implications for the generalizability of the results (see Section 2.5).

6.5   Repeated measures analysis of variance

Repeated measures ANOVA is a traditional method of modelling longitudinal data based on methods for factorial ANOVA and adapted for repeat measures. An advantage of this method is that the results are readily understood and easily communicated. However, a disadvantage is that no allowance is made for measurements taken closer together in time to be more correlated than measurements taken further apart. In practice, repeated measures ANOVA is most suited to data sets in which the outcome measurement has an equal variance at all time points and in which pairs of measurements from each participant are equally correlated regardless of the time interval between them.

In common with one- and two-way ANOVA, the variation in a repeated measures ANOVA model is partitioned into 'between-subject' and 'within-subject' factors (see Section 5.2.2). The within-subject factor, which is related to time, is generally of most interest as the outcome variable. However, differences in between-subject fixed factors such as gender or treatment group can also be tested. When a repeated measure ANOVA is requested in SPSS, the output includes both multivariate results (MANOVA) and univariate results (ANOVA). However, sometimes the results of the univariate and multivariate repeated measures tests will disagree. The multivariate test statistics are based on transformed variables, not the original variables. In addition, the presence of outliers, sample size and violations of the test assumption may influence the test results. If sphericity is present then the univariate test is more powerful.[4]

6.5.1 Assumptions of sphericity and homogeneity

When using repeated measures ANOVA, there is a core assumption of sphericity across the model. Sphericity requires that the variances of the differences for all pairs of repeated measures are constant. Sphericity should be checked for when there are three or more repeated measures conditions. The assumption of sphericity can be tested using Mauchly's test which gives an estimate of epsilon (ϵ), a measure of sphericity. This statistic has a value of 1 when sphericity is met and values less than 1 indicate further deviation from sphericity. However, the Mauchly's test is influenced by the sample size, in that, in small samples this test often fails to detect departures from sphericity and in large samples over detects sphericity.[5] If the P value is statistically significant ($P < 0.05$), this provides evidence that the variances of the differences are not equal and the assumption of sphericity is not met.

Another assumption is that the variances of the repeated measures are the same in each group, that is, there is homogeneity. This assumption is tested using Box's M which is very sensitive to non-normality. For this test, a P value larger than 0.001 provides evidence of homogeneity.

The F test of the univariate model is robust to some violations of the assumption of normality of residuals but not to the sphericity assumption. When sphericity is not met, the F value is inflated and the P value is biased towards significance. In this situation, the estimate of sphericity is adjusted using the Greenhouse-Geisser or the less conservative Huynh–Feldt methods. With these methods, the degrees of freedom are multiplied by the estimate of sphericity, consequently the degrees of freedom are decreased, making the F ratio more conservative. It is recommended that when the epsilon value is greater than 0.75 the Huynh–Feldt estimate is used and when the value is less than 0.75 the Greenhouse-Geisser is used.[5] If the F test is not significant then no adjustment is needed. Data that violate sphericity can be analyzed using MANOVA since the assumption of sphericity is not required for multivariate repeated measures.

6.5.2 Multivariate test

In SPSS, the repeated measures ANOVA commands automatically provide a MANOVA test. In MANOVA, the outcome variables are transformed into linear combinations of the differences between the repeated measures and the transformed scores are then weighted to form contrasts. Thus, the original outcome values across time are transformed to contrast values and the model is applied only to these variables. This method of transforming the data bypasses the problem of dealing with covariance between time points rather than addressing it directly as in a linear mixed model.

An advantage of MANOVA is that the test of sphericity does not need to be met. Thus, if the test of sphericity is violated, the P value obtained from the MANOVA can be used, but only if the results can be appropriately interpreted. A disadvantage of MANOVA is that the order of the data points has no influence on the results and therefore trends over time cannot be addressed. Using MANOVA may not be congruent with the study aims and, in some situations MANOVA is too general and may lack power to detect group differences when they exist (i.e. there is a high probability of type II error).

6.5.3   Univariate test

Univariate ANOVA is the test most commonly used for repeated measures data sets. When repeated measures ANOVA is requested in SPSS, interactions between the fixed factors and time (e.g. group × time interactions) are automatically included in the univariate tests although no centering is performed to exclude the effects of multicollinearity between the interaction and its derivatives. Interactions that are statistically significant indicate that the pattern of change over time is different between groups.

6.5.4   Missing values

Missing values limit the use of repeated measures ANOVA because participants with one or more missing values are excluded from the analysis. Thus missing values reduce the effective sample size, compromise statistical power and affect the generalizability of the results. If the number of missing values is small and the values are randomly missing, they can be replaced with a nominal value such as a mean value or the last value carried forward for each participant. However, as discussed earlier (see Section 1.14), these methods for replacing missing values may lead to biased results and other techniques should be considered.[6]

6.5.5   Data layout

In SPSS, for repeated measures ANOVA the data file needs to be in the 'wide' format with only one row per participant and each column is a repeated response for that participant organized along the same row.

6.5.6   Group comparisons

Several types of contrasts, that is, group comparisons can be undertaken in repeated measures ANOVA. The most appropriate test should be decided a priori. In SPSS, the following tests of contrasts are available:

- *Repeated*, which tests the means at adjacent time points against one another, for example, time 1 vs time 2, time 2 vs time 3 and so on.
- *Difference*, which tests the mean at each time point against the previous time point, for example, time 2 vs 1, time 3 vs 2 and so on.
- *Simple*, which tests each time point against the first or final time point, for example, time 1 vs the last time point, time 2 vs the last time point and so on.
- *Helmert*, which tests each time point against the mean of all later time points. This test is appropriate to test for an increase in values followed by a plateau. The time point at which the increase is no longer significant indicates where the plateau begins.

- *Polynomial*, which tests for a trend across the time points. Tests of significance for a linear trend through the data and for orders such as quadratic effects are included.
- *Deviation*, which tests each time point against the mean of all time points, for example, time 1 vs mean, time 2 vs mean and so on.

For pairwise post hoc comparisons, the Tukey's test is powerful when sphericity is met. When sphericity is violated, the Bonferroni is recommended since it maintains the type I error rate.[7]

6.5.7 Advantages and disadvantages of repeated measures ANOVA

The advantages of using repeated measures ANOVA are that:

- summary means plots can be requested to facilitate the interpretation of *P* values;
- tests of homogeneity and sphericity are automatically reported;
- an estimate of the effect size (eta-squared) can be requested;
- several types of contrasts are available to interpret between-group differences.

The disadvantages of repeated measures ANOVA analyses are that:

- participants with missing values for any time point are omitted;
- they only estimate and compare the group means, and do not provide information about individual growth;
- the correlation between repeated measures is not modelled;
- no allowance is made for the variance to change over time;
- the results become unreliable as the number of repeat measures relative to the number of participants increases.

Research question

The data set 'BMD_study_wide_file' contains the data from 60 elderly people who were enrolled in a randomized controlled trial in which the intervention group underwent a 4 week programme to increase bone density and the control group received a placebo treatment. Bone mineral density (BMD) was measured at three time points (baseline, 6 months and 1 year).

Question: Was the intervention effective in increasing BMD at 6 months and were any changes sustained at 1 year?

Null hypothesis: That there was no difference in BMD between the intervention and control groups at any time point.

Variables: Outcome variable = BMD measured over time (continuous); Explanatory variable = group (categorical)

The SPSS command sequence *Analyze* → *Descriptive Statistics* → *Frequencies* can be used to ascertain cell sizes.

Group

		Frequency	Per cent	Valid per cent	Cumulative per cent
Valid	Control	28	46.7	46.7	46.7
	Intervention	32	53.3	53.3	100.0
	Total	60	100.0	100.0	

The number of people in the two groups is almost equal at 28 and 32 so the cell ratio of approximately 1 does not violate the model assumptions. Boxplots using the SPSS command sequence *Graphs → Legacy Dialogs → Boxplot → Simple* can be used to examine how BMD is related to group at each time point to gain a working knowledge of the data. The boxplots in Figure 6.1 show that the median BMD was slightly lower in the intervention group than in the control group at baseline but the two groups have a similar range of values as would be expected in a randomized trial. At the 6-month and 1-year's follow-up, the median BMD is higher in the intervention group. There are no extreme univariate outliers in the data. The two outlying values with ID numbers of 52 and 49 have BMD values that are approximately 2.5 standard deviations from the mean and therefore are not of concern (see Section 2.5). Outlying values with common IDs across time periods such as ID number 52 suggest valid cases rather than recording errors. The outlying values are few and are not extreme and therefore the values are left unchanged in the analyses.

The command sequence to obtain repeated measures ANOVA is shown in Box 6.2. These commands require that the data set is structured in the 'wide' format.

Box 6.2 SPSS commands to obtain repeated measures ANOVA

SPSS Commands

BMD_study_wide file – IBM SPSS Statistics Data Editor
Analyze → General Linear Model → Repeated Measures
Repeated Measures Define Factor(s)
        Within-Subject Factor Name – change 'factor1' to 'Time'
        Number of Levels – enter '3'
        Click Add
        Click Define
Repeated Measures
        Highlight BMD.1, BMD.2 and BMD.3 and click into Within-Subjects
                Variables (Time) box
        Highlight Group and click into Between-Subjects Factor(s) box
Click on Plots
Repeated Measures: Profile Plots
        Highlight Time, click into Horizontal Axis

> *Highlight Group, click into Separate Lines, click Add*
> *Click Continue*
> *Repeated Measures*
>   *Click on Save*
> *Repeated Measures: Save*
>   *Select Standardized for Residuals*
>   *Click Continue*
> *Repeated Measures*
>   *Click on Options*
> *Repeated Measures: Options*
>   *Highlight Group, Time and Group*Time and click into 'Display Means for'*
>   *Tick 'Compare main effects'*
>   *Confidence interval adjustment: Bonferroni*
>   *Under Display, tick 'Estimates of effect size' and 'Homogeneity tests'*
>   *Click Continue*
> *Repeated Measures*
>   *Click OK*

The Between-Subjects Factors box shown below indicates that only 21 controls and 26 intervention participants have been included in the analysis. The remaining 13 participants have missing data and have been omitted. The Box's M test is significant at $P = 0.002$ indicating an unequal variance across groups in the model however the P value is not <0.001 and therefore the deviation from homogeneity is not a major concern. It can be seen in Figure 6.1 that the whiskers are larger in the intervention group than in the control group and the median is higher, so a significant P value is expected.

Between-Subjects Factors

		Value label	N
Group	1	Control	21
	2	Intervention	26

Box's Test of Equality of Covariance Matrices[a]

Box's M	22.186
F	3.424
df1	6
df2	12925.711
Sig.	0.002

Tests the null hypothesis that the observed covariance matrices of the dependent variables are equal across groups.
[a]Design: Intercept + Group.
Within-Subjects Design: time.

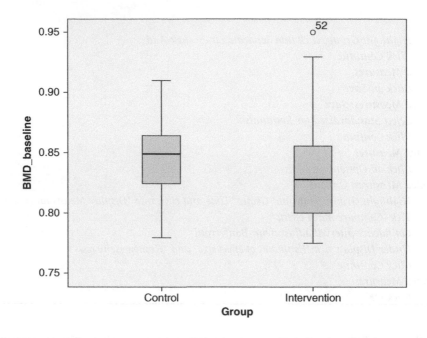

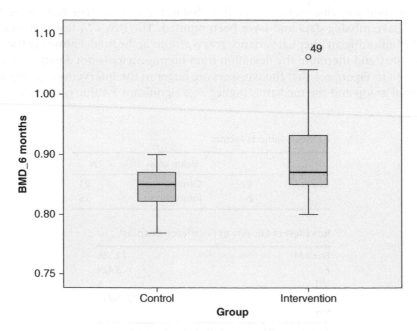

Figure 6.1 Boxplots of BMD.

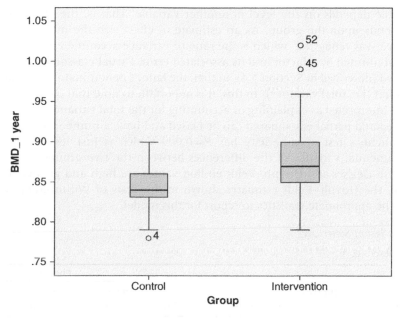

Figure 6.1 (*continued*)

Multivariate Tests[a]

Effect		Value	F	Hypothesis df	Error df	Sig.	Partial Eta-Squared
Time	Pillai's trace	0.490	21.137[b]	2.000	44.000	0.000	0.490
	Wilk's lambda	0.510	21.137[b]	2.000	44.000	0.000	0.490
	Hotelling's trace	0.961	21.137[b]	2.000	44.000	0.000	0.490
	Roy's largest root	0.961	21.137[b]	2.000	44.000	0.000	0.490
Time * Group	Pillai's trace	0.433	16.823[b]	2.000	44.000	0.000	0.433
	Wilk's lambda	0.567	16.823[b]	2.000	44.000	0.000	0.433
	Hotelling's trace	0.765	16.823[b]	2.000	44.000	0.000	0.433
	Roy's largest root	0.765	16.823[b]	2.000	44.000	0.000	0.433

Within-Subjects Design: Time.
[a] Design: Intercept + Group.
[b] Exact statistic.

The Multivariate Tests table shows four similar multivariate tests of the within-subjects effect, which is a form of MANOVA. In this example, all four tests have the same level of significance. Generally, the Wilk's lambda is reported. The values for Wilk's lambda indicate a significant effect of time on BMD ($P < 0.0001$) and also a significant interaction between time and group ($P < 0.0001$). A significant interaction indicates that effect of one variable depends on the level of another variable. That is, the effect of time on BMD depends upon the group. As an estimate of effect size the multivariate partial eta-squared was requested, which is the ratio of variance accounted by a factor to the variance accounted by a factor and its associated error. Partial eta-squared differs from eta-squared (described in Section 5.4), in that, the latter's denominator is the sum of the squares total (i.e. total variance). In this, it is important to note that partial eta-squared cannot be interpreted as explaining or accounting for the total variance. However, both eta-squared and partial eta-squared can be biased and have a number of limitations.[8]

The Mauchly's test of sphericity has $P = 0.009$ which is just less than 0.01 and indicates unequal variance of the differences between the two groups. However, the Greenhouse-Geisser and Huynh–Feldt epsilon values are high and greater than 0.75. Therefore, the Huynh–Feldt estimates shown in the Tests of Within-Subjects Effects table are the appropriate statistics to report for this model.

Mauchly's Test of Sphericity[b]

Measure:MEASURE_1

Within-subjects effect	Mauchly's W	Approx. chi-square	df	Sig.	Epsilon[a] Greenhouse-Geisser	Huynh-Feldt	Lower bound
Time	0.809	9.320	2	0.009	0.840	0.888	0.500

Tests the null hypothesis that the error covariance matrix of the orthonormalized transformed dependent variables is proportional to an identity matrix.
Within-subjects design: time.
[a]May be used to adjust the degrees of freedom for the averaged tests of significance. Corrected tests are displayed in the tests of Within-Subjects Effects table.
[b]Design: Intercept + Group.

Tests of Within-Subjects Effects

Measure:MEASURE_1

Source		Type III sum of squares	df	Mean square	F	Sig.	Partial eta-squared
Time	Sphericity assumed	0.024	2	0.012	28.237	0.000	0.386
	Greenhouse-Geisser	0.024	1.679	0.015	28.237	0.000	0.386
	Huynh–Feldt	0.024	1.776	0.014	28.237	0.000	0.386
	Lower bound	0.024	1.000	0.024	28.237	0.000	0.386
Time * Group	Sphericity assumed	0.018	2	0.009	21.198	0.000	0.320
	Greenhouse-Geisser	0.018	1.679	0.011	21.198	0.000	0.320
	Huynh–Feldt	0.018	1.776	0.010	21.198	0.000	0.320
	Lower bound	0.018	1.000	0.018	21.198	0.000	0.320
Error (Time)	Sphericity assumed	0.039	90	0.000			
	Greenhouse-Geisser	0.039	75.574	0.001			
	Huynh–Feldt	0.039	79.916	0.000			
	Lower bound	0.039	45.000	0.001			

In the univariate Tests of Within-Subject Effects table, it can be seen that the Huynh–Feldt correction has reduced the degrees of freedom by multiplying them by epsilon (e.g. time effect $2 \times 0.888 = 1.776$). With the adjustment, there is a significant effect of time on BMD ($P < 0.0001$) and a significant interaction between time and group ($P < 0.0001$). Since the interaction is significant, interpreting the main effects will not lead to an accurate understanding of the results. In general, a significant main effect should not be interpreted when there is a significant interaction that involves that main effect.

The Tests of Within-Subjects Contrasts table shows that there is a significant linear trend for BMD and there is a significant linear trend for the time by group interaction ($P < 0.0001$). Although the P values for the quadratic trends are also significant, the partial eta-squared is lower indicating that the linear trend is a better fit. The results of the trend contrasts should be interpreted with caution and the plots of the data should also be examined.

Tests of Within-Subjects Contrasts

Measure:MEASURE_1

Source	Time	Type III sum of squares	df	Mean square	F	Sig.	Partial eta-squared
Time	Linear	0.015	1	0.015	39.619	0.000	0.468
	Quadratic	0.009	1	0.009	19.259	0.000	0.300
Time * group	Linear	0.013	1	0.013	33.248	0.000	0.425
	Quadratic	0.006	1	0.006	11.693	0.001	0.206
Error (time)	Linear	0.017	45	0.000			
	Quadratic	0.022	45	0.000			

The Levene's test which can be used to check for homogeneity of variance, shows that the error variances pass the test of equality at baseline and 1 year in that the P values are not significant. However, the error variances are not equal at the 6 month time point. While ANOVA is relatively robust to non-normality, it is less robust to violations of homogeneity. This is a violation of the model assumptions and the results should be interpreted with caution. In reporting the results of the model, the violation of homogeneity should be reported. Alternatively, transformation of all data can be undertaken to stabilize the variances between the groups.

Levene's Test of Equality of Error Variances[a]

	F	df1	df2	Sig.
BMD_baseline	1.837	1	45	0.182
BMD_6 months	7.248	1	45	0.010
BMD_1 year	3.052	1	45	0.087

Tests the null hypothesis that the error variance of the dependent variable is equal across groups.
[a]Design: intercept + group.
Within Subjects Design: time.

The repeated measures Tests of Between-Subject ANOVA table shows that over time (i.e. averaged across all time points) there was a significant difference in BMD between the treatment groups with $P = 0.033$.

Tests of Between-Subjects Effects

Measure:MEASURE_1
Transformed variable: average

Source	Type III sum of squares	df	Mean square	F	Sig.	Partial eta-squared
Intercept	102.935	1	102.935	16781.865	0.000	0.997
Group	0.030	1	0.030	4.854	0.033	0.097
Error	0.276	45	0.006			

The SPSS commands for repeated measures ANOVA provides comparisons of the estimated marginal means of each group, at each time point and at the group by time interaction. These means are predicted means, not observed means, and are based on the specified linear model. The estimated marginal means below are for the main effect of group, with pairwise comparisons corrected for multiple comparisons using the Bonferroni adjustment. The Pairwise Comparisons table shows that there is a significant difference in overall BMD between the control and intervention group ($P = 0.033$), with the mean estimates indicating that the intervention group has a higher BMD than the control group. The Univariate Tests is an ANOVA test for the comparison and is similar to the result from the pairwise comparisons ($P = 0.033$) since there are only two groups.

Estimated marginal means

1. Group

Estimates

Measure: MEASURE_1

Group	Mean	Std. error	95% Confidence interval	
			Lower bound	Upper bound
Control	0.845	0.010	0.825	0.865
Intervention	0.874	0.009	0.856	0.892

Pairwise Comparisons

Measure: MEASURE_1

(I) Group	(J) Group	Mean difference (I − J)	Std. error	Sig.[a]	95% Confidence interval for difference[a]	
					Lower bound	Upper bound
Control	Intervention	−0.029[b]	0.013	0.033	−0.056	−.0003
Intervention	Control	0.029[b]	0.013	0.033	0.003	0.056

Based on estimated marginal means.
[a]Adjustment for multiple comparisons: Bonferroni.
[b]The mean difference is significant at the 0.05 level.

Univariate Tests

Measure: MEASURE_1

	Sum of squares	*df*	Mean square	*F*	Sig.	Partial eta-squared
Contrast	0.010	1	0.010	4.854	0.033	0.097
Error	0.092	45	0.002			

The *F* tests the effect of Group. This test is based on the linearly independent pairwise comparisons among the estimated marginal means.

The estimated marginal means below are for the main effect of time, that is, the levels of BMD at each time point which are averaged across the groups. The Pairwise Comparisons table shows there was a significant difference in BMD between Time 1 (baseline) and Time 2 (6 months) ($P < 0.0001$); and Time 1 (baseline) and Time 3 (1 year) ($P < 0.0001$). There was no significant difference between Time 2 and Time 3 ($P = 0.63$). The Multivariate Test also indicates that there is a significant time effect but does not provide information about which time points are different from one another.

2. Time

Estimates

Measure: MEASURE_1

Time	Mean	Std. error	95% Confidence interval	
			Lower bound	Upper bound
1	0.841	0.006	0.828	0.853
2	0.871	0.008	0.854	0.888
3	0.866	0.007	0.853	0.880

Pairwise Comparisons

Measure: MEASURE_1

(*I*) Time	(*J*) Time	Mean difference (*I − J*)	Std. error	Sig.[b]	95% Confidence interval for difference[b]	
					Lower bound	Upper bound
1	2	−0.030[a]	0.005	0.000	−0.043	−0.017
	3	−0.026[a]	0.004	0.000	−0.036	−0.015
2	1	0.030[a]	0.005	0.000	0.017	0.043
	3	0.005	0.004	0.626	−0.004	0.014
3	1	0.026[a]	0.004	0.000	0.015	0.036
	2	−0.005	0.004	0.626	−0.014	0.004

Based on estimated marginal means.
[a]The mean difference is significant at the 0.05 level.
[b]Adjustment for multiple comparisons: Bonferroni.

The Group by Time table indicates the estimated marginal means of each group at each time point.

Multivariate Tests

	Value	F	Hypothesis df	Error df	Sig.	Partial eta-squared
Pillai's trace	0.490	21.137[a]	2.000	44.000	0.000	0.490
Wilk's lambda	0.510	21.137[a]	2.000	44.000	0.000	0.490
Hotelling's trace	0.961	21.137[a]	2.000	44.000	0.000	0.490
Roy's largest root	0.961	21.137[a]	2.000	44.000	0.000	0.490

Each F tests the multivariate effect of Time. These tests are based on the linearly independent pairwise comparisons among the estimated marginal means.
[a] Exact statistic.

3. Group * Time

Measure: MEASURE_1

Group	Time	Mean	Std. error	95% Confidence interval	
				Lower bound	Upper bound
Control	1	0.842	0.009	0.824	0.861
	2	0.847	0.012	0.822	0.872
	3	0.844	0.010	0.825	0.864
Intervention	1	0.839	0.008	0.823	0.856
	2	0.895	0.011	0.872	0.917
	3	0.888	0.009	0.870	0.906

To interpret the significant interaction between time and group, simple effects tests (or simple main effects) are conducted. This test examines the main effect of one explanatory variable at a fixed level of the other explanatory variable (as discussed in Section 5.8.1). A simple effects test can be used to examine the effect of group at each level of time, that is, whether there is a difference between the groups at each time point. This comparison is usually of most interest. Simple effects analysis in SPSS cannot be tested directly in SPSS and command syntax has to be used. This analysis can be obtained by using the '*Paste*' option in the SPSS dialog box to save the syntax from the SPSS command sequence shown in Box 6.2 and then replacing the EMMEANS lines with the following:

/EMMEANS = TABLES(Group*Time) COMPARE(Group)

When the SPSS syntax is run (by clicking on the green arrow), the SPSS output will include the Pairwise Comparisons table shown below which compares group differences within each time point, as well as the Univariate Tests which report the F values for the tests of simple effects. Another simple effects test is to compare time points within each group. This can be obtained by the using following syntax line (SPSS output not included):

/EMMEANS = TABLES(Group*Time) COMPARE(Time).

Estimated marginal means

Group * time

Estimates

Measure:MEASURE_1

Group	Time	Mean	Std. error	95% Confidence interval	
				Lower bound	Upper bound
Control	1	0.842	0.009	0.824	0.861
	2	0.847	0.012	0.822	0.872
	3	0.844	0.010	0.825	0.864
Intervention	1	0.839	0.008	0.823	0.856
	2	0.894	0.011	0.872	0.917
	3	0.888	0.009	0.870	0.906

Pairwise Comparisons

Measure: MEASURE_1

	(I)	(J)	Mean difference			95% Confidence Interval for Difference[a]	
Time	Group	Group	(I−J)	Std. error	Sig.[a]	Lower bound	Upper bound
1	Control	Intervention	0.003	0.012	0.796	−0.021	0.028
	Intervention	Control	−0.003	0.012	0.796	−0.028	0.021
2	Control	Intervention	−0.047[b]	0.017	0.007	−0.081	−0.014
	Intervention	Control	0.047[b]	0.017	0.007	0.014	0.081
3	Control	Intervention	−0.044[b]	0.013	0.002	−0.070	−0.017
	Intervention	Control	0.044[b]	0.013	0.002	0.017	0.070

Based on estimated marginal means.
[a] Adjustment for multiple comparisons: least significant difference (equivalent to no adjustments).
[b] The mean difference is significant at the 0.05 level.

Univariate Tests

Measure: MEASURE_1

	Time	Sum of squares	df	Mean square	F	Sig.	Partial eta-squared
1	Contrast	0.000	1	0.000	0.068	0.796	0.001
	Error	0.078	45	0.002			
2	Contrast	0.026	1	0.026	8.069	0.007	0.152
	Error	0.145	45	0.003			
3	Contrast	0.022	1	0.022	10.799	0.002	0.194
	Error	0.092	45	0.002			

Each *F* tests the simple effects of Group within each level combination of the other effects shown. These tests are based on the linearly independent pairwise comparisons among the estimated marginal means.

In the Pairwise Comparisons table, the mean differences are computed from the marginal (predicted) means and provide a guide to relative differences between the groups at each time point. This table shows that BMD was not significantly different between groups at baseline (time 1) with a small mean difference of 0.003 and $P = 0.796$. In a randomized trial such as this, baseline values are expected to be balanced between the groups. However, the mean BMD is significantly different between groups at 6 months post-intervention (time 2) with $P = 0.007$ indicating treatment efficacy and the difference is maintained at 1 year (time 3) with $P = 0.002$. This P value is slightly more significant than at 6 months even though the mean difference is slightly smaller because the standard error is smaller. In this table, no adjustment has been made for multiple comparisons. A multiple comparisons procedure such as the Holm (a modified Bonferroni procedure), which is uniformly better and more powerful than the Bonferroni can be used.[9]

Examination of the P values for the simple effects shown in the Univariate Tests table indicates that at baseline (time 1) there was no significant difference between the intervention and control group. There is a significant difference between the groups at post-intervention and 1 year follow-up. In this example, with only two groups in a factor and only one factor, the P values shown in the Univariate Tests table are the same as shown in the Pairwise Comparisons table (see Section 5.2.2). The F values and corresponding P values are used to report the simple effects tests.

The profile plot (see Figure 6.2) obtained from the SPSS commands in Box 6.2 can also be used to interpret the data. Figure 6.2 shows the marginal means at each time point and indicates balanced groups at time 1, little change in BMD in the control group over time and an increase in BMD in the intervention group which was sustained to one year follow-up. The profile plot shows that the lines cross and are not parallel indicating an interaction.

The residuals are saved to the spreadsheet with a separate residual for each time point. The distribution of the residuals for all three time points (denoted as ZRE_1, ZRE_2 and ZRE_3 in the SPSS spreadsheet) should be checked for normality to ensure that the model is valid. The residuals can be plotted using the command sequence *Graphs → Legacy Dialogs → Histogram*. The residuals for BMD at time 1 are shown in Figure 6.3. The residuals are approximately normally distributed conforming to a bell-shaped curve and importantly with no data points more than 3 standard deviations. The residuals at time points 2 and 3 are similar (histograms not shown).

Reporting the results of repeated measures ANOVA

There are many mean values and P values that can be reported from a repeated measures ANOVA analysis. In this example, the research question was to explore whether there were any differences between the control and intervention groups at the three time points and therefore it is appropriate to report the within group differences at each time point as shown in Table 6.1. The P values for the group by time interaction can be reported in the text or as a footnote to the table.

When reporting the results of a repeated measures ANOVA, the means and standard deviation (or standard error), sample size, the significant main effects or interactions are generally included. In addition, the results of the simple effects tests with corresponding F and P values are reported with any post hoc comparisons. In this example, the results

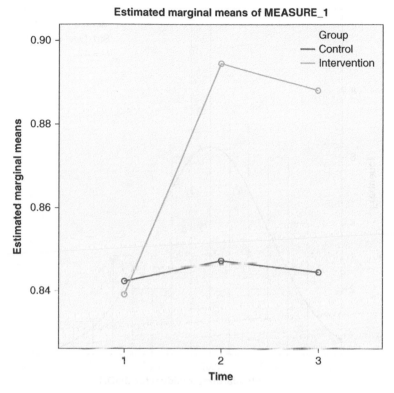

Figure 6.2 Profile plot of BMD by time and group.

Table 6.1   Results of repeated measures ANOVA

Time point	Control group BMD Mean (SE) $n=21$	Intervention group BMD Mean (SE) $n=26$	Mean difference (95% CI)	P value
Baseline	0.84 (0.01)	0.84 (0.01)	−0.003 (−0.028, 0.021)	0.80
6 months	0.85 (0.01)	0.89 (0.01)	0.047 (0.014, 0.081)	0.007
1 year	0.84 (0.01)	0.89 (0.01)	0.044 (0.017, 0.070)	0.002

Note: Estimated marginal means reported.

of the simple effects tests are not reported since the post hoc comparisons have the same *P* values and provide additional information on the direction and size of the difference.

Alternatively, the results could be reported as 'A repeated measures ANOVA was conducted to compare the BMD of elderly people who received an intervention programme to those who received the placebo treatment. A total of 60 elderly people were randomized to receive either the 4 week intervention or placebo. BMD was measured at baseline, 6 months and 1 year later. Complete data was available at all time points

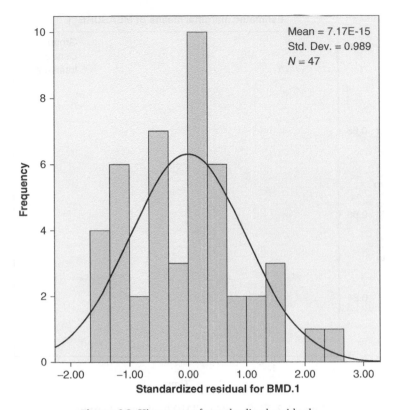

Figure 6.3 Histogram of standardized residuals.

for 21 people who received the placebo treatment and 26 people who received the intervention. Mauchly's test indicated that the assumption of sphericity had been violated, therefore the Huynh–Feldt corrected tests are reported. There was a significant interaction between time and group ($F(1.78, 79.92) = 21.20$, $P < 0.0001$). Post hoc comparisons indicated that that there was no difference between the two groups at baseline ($P = 0.80$). There was a significant difference between the two groups at 6 months and 1 year, with intervention group having higher BMD levels than the control group ($P = 0.007$ and $P = 0.002$ respectively)'.

The profile plot shown in Figure 6.2 can be redrawn to publication quality in SigmaPlot with error bars included. The SigmaPlot commands for producing the plot with error bars are shown in Box 6.3. The spreadsheet for the summary data that are entered into SigmaPlot are as shown below where column 2 shows the mean values for the control group, column 3 is the width of the 95% CI for the control group, column 4 is the mean values for the intervention group and column 5 is the width of the 95% CI for the intervention group:

Column 1	Column 2	Column 3	Column 4	Column 5
Baseline	0.842	0.0158	0.839	0.0188
6 months	0.847	0.0162	0.895	0.0288
1 year	0.845	0.0153	0.888	0.0213

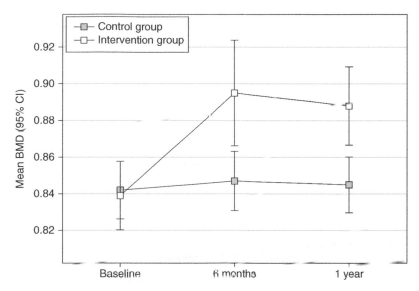

Figure 6.4 Mean (SE) BMD levels from baseline to 1 year for the intervention and control group.

Once the plot is obtained using the command sequence shown in Box 6.3 it can be customized using the options to produce the plot shown in Figure 6.4. Because the data are longitudinal and are collected from a single cohort, it is valid to link the mean values with lines to show how the mean values in the cohort change over time. By comparing the 95% confidence intervals, it can clearly be seen that there is no significant difference between the groups at baseline but that the mean values are significantly different for the two groups at both the 6 months and 1 year follow-up times.

Box 6.3 SigmaPlot commands for drawing a line and dot plot

SigmaPlot commands

Data 1*

> *At top of the screen Click on Graph → Create Graph*
> *Click on Line/Scatter Plot in sub-menu*
> *Click on Simple Line and Scatter – Error Bars in Scatter Group*

Create Graph – Error Bars

> *Symbol Values = Worksheet Columns (default), click Next*

Create Graph – Data Format

> *Highlight XY pair, click Next*

Create Graph – Select Data

> *Data for X = use drop box and select Column 1*
> *Data for Y = use drop box and select Column 2*
> *Data for Error = use drop box and select Column 3*
> *Click Finish*

Graph Page

> Click on Add Plot
> Add Plot - Type
> Click on Line and Scatter Plot in sub-menu
> Add Plot - Style
> Click on Line and Simple Scatter – Error Bars in Scatter Group
> Add Plot - Style
> Click on Simple Error Bars
> Add plot – Error Bars
> Symbol Values = Worksheet Columns (default), click Next
> Add Plot – Data Format
> Highlight XY pair, click Next
> Add Plot – Select Data
> Data for X = use drop box and select Column 1
> Data for Y = use drop box and select Column 4
> Data for Error = use drop box and select Column 5
> Click Finish

6.6 Linear mixed models

A core feature of longitudinal data is that the measurements for each participant are almost always positively correlated with each another. When modelling changes over time, these within-subject correlations can be taken into account. If within-subject correlations are ignored, as in repeated measures ANOVA, then the statistical power of the study may be reduced and the P value may be biased towards non-significance.

In mixed models, within-subject correlations are modelled using the covariance structure. The covariance structure is built on the variance around the outcome measurement at each time point and on the correlations between measurements taken at different times from the same participant. Obviously, two measurements from the same participant would be expected to be correlated because they share common contributions. In addition, measurements taken closer together are expected to be more correlated than measurements taken further apart because influential factors are likely to be similar at close time points but may change over longer periods of time.

In general, linear mixed models are both more theoretically correct and more flexible than repeated measures ANOVA for analysing longitudinal data. The term 'mixed' is used because both fixed and random factors are included. Fixed factors are assumed to have the same effect for all subjects whereas the effects of random factors such as the individual regression intercepts are assumed to vary from subject to subject. Other random factors can be factors used in sampling, for example, when a school is the unit of sampling children or a hospital is the unit of sampling patients. In this chapter, such random factors are not discussed. A fixed factor is a factor in which all possible groups or all levels of the factor are included; for example, males and females or number of siblings (see Section 5.9.1).

Mixed models are adapted from regression methods in which variances in the intercepts and slopes from individual participants are modelled using maximum likelihood (ML) methods. Because the data for each participant is summarized using a regression approach, the number of time points for each participant can be unequal.

An appealing aspect of mixed models is that they are more flexible than ANOVA methods for accommodating study designs with unequal numbers of participants in each group (or cell). Also, there is no requirement that each participant has the same number of observations and there are no requirements for sphericity or homogeneity of variance across time intervals. However, for valid results that can be generalized to a population, any missing data must ideally be 'missing completely at random (MCAR)', or at least, missing at random (MAR). For MCAR, the probability of an observation missing is not related to observed or unobserved measurements; for example, a person moving to another city. For MAR, the missing of an observation is related to the observed data; for example, in measuring the weight of participants, it is found that females are less likely to report their weight. That is, the probability that weight is missing depends on the gender of the person.

6.6.1 Covariance structures

Before undertaking the analysis, a covariance structure that is appropriate for the data set needs to be selected. Because covariance patterns vary widely, the first step in building the model is to find an appropriate covariance structure to fit the data. Even if a reasonable assumption about the covariance structure can be made, it is a good idea to test the model against one with a standard structure; for example, 'variance components' or 'unstructured' covariance.

Some covariance structures that are commonly used are as follows:

- Variance components comprise one of the simplest covariance structures. This structure assumes that the random effects are independent and the variances of the random effects are equal.
- Unstructured (UN) is a general structure that makes no assumptions about equal variances or correlations in the data. However, this structure is often too general and is best used when the data are balanced and complete and when there is equal spacing between time points;
- Autoregressive first order (AR(1)) assumes that measurements taken close together in time are more correlated than measurements taken far apart. That is, the correlation between measurements will decrease as the time between them increases. This is often the case in studies such as randomized controlled trials in which the outcome changes over time;
- Compound symmetry (CS) specifies that the measurements have the same variance at all times and that all pairs of measurements from the same person have the same correlation, that is, there is constant variation and covariance. This structure is equivalent to repeated measures ANOVA when the data are complete. This is a restrictive covariance structure and is best suited for when there is large between-subject variation.

The best structure to use is ascertained by running models with different covariance structures and then comparing the -2 log likelihood ($-2LL$) value, which is an estimate of the fit of a model. Because $-2LL$ is the sum of the squared errors, a smaller $-2LL$ indicates a better fit. When models have the same variables, subtracting the $-2LL$ values between models is equivalent to a chi-square value with 1 degree of freedom.

A significant chi-square value indicates that the model with the lower −2LL is a significantly better fit. This method is similar to using the 'R square change' option in multiple regression (see Section 7.3). Once the most appropriate covariance structure is identified, the time and factor effects in the model can be tested.

6.6.2 Advantages and disadvantages of mixed models

The advantages of linear mixed models are that:

- Within-subject correlations in data from the same participant and variances that change over time (i.e. unequal variances) can be modelled in the covariance structure;
- Estimates of standard errors are valid;
- Cell imbalance is not a problem;
- Missing data points do not exclude participants from the analysis;
- Interactions are not automatically included;
- There is no requirement for sphericity or homogeneity of variance across the model.

The disadvantages of using mixed models in SPSS are that:

- No estimate of effect size such as eta-squared is available;
- No means plots are directly available.

6.6.3 Data layout

Linear mixed models are accessed via the SPSS command sequence *Analyze → Mixed Model → Linear* and the data file needs to be in the 'long' format with each time point for a participant on a separate line and the lines for the same participant linked by a common factor such as an identification (ID) number. The data set can be converted from the 'wide' to the 'long' format (or vice versa) using the SPSS command sequence *Data → Restructure*.

Before undertaking a linear mixed model analysis, the 'BMD_study_wide_file' previously used, which is in the 'wide' format has to be restructured into the 'long' format with each BMD value on a separate line using the SPSS commands shown in Box 6.4.

Box 6.4 SPPS commands to restructure data from wide format to long format

SPSS Commands

BMD_study_wide_file.sav – IBM SPSS Statistics Data Editor
Data → Restructure
Restructure Data Wizard
      What do you want to do? Select 'Restructure selected variables to cases'
      Click Next

Restructure Data Wizard – Step 2 of 7
>   *How many variables do you want to restructure? Select 'One'*
>   *(for example, w1,w2, and w3)*
>   *Click Next*
Restructure Data Wizard – Step 3 of 7
>   *Case Group Identification: select 'Use case number'; Name:'id'*
>   *Variables to be Transposed: change 'trans1' to 'BMD' in the Target Variable box*
>   *Highlight BMD.1, BMD.2 and BMD.3 and click into the area below the*
>   *Target Variable box*
>   *Highlight Group and click into Fixed Variable(s)*
>   *Click Next*
Restructure Data Wizard – Step 4 of 7
>   *How many variables do you want to create? Select 'One'*
>   *Click Next*
Restructure Data Wizard – Step 5 of 7
>   *What kind of index values? Select Sequential numbers: Index Values: 1,2.3*
>   *Click Next*
Restructure Data Wizard – Step 6 of 7
>   *Handling of Variables not Selected: select Drop variable(s) from the new data file*
>   *System Missing or Blank Values in all Transposed Variables: select Create a case in the*
>   *new file Click Next*
Restructure Data Wizard - Finish
>   *What do you want to do? Select Restructure the data now*
>   *Click Finish, Click OK*

Once the restructure is complete, use the SPSS commands *'File → Save As'* to save the data file under a new name: 'BMD_study_long_file'. Using *'File → Save'* will overwrite the original wide data file. In the 'long' format, each repeat measure is located on a new row. Since the BMD of participants was assessed on three occasions, there are three data rows for each participant. The fixed variable labels will be transferred to the new 'long' file but the restructured variables will need to be relabelled. This data file now has 180 lines and only the single data points with missing values will be excluded from the analysis. The 'time' variable is now labelled as a variable named 'Index1' with values 1, 2 and 3. These can be relabelled with the variable name 'Time' and the variable labels as BMD_baseline, BMD_6 month and BMD_1 year respectively under the SPSS Variable View.

6.6.4   Obtaining a plot

The SPSS linear mixed model procedure does not produce a plot of the data however one can be obtained for a file in long format using the command sequence shown in Box 6.5.

Box 6.5 SPSS Commands to obtain an error bar graph for data in the long format

SPSS Commands

BMD_study_long_file.sav – IBM SPSS Statistics Data Editor
Graphs → Legacy Dialogs → Error Bar
Error Bar
     Select 'Clustered'
     Data in Chart Are: select Summaries for groups of cases
     Click 'Define'
Define Clustered Error Bar: Summaries for Groups of Cases
     Highlight BMD and click into Variable
     Highlight Time and click into Category Axis
     Highlight Group and click into Define Clusters by
     Bars Represent: Confidence interval for mean; Level 95%
     Click OK

Figure 6.5 is similar to the SigmaPlot figure shown in Figure 6.4. In these figures, the 95% confidence intervals convey additional information that is not provided in Figure 6.2. The mean BMD in the intervention group has significantly increased in that the 95% CIs at 6 months and 1 year do not overlap with those at baseline. However, there has been no change in the control group with the 95% CI at each time point overlapping. It is important to obtain a figure such as this so that the P values from the post hoc tests in the linear mixed model can be correctly interpreted. At baseline, the mean BMD values are not very different between groups and the large overlap of 95% CIs show that the means are not significantly different. However, at both 6 months and 1 year, the two groups have significantly different mean BMD values with confidence intervals that do not overlap.

6.6.5 Building a mixed model

The type of covariance structure used can either be selected on theoretical grounds or different covariance structures can be tested to determine which one provides a model with the best fit. For this, a good model building strategy is to begin with a model using a basic covariance structure and then to test whether different covariance structures improve the fit. Once the covariance structure that provides the best fit is decided, the effects of adding further variables can be tested in subsequent models.

There are two options in SPSS for estimating parameters in the model: ML and restricted maximum likelihood (REML). In ML, the regression coefficients and the variance components are included in the likelihood function so the fit of entire model is described. In REML, variance components are calculated after the fixed effects have been removed from the model and describe the fit of the random effects.[10] In estimating

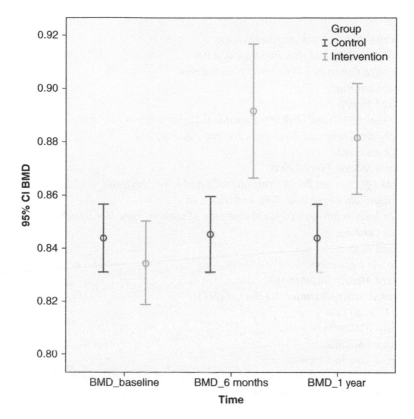

Figure 6.5 Error bar graphs (95% CI) of BMD by time and group.

the variance components, REML is less biased than ML. In most cases, the difference between the estimates produced by the two methods is minimal.[10] However, for small samples or when the number of fixed effects is large, REML is preferred.[11] When comparing models with different fixed effects and variance components, ML must be used.[5]

The SPSS command sequence shown in Box 6.6 can be used to obtain a linear mixed model on the BMD data to test for differences between times and groups, as well as interactions. Since there are three measurements for each participant it is appropriate to include time as a repeated measure and also as a fixed factor.

Box 6.6 SPSS commands to conduct a linear mixed model

SPSS Commands

BMD_study_long_file.sav – IBM SPSS Statistics Data Editor
        Analyze → Mixed Models → Linear
Linear Mixed Models: Specify Subjects and Repeated

> *Highlight id and click into Subjects box*
> *Highlight Time and click into Repeated box*
> *Repeated Covariance Type: select Unstructured*
> *Click Continue*
> *Linear Mixed Models*
> *Highlight BMD and click into Dependent Variable box*
> *Highlight Group and Time and click into Factor(s) box*
> *Click on Fixed*
> *Linear Mixed Models: Fixed Effects*
> *Fixed Effects: select Build terms (default) and select 'Factorial' (default) and*
>   *highlight Group and Time and click Add*
> *Click Include intercept (default) and Sum of squares: Type III (default)*
> *Click Continue*
> *Linear Mixed Models*
> *Click on Estimation*
> *Linear Mixed Models: Estimation*
> *Method: select Maximum Likelihood (ML)*
> *Click Continue*
> *Linear Mixed Models*
> *Click on Statistics*
> *Linear Mixed Models: Statistics*
> *Model Statistics: tick Parameter estimates and Tests for covariance parameters*
> *Confidence interval: 95% (default)*
> *Click Continue*
> *Linear Mixed Models*
> *Click on EM Means*
> *Linear Mixed Models: EM Means*
> *Highlight Group, Time and Group*Time and click into Display Means for*
> *Click Continue*
> *Linear Mixed Models*
> *Click on Save*
> *Linear Mixed Models: Save*
> *Predicted Values & Residuals: tick Residuals, click Continue*
> *Linear Mixed Models*
> *Click OK*

In the Model Dimension table the number of levels in the model is displayed, which is similar to the degrees of freedom. The number of parameters in the model will vary according to the covariance structure selected. The Number of Subjects column shows that 60 patients are included in the model compared with only 47 who were included in the repeated measures ANOVA model.

Mixed model analysis

Model Dimension[a]

		Number of levels	Covariance structure	Number of parameters	Subject variables	Number of subjects
Fixed Effects	Intercept	1		1		
	Group	2		1		
	Time	3		2		
	Group * Time	6		2		
Repeated Effects	Time	3	Unstructured	6	id	60
Total		15		12		

[a]Dependent variable: BMD.

Information Criteria[a]

−2 log likelihood	−705.284
Akaike's Information Criterion (AIC)	−681.284
Hurvich and Tsai's Criterion (AICC)	−679.258
Bozdogan's Criterion (CAIC)	−631.868
Schwarz's Bayesian Criterion (BIC)	−643.868

The information criteria are displayed in smaller-is-better forms.
[a]Dependent variable: BMD.

The Information Criteria table allows different models to be compared and displays fit indices. For these indices, the lower the number, the better the model fits the data. The −2 restricted log likelihood (−2LL) which is −705.284 is a basic estimate of fit. The other criterion measures shown in this table are modifications to the −2LL value made for more complex models. When fitting models, the likelihood value can be increased by adding parameters; however, this may result in overfitting. To overcome this, a penalty adjustment is made to the likelihood for the number of parameters included in the model. Akaike's Information Criterion (AIC) adjusts the −2LL by twice the number of parameters in the model and should be used if the sample size is large. When the sample size is small, the corrected Akaike's Information Criterion (AICC) should be used. As the sample size increases, the AIC will be similar to the AICC. The Bozdogan's Criterion (CAIC) adjusts the −2LL by the number of parameters times one plus the log of the number of cases. The Schwarz's Bayesian Criterion (BIC) adjusts the −2LL by the number of parameters times the log of the number of cases. Both the BIC and CAIC make a greater penalty adjustment to the −2LL than the AIC.

This basic model can then be rerun with a different covariance structure to determine whether the fit can be improved. When the model was rerun with an autoregressive covariance structure (AR(1)) or using compound symmetry, the −2LL indicated a loss of fit. When a model has a higher −2LL and therefore a poorer fit, the standard errors around estimated mean values will be larger and therefore less precise.

The Type III Tests of Fixed Effects are overall tests of significance for the predictor variables included in the model, accounting for the other predictors in the model. The Fixed Effects table shows that there is a significant difference between the groups

($P=0.041$), that BMD changes significantly with time ($P<0.0001$) and that there is a significant interaction between group and time ($P<0.0001$). As with the repeated measures ANOVA, the significant interaction between group and time are the more important findings. The significant interaction was expected following the error bar graph (Figure 6.4), which shows that the two groups have very different changes over time. If the interaction was not significant, it could be removed and the linear mixed model rerun.

Fixed effects

Type III Tests of Fixed Effects[a]

Source	Numerator df	Denominator df	F	Sig.
Intercept	1	60.256	24733.683	0.000
Group	1	60.256	4.341	0.041
Time	2	55.199	20.478	0.000
Group * Time	2	55.199	21.580	0.000

[a]Dependent variable: BMD.

Estimates of fixed effects[a]

Parameter	Estimate	Std. error	df	t	Sig.	95% Confidence interval Lower bound	95% Confidence interval Upper bound
Intercept	0.879760	0.007638	61.115	115.186	0.000	0.864488	0.895032
[Group = 1]	−0.037278	0.011189	61.261	−3.332	0.001	−0.059650	−0.014906
[Group = 2]	0[b]	0	.	.	.	.	.
[Time = 1]	−0.045166	0.004957	58.793	−9.112	0.000	−0.055085	−0.035247
[Time = 2]	0.005786	0.004484	53.584	1.290	0.202	−0.003205	0.014778
[Time = 3]	0[b]	0	.	.	.	.	.
[Time = 1] * [Group = 1]	0.046685	0.007269	59.005	6.422	0.000	0.032139	0.061230
[Time = 2] * [Group = 1]	−0.002835	0.006681	54.046	−0.424	0.673	−0.016229	0.010559
[Time = 3] * [Group = 1]	0[b]	0	.	.	.	.	.
[Time = 1] * [Group = 2]	0[b]	0	.	.	.	.	.
[Time = 2] * [Group = 2]	0[b]	0	.	.	.	.	.
[Time = 3] * [Group = 2]	0[b]	0	.	.	.	.	.

[a]Dependent variable: BMD.
[b]This parameter is set to zero because it is redundant.

In the Estimates of Fixed Effects table, the maximum likelihood estimates of the fixed effect parameters (or regression coefficients) are reported in the column labelled Estimate. In SPSS, the highest value of a 'group' variable or the last value of the 'time' variable is the default reference group. In this table, the reference group is the control group. Therefore, the estimate of group 1 indicates that on average, the value of BMD value is 0.037 units lower in Group 1 (control) than in Group 2 (intervention). For time, the reference category is time 3, which is BMD at 1 year. The P value of 0.202 indicates that the predicted mean for 6 months (time 2) was not significantly different from the predicted mean at 1 year. The predicted mean at baseline (time 1) is significantly lower than at 1 year with $P < 0.0001$. On average, the BMD value at baseline is 0.045 lower than that at 1 year, with the 95% CI for the difference −0.055 to −0.035 units.

There was also a significant interaction of Time 1 by Group 1 with a P value <0.0001 indicating that the difference in the slope between the control group and intervention group is significantly different from baseline to 1 year. There was no significant interaction of Time 2 by Group 1 with a P value of 0.67 indicating that the rate of change over time from 6 months to 1 year was similar for the groups. This is shown in Figure 6.4 where the lines from 6 months to 1year are approximately parallel.

The degrees of freedom are an approximation and therefore do not have integer values. The Estimates of Fixed Effects table is useful for estimating effect sizes. The coefficients can be interpreted much like regression coefficients in that the predicted BMD for a patient in Group 1 at Time 1 (baseline) is calculated from the values in the Estimate column as follows:

$$\text{Predicted BMD} = \text{Intercept} + [\text{Group} = 1] + [\text{Time} = 1] + [\text{Time 1}] * [\text{Group 1}]$$

$$= 0.8798 + (-0.0373) + (-0.0452) + (0.0467)$$

$$= 0.844$$

This is the value shown in the following Estimated Marginal Means table for Group * Time.

The Estimates of Covariance Parameters table displays the estimates of variance parameters which define an unstructured 3×3 variance-covariance matrix. [12] UN (1,1) corresponds to the value in the first row and first column of the matrix is the variance for the error term at time 1 (baseline). Similarly, UN (2,2) and UN (3,3) are the estimated variance at time 2 (6 months) and time 3 (1 year). The other estimates in the table represent the covariances between time points. UN (2,1) is the covariance between error terms at the second (6 month) and first (baseline) time points. UN (3,1) is the covariance between the third (1 year) and first (baseline) time points. Similarly, UN (3,2) is the covariance between the third (1 year) and second (baseline) time points.

Covariance parameters

Estimates of Covariance Parameters[a]

Parameter		Estimate	Std. error	Wald Z	Sig.	95% Confidence interval	
						Lower bound	Upper bound
Repeated Measures	UN (1,1)	0.001468	0.000268	5.477	0.000	0.001026	0.002099
	UN (2,1)	0.001544	0.000330	4.680	0.000	0.000897	0.002190
	UN (2,2)	0.002793	0.000521	5.365	0.000	0.001938	0.004024
	UN (3,1)	0.001274	0.000269	4.736	0.000	0.000747	0.001801
	UN (3,2)	0.002037	0.000396	5.142	0.000	0.001261	0.002814
	UN (3,3)	0.001834	0.000336	5.451	0.000	0.001280	0.002628

[a]Dependent variable: BMD.

In the Covariance Parameters table, SPSS also reports the Wald tests of the null hypotheses that each parameter is equal to 0. All diagonal elements of the matrix UN (1,1), UN (2,2) and UN (3,3) are all significantly different from 0 indicating that the measurements at each time point are not independent. However, likelihood ratio tests may be more suitable for testing covariance parameters, assuming the sample size is large.[12] The Estimate values in the table can also be used to calculate the correlation between time points. For example, the covariance UN (2,1) can by divided by the square root of UN (1,1) $\times$ UN (2,2) to provide an estimate of the correlation between the time points. Here the correlation equals $0.001544/\sqrt{(0.001468 \times 0.002793)} = 0.76$ indicating a high degree of correlation between the first and second time point. Similarly, a correlation value of 0.90 can be obtained for UN (3,2) by dividing this value by the square root of UN (3,3) multiplied by UN (2,2). This high correlation value suggests that there is very little change from 6 months to 1 year. The estimated marginal means are also reported for each group, at each time point and group by time interaction. As with repeated measures ANOVA, these are the means that are predicted from the model and are not the actual means.

Estimated marginal means

1. Group[a]

Group	Mean	Std. error	df	95% Confidence interval	
				Lower bound	Upper bound
Control	0.844	0.008	60.365	0.828	0.860
Intervention	0.867	0.007	60.130	0.852	0.881

[a]Dependent variable: BMD.

2. Time[a]

Time	Mean	Std. error	df	95% Confidence interval	
				Lower bound	Upper bound
BMD_baseline	0.839	0.005	60.000	0.829	0.849
BMD_6 month	0.865	0.007	59.839	0.852	0.879
BMD_1 year	0.861	0.006	61.261	0.850	0.872

[a]Dependent variable: BMD.

3. Group * Time[a]

Group	Time	Mean	Std. error	df	95% Confidence interval	
					Lower bound	Upper bound
Control	BMD_baseline	0.844	0.007	60.000	0.830	0.858
	BMD_6 month	0.845	0.010	60.324	0.825	0.866
	BMD_1 year	0.842	0.008	61.389	0.826	0.859
Intervention	BMD_baseline	0.835	0.007	60.000	0.821	0.848
	BMD_6 month	0.886	0.009	59.281	0.867	0.904
	BMD_1 year	0.880	0.008	61.115	0.864	0.895

[a]Dependent variable: BMD.

As with repeated measures ANOVA, a significant interaction can be examined further by conducting simple effects tests that compare groups at each time point. The SPSS command syntax can be obtained by using the 'Paste' option in the SPSS dialog box and then replacing the EMMEANS line with the following:

/EMMEANS = TABLES(Group*Time) COMPARE(Group)

When the model is run using the syntax, the comparison tables shown below which compare group differences within each time point will be obtained. To compare time points within each group the following line can be added (SPSS output not displayed here):

/EMMEANS = TABLES(Group*Time) COMPARE(Time).

Pairwise Comparisons[a]

Time	(I) Group	(J) Group	Mean difference (I − J)	Std. error	df	Sig.[b]	95% Confidence interval for difference[b] Lower bound	Upper bound
BMD_baseline	Control	Intervention	0.009	0.010	60.000	0.347	−0.010	0.029
	Intervention	Control	−0.009	0.010	60.000	0.347	−0.029	0.010
BMD_s6 month	Control	Intervention	−0.040[c]	0.014	59.839	0.005	−0.068	−0.012
	Intervention	Control	0.040[c]	0.014	59.839	0.005	0.012	0.068
BMD_1 year	Control	Intervention	−0.037[c]	0.011	61.261	0.001	−0.060	−0.015
	Intervention	Control	0.037[c]	0.011	61.261	0.001	0.015	0.060

Based on estimated marginal means.
[a] Dependent variable: BMD.
[b] Adjustment for multiple comparisons: least significant difference (equivalent to no adjustments).
[c] The mean difference is significant at the 0.05 level.

Univariate Tests[a]

Time	Numerator df	Denominator df	F	Sig.
BMD_baseline	1	60.000	0.900	0.347
BMD_6 month	1	59.839	8.395	0.005
BMD_1 year	1	61.261	11.100	0.001

Each F tests the simple effects of Group within each level combination of the other effects shown. These tests are based on the linearly independent pairwise comparisons among the estimated marginal means.
[a] Dependent variable: BMD.

As with repeated measures ANOVA, the means and pairwise comparisons are predicted values. However, they are important for interpreting relative differences between the groups. The Pairwise Comparisons table shows the mean difference between the groups at each time point and indicates that there was no significant difference between groups at baseline (mean difference 0.009, 95% CI −0.010, 0.029, $P = 0.35$). However, the difference between the two groups is statistically significant at the 6 month follow-up (mean difference −0.040, 95% CI −0.068, −0.012, $P = 0.005$) and 1 year follow-up (mean difference −0.037, 95% CI −0.060, −0.015, $P = 0.001$).

In the Univariate Tests table the P values of the simple effects tests are the same as shown in the Pairwise Comparisons table (see Section 5.2.2).

The residuals should be checked for normality to ensure that the model is valid. Because each covariance matrix provides different residuals, the residuals should be checked after the most appropriate covariance matrix has been decided. Each residual is the observed data value minus the predicted value. The residuals can be saved to the sheet while running the model and plotted as a histogram shown in Figure 6.6 using the SPSS command sequence *Graphs → Legacy Dialogs → Histogram* with Residuals as the variable and selecting Display normal curve.

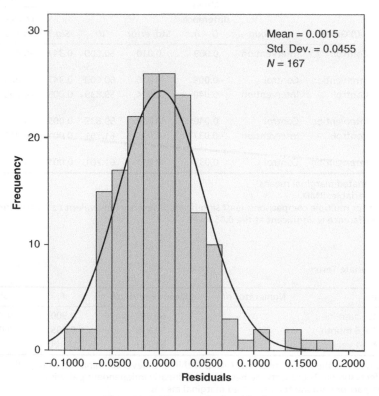

Figure 6.6 Histogram of residuals.

In this model, there are no residuals that are univariate outliers. Although the distribution is slightly skewed to the left, this should not bias the model or violate the assumptions.

6.6.6   *Reporting the results of a linear mixed model*

The results of a linear mixed model can be reported in a similar format as a repeated measures ANOVA (see Table 6.1 and Figure 6.4).

6.6.7   *Comparison of results: Repeated measures ANOVA and mixed model*

Although both repeated measures ANOVA and mixed models may use some similar terms and produce some common results, the methods in which the data are modelled is essentially quite different. If there are no missing data, the cell size ratio is low and the variances and correlations between time points are equal then repeated measures ANOVA and mixed models give the same results. However, when the cell size ratio is large or an inappropriate correlation structure is used in the mixed model, the results from the two methods are unlikely to agree. The P values between the two models may also differ because the models use a different subset of participants. Only 47 participants were included in the ANOVA but 60 are included in the mixed model. Linear mixed models are the preferred method for analyzing data from randomized trials because the inclusion of all available data from participants maintains the balance of confounders that the randomization process was designed to achieve.

Mixed model results with an appropriate covariance structure are preferred because repeated measures ANOVA is only optimal when the assumptions are met. In general, a linear mixed model with an appropriate covariance structure has higher statistical power to test for effects. Because the output from all types of models that are used to analyze longitudinal data can be difficult to interpret, it is important that the interpretation of between-group differences and P values is also based on the transparent effects that can be demonstrated using summary plots and post hoc analyses.

6.7   Notes for critical appraisal

For repeated measures ANOVA and linear mixed models, it is important that the assumptions for each test are met to avoid inaccurate results. When critically appraising a journal article in which the results from an analysis of longitudinal data are reported, some of the most important questions to ask are shown in Box 6.7.

Box 6.7 Questions for critical appraisal

The following questions should be asked when appraising published results from analyses in which repeated measures ANOVA or linear mixed mode has been used:

- Does each cell have an adequate number of participants?
- Are there any variables in the model that are collinear with other independent variables?
- Are there any outliers that would tend to inflate or reduce differences between groups or that would distort the model and therefore the P values?
- Are the residuals normally distributed?
- Have plots been included to help interpret the P values produced by the post hoc tests?
- Do the P values reflect the differences between cell means and the group sizes?

For repeated measures ANOVA:

- Have the requirements of sphericity and homogeneity been met?
- Does the omission of people with missing data values affect the generalizability of the results?

For linear mixed models:

- Has an appropriate covariance structure been used?

References

1. Maxwell S, Delaney H. *Designing experiments and analyzing data*. Wadsworth: Belmont, CA, 1990.
2. De Klerk NH. Repeated warnings re repeated measures. *Aust NZ J Med* 1986; **16**: 637–638.
3. Tabachnick BG, Fidell LS. *Using multivariate statistics*. Allyn & Bacon, 2001.
4. Stevens J *Applied multivariate statistics for the social sciences*, 3rd edn. Lawrence Erlbaum Associates: Mahway, NJ, 1996.
5. Field A. *Discovering statistics*, 3rd edn. Sage Publications: London, 2013
6. Fairclough DL. *Design and analysis of quality of life studies in clinical trials*, 2nd edn. Chapman & Hall/CRC: Boca Raton, FL, 2010.
7. Maxwell SE. Pairwise multiple comparisons in repeated measures design. *J Educ Stat* 1980; **5**: 269–287.
8. Richardson JTE. Eta squared and partial eta squared as measures of effect size in educational research. *Educ Res Rev* 2011; **6**: 135–147
9. Aickin M, Gensler H. Adjusting for multiple testing when reporting research results: the Bonferroni vs Holm methods. *Am J Public Health* 1996; **86**: 726–728.
10. Hox J. *Multilevel analysis: techniques and applications*, 2nd edn. Routledge: New York, 2010.
11. Hayes AF. A primer on multilevel modeling. *Hum Commun Res* 2006; **32**: 385–410.
12. West BT. Analyzing longitudinal data with the linear mixed models procedure in SPSS. *Eval Health Prof* 2009; **32**: 207–228.

CHAPTER 7

Correlation and regression

Angling may be said to be so like mathematics that it can never be fully learnt.
IZAAK WALTON (1593–1683)

Objectives

The objectives of this chapter are to explain how to:
- examine a linear relationship between two continuous variables
- interpret parametric and non-parametric correlation coefficients
- build a regression model that satisfies the assumptions of regression
- use a regression model as a predictive equation
- include binary and dummy group variables in a multivariate model
- plot regression equations that include binary group variables
- include more than one continuous variable in a multivariate model
- test for multicollinearity and interactions between variables
- identify and deal with outliers and remote points
- explore non-linear fits for regression models
- understand sample size requirements
- calculate effect size
- critically appraise the literature when regression models are reported

7.1 Correlation coefficients

A correlation coefficient describes how closely two variables are related, that is, the amount of variability in one measurement that is explained by another measurement. The range of a correlation coefficient is from −1 to +1, where the maximum values indicate that one variable has a perfect linear association with the other variable and that both variables are measuring the same entity without error. In practice, this rarely occurs because even if two instruments are intended to measure the same entity both usually have some degree of measurement error.

A positive correlation coefficient indicates that both variables increase in value together and a negative coefficient indicates that one variable decreases in value as the other variable increases. It is important to note that a significant association between two variables does not imply that they have a causal relationship. A

Medical Statistics: A Guide to SPSS, Data Analysis and Critical Appraisal, Second Edition.
Belinda Barton and Jennifer Peat.
© 2014 John Wiley & Sons, Ltd. Published 2014 by John Wiley & Sons, Ltd.
Companion website: www.wiley.com/go/barton/medicalstatistics2e

correlation coefficient of zero indicates a random relationship and the absence of a linear association. However, a correlation coefficient that is not significant does not imply that there is no relationship between the variables because there may be a non-linear relationship such as a curvilinear or cyclical relationship.

Correlation coefficients are rarely used as important statistics in their own right. An inherent limitation is that correlation coefficients reduce complex relationships to a single number that does not adequately explain the relationship between the two variables. Another inherent problem is that the statistical significance of the test is often over-interpreted. The P value is an estimate of whether the correlation coefficient is significantly different from zero so that a small correlation of no clinical importance can become statistically significant, especially when the sample size is large. In addition, outliers, the range of the data as well as the relationship between the two variables influence the correlation coefficient.

7.1.1 Types of correlation coefficients

There are three types of bivariate correlations. The type of correlation that is used to examine a linear relationship is determined by the nature of the variables.

Pearson's correlation coefficient (r) is a parametric correlation coefficient that is used to measure the linear association between two continuous variables that are both normally distributed. The Pearson's correlation coefficient (also known as the Pearson product-moment correlation coefficient) for a sample is denoted as r and represented in the population as ρ. The sample correlation coefficient can be squared to give the coefficient of determination (R^2), which is an estimate of the per cent of variation in one variable that is explained by the other variable.

The assumptions for using Pearson's correlation coefficient are shown in Box 7.1

Box 7.1 Assumptions for using Pearson's correlation coefficient

The assumptions that must be satisfied to use Pearson's correlation coefficient are:
- both variables must be continuous and normally distributed
- the sample must have been selected randomly from the general population
- the observations are independent of one another
- the relationship between the two variables is linear
- the variance is constant over the length of the data

If the assumption of random selection is not met, the correlation coefficient does not describe the true association between two variables that would be found in the general population. In this case, it would not be valid to generalize the association to other populations or to compare the r value with results from other studies.

Spearman's ρ (rho) is a rank correlation coefficient that is used for two ordinal variables or when one variable has a continuous normal distribution and the other variable is categorical or non-normally distributed. When this statistic is computed, the categorical or non-normally distributed variable is ranked, that is, sorted into ascending order and numbered sequentially, and then a correlation of the ranks with the continuous variable that is equivalent to Pearson's r is calculated. This test is a non-parametric test, so it can be used with variables that have a non-normal distribution.

Kendall's τ (tau) is used for correlations between two categorical or non-normally distributed variables. This test is non-parametric test of the measure of correlation between two ranked variables. In this test, Kendall's τ is calculated as the number of concordant pairs minus the number of disconcordant pairs divided by the total number of pairs. Kendall's tau-b is then adjusted for the number of pairs that are tied.

Research question

The spreadsheet **weights.sav,** which was used in Chapter 5, contains the data from a population sample of 550 term babies who had their weight recorded at 1 month of age.

Question: Is there a linear association between the weight, length and head circumference of 1-month-old babies?

Null hypothesis: That there is no linear association between weight, length and head circumference of babies at 1 month of age.

Variables: Weight, length and head circumference (continuous)

The variables weight, length and head circumference are all continuous variables that have an approximately normal distribution. Therefore their relationships to one another can be examined using Pearson's correlation coefficients. The null hypothesis is that the population correlation coefficients from which the sample was derived from are equal to zero, indicating no linear relationship between the variables. The alternative hypothesis (two-tailed) is that the correlation coefficients do not equal zero, so they may be greater than or less than zero.

Before computing any correlation coefficient, it is important to obtain scatter plots to obtain an understanding of the nature of the relationships between the variables. Box 7.2 shows the SPSS commands to obtain the matrix of scatter plots.

Box 7.2 SPSS commands to obtain scatter plots between variables

SPSS Commands

weights.sav – IBM SPSS Statistics Data Editor
       Graphs → Legacy Dialogs → Scatter/Dot
Scatter/Dot
       Click on Matrix Scatter and click on Define
Scatterplot Matrix
       Highlight Weight, Length, Head circumference, click over into Matrix Variables
       Click OK

The matrix in Figure 7.1 shows each of the variables plotted against one another. The number of rows and columns is equal to the number of variables selected. Each variable is shown once on the x-axis and once on the y-axis to give six plots, three of which are

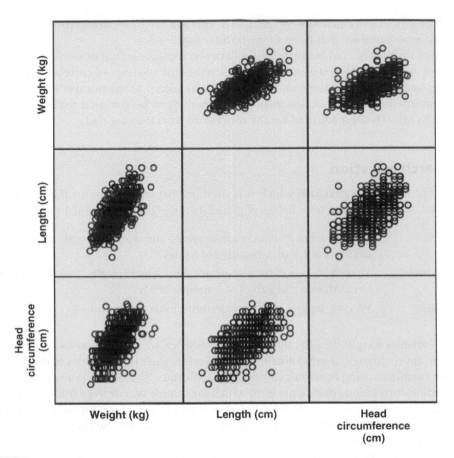

Figure 7.1 Scatter plot of weight by length by head circumference.

mirror images of the other three plots. In Figure 7.1, the scatter plot between weight and length is shown in the middle box on the top row, the scatter plot between weight and head circumference is in the right hand box on the top row, and the scatter plot between length and head circumference is in the third column of the middle row. All scatter plots in Figure 7.1 slope upwards to the right indicating a positive association between the two variables. If an association was negative, the scatter plot would slope downwards to the right.

The scatter plots indicate that there is a reasonable, positive linear association for all bivariate combinations of the three variables. It is clear that weight has a closer relationship with length than with head circumference in that the scatter around the plot is narrower.

7.1.2 Obtaining correlations in SPSS

To obtain the correlation coefficients (two-tailed) between the three variables, the SPSS commands shown in Box 7.3 can be used. Normally only one type of coefficient would be requested but to illustrate the difference between the correlation coefficients, all three are requested in this example. In the SPPS output, the correlation matrix shown below reports the *r* values, *P* values and sample size for each correlation. If a left diagonal line was drawn through the matrix, it can be seen that the information above the diagonal line is the same as the information below the line.

Box 7.3 SPSS commands to obtain correlation coefficients

SPSS Commands

weights.sav – IBM SPSS Statistics Data Editor
 Analyze → Correlate → Bivariate
Bivariate Correlations
 Highlight Weight, Length, Head circumference, click over into Variables
 Under Correlation Coefficients, tick Pearson (default), Kendall's tau-b and Spearman
 Under Test of Significance, tick Two-tailed (default)
 Tick Flag significant correlations (default)
 Click OK

Correlations

Correlations

		Weight (kg)	Length (cm)	Head circumference (cm)
Weight (kg)	Pearson correlation	1	0.713**	0.622**
	Sig. (two-tailed)		0.000	0.000
	N	550	550	550
Length (cm)	Pearson correlation	0.713**	1	0.598**
	Sig. (two-tailed)	0.000		0.000
	N	550	550	550
Head circumference (cm)	Pearson correlation	0.622**	0.598**	1
	Sig. (two-tailed)	0.000	0.000	
	N	550	550	550

**Correlation is significant at the 0.01 level (two-tailed).

If the *P* value is less than the level of significance, typically 0.05, the null hypothesis is rejected and we can conclude that there is a linear relationship between the two variables. The correlation values would have a single asterisk if they were significant at the $P < 0.05$ level. In the table, the coefficients that are significant at the $P < 0.01$ level are identified with two asterisks.

A comparison of the Pearson correlations (*r* values) in the Correlations table shows that the best predictor of weight is length with an *r* value of 0.713 compared to a weaker, but moderate association between weight and head circumference with an *r* value of 0.622. Head circumference is related to length with a slightly lower *r* value of 0.598. Despite their differences in magnitude, the correlation coefficients are all highly significant at the $P < 0.0001$ level emphasizing the insensitive nature of the *P* values for selecting the most important predictors of weight.

The correlation coefficient, r, can be squared to obtain the coefficient of determination, R^2, which indicates the per cent of variance in one variable that can be explained by the other variable. R^2 will be discussed in more detail later in this chapter.

In the Non-parametric Correlations table, the Kendall's tau-b coefficients are all lower than the Pearson's coefficients indicating that there are some tied ranks in the data set, that is, babies with the same weight and length as one other. A value of 0.540 for the correlation between weight and length indicates that 54% of ranks are concordant and 46% are discordant. The Spearman's coefficients are similar in magnitude to the Pearson's correlation coefficients.

Non-parametric Correlations

Correlations

			Weight (kg)	Length (cm)	Head circumference (cm)
Kendall's tau-b	Weight (kg)	Correlation coefficient	1.000	0.540**	0.468**
		Sig. (two-tailed)		0.000	0.000
		N	550	550	550
	Length (cm)	Correlation coefficient	0.540**	1.000	0.454**
		Sig. (two-tailed)	0.000		0.000
		N	550	550	550
	Head circumference (cm)	Correlation coefficient	0.468**	0.454**	1.000
		Sig. (two-tailed)	0.000	0.000	
		N	550	550	550
Spearman's Rho	Weight (kg)	Correlation coefficient	1.000	0.711**	0.626**
		Sig. (two-tailed)		0.000	0.000
		N	550	550	550
	Length (cm)	Correlation coefficient	0.711**	1.000	0.596**
		Sig. (two-tailed)	0.000		0.000
		N	550	550	550
	Head circumference (cm)	Correlation coefficient	0.626**	0.596**	1.000
		Sig. (two-tailed)	0.000	0.000	
		N	550	550	550

**Correlation is significant at the 0.01 level (two-tailed).

Partial correlations can also be conducted using the following SPSS commands, *Analyze → Correlate → Partial*. With this type of correlation, the linear relationship between two variables can be examined, while controlling or holding constant the effects of another confounding variable. The null hypothesis for a partial correlation is that there is no linear relationship between two variables after controlling for the effects of a confounding variable. For example, partial correlations could be conducted for the association between weight and head circumference after controlling for body length. The assumptions for a partial correlation are the same as for Pearson's correlation shown in Box 7.1.

7.1.3 *Effect size for correlations*

The absolute value of the Pearson's correlation coefficient indicates the strength of the relationship between two variables. Cohen defines an r value of 0.1 as a small effect

Table 7.1 Total sample size required for detecting a significant correlation coefficient value (two-tailed)

Correlation coefficient (r)	$\alpha = 0.05$, Power = 80% N required
0.1	780
0.2	200
0.3	85
0.4	50
0.5	30
0.6	20
0.7	15

size, an r value of 0.3 a medium effect size and an r value of 0.5 as a large effect size.[1] It is important to note that the P value is influenced by the size of the effect and the sample size. Therefore, both the effect size and the sample size should be considered when interpreting P values and statistical significance. A relatively small effect size of 0.2 will be statistically significant with a large sample size, but may not be clinically important. Conversely, a large effect size will be statistically significant with a relatively small sample size. Table 7.1 shows the sample size required to detect a correlation coefficient, r, which is statistically different from zero (two-tailed), with power equal to 80% and $P < 0.05$.[2]

7.1.4   Influence of the range of the variable

The influence on r values when using a selected sample with a smaller range of values rather than a random sample can be demonstrated by repeating the analysis using only part of the data set. Using the following SPSS commands *Analyze → Descriptive Statistics → Descriptives* shows that length ranges from a minimum value of 48.0 cm to a maximum value of 62.0 cm. To examine the correlation in a selected sample, the data set can be restricted to babies less than 55.0 cm in length using the commands shown in Box 7.4.

Box 7.4 SPSS commands to calculate a correlation coefficient for a subset of the data

SPSS Commands

weights.sav – IBM SPSS Statistics Data Editor
      Data → Select Cases

> *Select Cases*
> > *Select If condition is satisfied → Click on If box*
> *Select Cases: If*
> > *Highlight Length and click over into white box*
> > *Type in <55 following length*
> > *Click Continue*
> *Select Cases*
> > *Click OK*

When *Select Cases* is used, the row number of cases that are not selected to be included in the analysis appear in the SPSS Data View with a diagonal line through them. In addition, a filter variable to indicate the status of each case in the analysis is generated at the end of the spreadsheet with the coding 0 = not selected and 1 = selected. Also the text *Filter On* is shown in the bottom right hand side of the SPSS Data View screen.

To examine the relationship between the variables for only babies less than 55.0 cm in length, Pearson's correlation coefficients can be obtained by reusing the commands shown in Box 7.2.

Correlations

Correlations

		Weight (kg)	Length (cm)	Head circumference (cm)
Weight (kg)	Pearson correlation	1	0.494**	0.504**
	Sig. (two-tailed)		0.000	0.000
	N	272	272	272
Length (cm)	Pearson correlation	0.494**	1	0.390**
	Sig. (two-tailed)	0.000		0.000
	N	272	272	272
Head circumference (cm)	Pearson correlation	0.504**	0.390**	1
	Sig. (two-tailed)	0.000	0.000	
	N	272	272	272

**Correlation is significant at the 0.01 level (two-tailed).

When compared with Pearson's *r* values from the full data set, the correlation coefficient between weight and length is substantially reduced from 0.713 to 0.494 when the upper limit of length is reduced from 62 cm to 55 cm. However, the top centre plot in Figure 7.1 shows that the relationship between weight and length in the lower half of the data is similar to the total sample. In general, *r* values are higher when the range of the explanatory variable is wider even though the relationship between the two variables is unchanged. For this reason, only the coefficients from random population samples have an unbiased value and can be compared with one another.

Once the correlation coefficients are obtained, the full data set can be reselected using the command sequence *Data → Select Cases → All cases.*

7.1.5   *Reporting correlation coefficients*

In reporting correlation coefficients for publication, the type of correlation conducted, the value of the correlation coefficient (2 or 3 decimal places), the P value and the sample size should be reported. In reporting Pearson's correlation coefficient in this example, it could be reported as 'The weight of babies at 1 month was significantly related to their length ($r = 0.71$, $P < 0.001$, $n = 550$) and also to their head circumference ($r = 0.32$, $P < 0.001$, $n = 550$). There was also a significant association between the length of babies and their head circumference ($r = 0.60$, $P < 0.001$, $n = 550$). These results indicate that as the length of babies increases, so does their head circumference and weight'.

7.2   **Regression models**

Regression models are used to measure the extent to which one or more explanatory variables predict an outcome variable. In this, a regression model is used to fit a straight line through the data, where the regression line is the best predictor of the outcome variable using one or more explanatory variables.

There are two principal purposes for building a regression model. The most common purpose is to build a predictive model, for example, in situations in which age and gender are used to predict normal values in lung size or body mass index (BMI). Normal values are the range of values that occur naturally in the general population. In developing a model to predict normal values, the emphasis is on building an accurate predictive model.

The second purpose of using a regression model is to examine the effect of an explanatory variable on an outcome variable after adjusting for other important explanatory factors. These types of models are used for hypothesis testing. For example, a regression model could be built using age and gender to predict BMI and could then be used to test the hypothesis that groups with different exercise regimes have different BMI values.

7.2.1   *Relationship between regression and ANCOVA*

The mathematics of regression is identical to the mathematics of analysis of covariance (ANCOVA). However, regression provides more information than ANCOVA in that a linear equation is generated that explains the relationship between the explanatory variables and the outcome. By using regression, additional information about the relationships between variables and the between-group differences is obtained. Regression can also be a more flexible approach because some of the assumptions such as those relating to cell and variance ratios are not as restrictive as the assumptions for ANCOVA (see Chapter 5). However, in common with ANCOVA, it is important to remember that regression gives a measure of association at one point in time only, that is, at the time the measurements were collected, and a significant association does not infer causality.

Although the mathematics of regression is similar to ANOVA in that the explained and unexplained variations are compared, some terms are labelled differently. In regression, the distance between an observed value and the overall mean is partitioned into two components – the variation about the regression, which is also called the residual

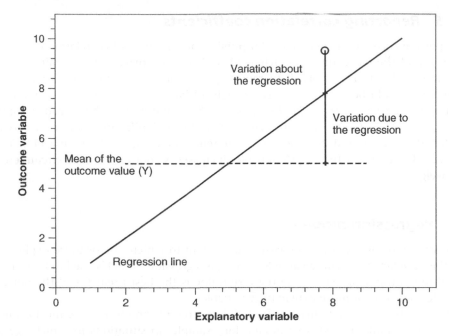

Figure 7.2 Calculation of the variation in regression.

variation, and the variation due to the regression.[3] Figure 7.2 shows how the variation for one data point, shown as a circle, is calculated.

The variation about the regression is the explained variation and the variation due to the regression is the unexplained variation. As in ANOVA, these distances are squared and summed and the mean square is calculated. The *F* value, which is calculated as the regression mean square divided by the residual mean square, ranges from 1 to a large number. If the two sources of variance are similar, there is no association between the variables and the *F* value is close to 1. If the variation due to the regression is large compared to the variation about the regression, then the *F* value will be large indicating a strong association between the outcome and explanatory variables.

When there is only one explanatory variable, the equation is called a simple linear regression. When there is more than one explanatory variable in the model, the equation is called a multiple linear regression.

7.2.2 The regression equation

When there is only one explanatory variable, the equation of the best fit for the regression line is as follows:

$$y = a + bx$$

where '*y*' is the value of the outcome variable, '*x*' is the value of the explanatory variable, '*a*' is the intercept of the regression line and '*b*' is the slope of the regression line. This is a classic equation for a straight line. With a regression model, an estimation of the best fitting straight line through the data that minimizes the residual variation is calculated.

In practice, the slope of the line, as estimated by 'b', represents the unit change in the outcome variable 'y' with each unit change in the explanatory variable 'x'. If the slope is positive, 'y' increases as 'x' increases and if the slope is negative, 'y' decreases as 'x' increases. The intercept is the point at which the regression line intersects with the y-axis when the value of 'x' is zero. This value is part of the regression equation but does not usually have any clinical meaning. The fitted regression line passes through the mean values of both the explanatory variable 'x' and the outcome variable 'y'.

When using regression, the research question must be framed so that the explanatory and outcome variables are classified correctly. An important concept is that regression predicts the mean y value given the observed x value and in this, the error around the explanatory variable is not taken into account. Therefore, measurements that can be taken accurately, such as age and height, are good explanatory variables. Variables that are difficult to measure accurately or are subject to bias, such as birth weight recalled by parents when the baby has reached school age, should be avoided as explanatory variables.

7.2.3 Assumptions for regression

To avoid bias in a regression model or a lack of precision around the regression coefficients, the assumptions for using regression that are shown in Box 7.5 must be tested and met. In regression, mean values are not compared as in ANOVA so that any bias between groups as a result of non-normal distributions is not as problematic. Regression models are robust to moderate degrees of non-normality provided that the sample size is large and that there are few multivariate outliers in the final model. In general, the residuals but not the outcome variable have to be normally distributed. Also, the sample does not have to be selected randomly because the regression equation describes the relation between the variables and is not influenced by the spread of the explanatory variable. However, it is important that the final prediction equation is only applied to populations with the same characteristics as the study sample.

Box 7.5 Assumptions for using regression

The assumptions that must be met when using regression are as follows:

Study design

- The sample is representative of the population to which inference will be made.
- The sample size is sufficient to support the model.
- The data have been collected in a period when the relationship between the outcome and the explanatory variable/s remains constant.
- All important explanatory variables (covariates) are included.

Independence

- All observations are independent of one another.
- There is low multicollinearity between explanatory variables.

> **Model building**
> - The relation between the explanatory variable/s and the outcome variable is approximately linear.
> - The explanatory variables correlate with the outcome variable.
> - The residuals are normally distributed.
> - The variance is homoscedastic, that is, constant over the length of the model.
> - There are no multivariate outliers that bias the regression estimates.

Under the study design assumptions shown in Box 7.5, one assumption is that the data are collected in a period when the relationship remains constant. For example, in building a model to predict normal values for blood pressure, the data must be collected when the participants have been resting rather than exercising and participants taking anti-hypertensive medications should be excluded. It is also important that all known covariates such as age and gender are included in the model before testing the effects of new variables in the model.

The two assumptions of independence between observations and explanatory variables are important. When explanatory variables are significantly related to each other, a decision needs to be made about which variable to include and which variable to exclude.

The remaining assumptions about the nature of the data can be tested when building the model. In this chapter, the assumptions are tested after obtaining a parsimonious model but in practice the assumptions should be tested at each step in the model building process.

7.2.4   R value and effect size

In linear regression, the R value which is calculated is the multiple correlation coefficient and is the correlation between the observed and predicted values of the outcome variable. The value of R will range between 0 and 1. R can be interpreted in a similar way to Pearson's correlation coefficient. In simple linear regression, R is the absolute value of Pearson's correlation coefficient between the outcome and explanatory variable.

The R square (R^2) value is the square of the R value (i.e. $R \times R$) and is called the coefficient of determination. R square has a valuable interpretation in that it indicates the per cent of the variance in the outcome variable that can be explained or accounted for by the explanatory variables. Hence, it is a measure of the 'goodness of fit' of the regression line to the data. The adjusted R square value is the R value adjusted for the number of explanatory variables included in the model and can therefore be compared between models that include different numbers of explanatory variables.

The R value for the model is equivalent to r when there is one explanatory variable in the model and can be used as a measure of effect size. Alternatively, Cohen's f discussed in Chapter 5 can be extended to simple linear and multiple regressions using the R^2 value rather than an eta squared value as follows:

$$\text{Cohen's} f = \sqrt{\frac{R^2}{(1 - R^2)}}$$

7.2.5 Sample size required

One of the assumptions is that the sample size is sufficient to support the regression model. The sample size required to support a model depends on both the R value of the model and the number of variables that are included. Table 7.2 shows the number of participants required in models with 1 to 4 independent predictors. The sample size requirement increases with the number of predictor variables. More detailed estimates are available in web-based programs; for example, the StatsToDo website detailed in the 'Useful Websites' section.

Table 7.2 Sample size requirement for regression analyses

R value	1 predictor variable	2 predictor variables	3 predictor variables	4 predictor variables
0.2	190	230	265	290
0.3	80	100	115	125
0.4	45	55	65	70

Research question

Using the spreadsheet **weights.sav**, regression analysis can be used to answer the following research question:

Question:	Can body length be used to predict weight at 1 month of age?
Null hypothesis:	That there is no relationship between length and weight at 1 month.
Variables:	Outcome variable = weight (continuous),
	Explanatory variable = length (continuous)

The SPSS commands to obtain a regression equation for the relationship between length and weight are shown in Box 7.6.

Box 7.6 SPSS commands to obtain regression estimates

SPSS Commands

weights.sav – IBM SPSS Statistics Data Editor
        Analyze → Regression → Linear
Linear Regression
        Highlight Weight, click into Dependent box
        Highlight Length, click into Independent(s) box
        Method = Enter (default)
        Click OK

In the Model Summary table it can be seen that the R square value is approximately equal to the square of the R value, that is, 0.713×0.713, which is the coefficient of determination. The R square value of 0.509 indicates a modest relationship in that 50.9% of the variation in weight is explained by length. On the basis of Cohen's classification described in Section 7.1, the value of 0.713 would be a large effect size.

Converting R square to Cohen's $f = \sqrt{0.509/(1 - 0.509)} = 1.02$. This is also a large effect size and from this, it can be concluded that body length has an important association with weight at 1 month. In the Model Summary table, the standard error of the estimate of 0.42229 is the standard error around the outcome variable weight at the mean value of the explanatory variable length and as such gives an indication of the precision of the model. Generally, the more precise the model is, the smaller the standard error.

Regression

Model Summary

Model	R	R square	Adjusted R square	Std. error of the estimate
1	0.713[a]	0.509	0.508	0.42229

[a] Predictors: (constant), length (cm).

In the ANOVA table, the F value is calculated as the unexplained variation due to the regression divided by the explained variation about the regression, or the residual variation. Thus, F is the regression mean square of 101.119 divided by the residual mean square of 0.178, or 568.08. The resulting F value of 567.043 in the table is slightly different as a result of rounding errors and is highly significant at $P < 0.0001$ indicating that there is a significant linear relationship between length and weight. This also indicates that the regression model overall significantly predicts weight.

ANOVA[a]

Model		Sum of squares	df	Mean Square	F	Sig.
1	Regression	101.119	1	101.119	567.043	0.000[b]
	Residual	97.723	548	0.178		
	Total	198.842	549			

[a] Dependent variable: weight (kg).
[b] Predictors: (constant), length (cm).

In the Model table, the null hypotheses being tested are firstly that the Constant value (the Intercept or value a in the regression model) is equal to zero and secondly, that the regression coefficient or slope of the line (the value b in the regression model) is equal to zero. The t values, which are calculated by dividing the beta values (unstandardized coefficient B) by their standard errors, are a test of whether each regression coefficient is significantly different from zero and as such are equivalent to a one-sample t-test. If the regression coefficient is equal to zero this means that for a unit change in the explanatory variable, the predicted value of the outcome variable remains the same. That is, the explanatory variable does not significantly predict the outcome variable.

In this example, both the constant (intercept) and slope of the regression line are significantly different from zero at $P < 0.0001$ which is shown in the column labelled 'Sig'.

The Coefficients table shows the unstandardized coefficients that are used to formulate the regression equation in the form of $y = a + bx$ as follows:

$$\text{Weight} = -5.412 + (0.178 \times \text{Length})$$

The Constant value of -5.412 is the y intercept, that is, the predicted value of weight is when x (length) equals zero. The regression coefficient, b equals 0.178 and indicates that for each unit increase in length, weight will increase by 0.178 kg since the regression coefficient b is a positive value.

Coefficients[a]

| Model | Unstandardized coefficients | | Standardized coefficients | | |
	B	Std. error	Beta	T	Sig.
1 (Constant)	−5.412	0.411		−13.167	0.000
Length (cm)	0.178	0.007	0.713	23.813	0.000

[a]Dependent variable: weight (kg).

Because length is the only explanatory variable in the model, the standardized beta coefficient, which indicates the relative contribution of a variable to the model, is the same as the R value shown in the first table. For length, the square of the t value is equal to the F value in the ANOVA table, that is, the square of 23.813 is equal to 567.043.

7.2.6   *Generalizability of regression*

Regression equations can only be generalized to samples with the same characteristics as the study sample. Thus, this regression model only describes the relation between weight and length in 1-month-old babies who were term births because premature birth was an exclusion criterion for study entry. The model could not be used to predict normal population values because the data are not from a random population sample, which would include premature births. However, the model could be used to predict the normal birth weight values for term babies.

7.2.7   *Plotting a regression line*

The SPSS commands shown in Box 7.7 can be used to obtain a scatter plot of the observed values of weight plotted against length and to draw the regression line with mean prediction intervals.

In Figure 7.3, the 95% mean prediction interval around the regression line is a 95% confidence interval, that is, the area in which there is 95% certainty that the true regression line lies. This interval band is slightly curved because the errors in estimating the intercept and the slope are included in addition to the error in predicting the outcome variable.[4] The error in estimating the slope increases as the difference between the predicted value and the actual value of the explanatory variable increases, resulting in a curved 95% confidence band around the sample regression line. In Figure 7.3, the 95% confidence interval is narrow as a result of the large sample size.

Box 7.7 SPSS commands to obtain a scatter plot with a regression line

SPSS Commands

weights.sav – IBM SPSS Statistics Data Editor
        Graphs → Legacy Dialogs → Scatter/Dot
Scatter/Dot
        Select Simple Scatter and click Define
        Highlight Weight and click into Y Axis box
        Highlight Length and click into X Axis box
        Click OK
Output 1 [Document 1] – IBM SPSS Statistics Viewer
        Double click on the scatter plot
Chart Editor
        Select Elements and select Fit Line at Total
Properties
        Click the Fit Line tab and select Linear for Fit Method
        Confidence Intervals: select Mean and enter 95% (default)
        Select Attach label to line (default)
        Click Apply
        Click Close

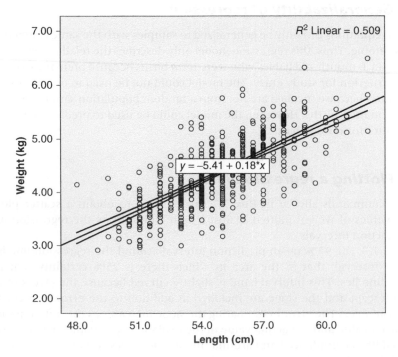

Figure 7.3 Scatter plot of weight on length with regression line and 95% mean confidence interval.

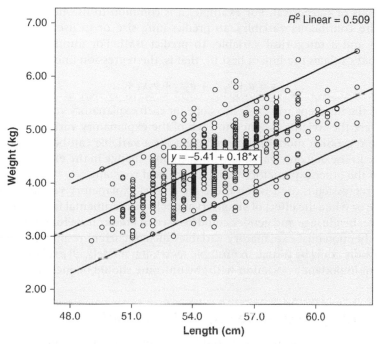

Figure 7.4 Scatter plot of weight on length with regression line and 95% individual confidence interval.

By repeating the same commands shown in Box 7.7 and in the Fit Line tab, selecting *Confidence Intervals: Individual* Figure 7.4 can be obtained. The 95% individual prediction interval is in which 95% of the data points lie is the distance between the 2.5 and 97.5 percentiles. This interval is used to predict normal values. Clearly, any definition of normality is specific to the context but normal values should only be based on large sample sizes, preferably of at least 200 participants.[5]

7.2.8 Reporting a simple linear regression

If the regression model assumptions have been satisfied, the results of the simple linear regression can be reported as the plot shown in Figure 7.3 in addition to the equation that defines the relationship, that is,

$$\text{Weight} = -5.412 + (0.178 \times \text{Length})$$

In addition it would be important to report that the R^2 of the model is 0.51, and that the effect size Cohen's f is equal to 1.02.

7.3 Multiple linear regression

A regression model in which the outcome variable is predicted from two or more explanatory variables is called a multiple linear regression. Explanatory variables may be continuous or categorical. For example, it is common to use height and age, both of which are continuous variables, to predict lung size or to use age and gender, a continuous and a categorical variable, to predict BMI. For multiple regression, the equation that explains the line of best fit, that is, the regression line, is

$$y = a + b_1x_1 + b_2x_2 + b_3x_3 + \ldots$$

where 'a' is the intercept and 'b_i' is the slope for each explanatory variable. In effect, b_1, b_2, b_3, etc. are the weights assigned to each of the explanatory variables in the model. In multiple regression models, the coefficient for a variable can be interpreted as the unit change in the outcome variable with each unit change in the explanatory variable, when all of the other explanatory variables are held constant.

Multiple regression is used when there are several explanatory variables that predict an outcome or when the effect of an observational or experimental factor is being tested. For example, height, age and gender could be used to predict lung function and then the effects of other potential explanatory variables such as current respiratory symptoms or smoking history could be tested. In multiple regression models, all explanatory variables that have an important association with the outcome should be included.

7.3.1   Building a multiple regression model

Multiple linear regression models should be built up gradually through a series of uni-variate, bivariate, and multivariate methods. In multiple regression, each explanatory variable should ideally have a significant correlation with the outcome variable but the explanatory variables should not be highly correlated with one another, that is collinear. In addition, models should not be over-fitted with a large number of variables that increase the R square by small amounts. In over-fitted models, the R square may decrease when the model is applied to other data.

Decisions about which variables to remove or include in a model should be based on expert knowledge and biological plausibility in addition to statistical considerations. These decisions often need to take cost, measurement error and theoretical constructs into account in addition to the strength of association indicated by R values, P values and standardized coefficients. The ideal model should be parsimonious, that is comprised of the smallest number of variables that predict the largest amount of variation.

Once a decision has been made about which explanatory variables to test in a model, the distribution of both the outcome and the continuous explanatory variables should be examined using methods outlined in Chapter 2, largely to identify any univariate outliers. The assumptions of regression should also be checked. The order in which the explanatory variables are entered into the regression model is important because this can make a difference to the amount of variance that is explained by each variable, especially when explanatory variables are significantly related to each other.[6]

7.3.2   Methods of multivariate modelling

There are three major methods of entering the explanatory variables that include standard, stepwise or sequential (forward or backward).[7] In standard (or forced entry) multiple regression, called the 'enter' method in SPSS, all variables are entered into the model together and the unique contribution of each variable to the outcome variable is calculated. However, an explanatory variable that is correlated with the outcome variable may not be a significant predictor when the other explanatory variables have accounted for a large proportion of the variance so that the remaining variance is small.[5] Therefore, it is important to consider the overall correlation and also the unique contribution of the explanatory variable.[7]

In stepwise multiple regression, the order of the explanatory variables is determined by the strength of their correlation with the outcome variable or by predetermined statistical criteria. The stepwise procedure can be forward selection, backward deletion or stepwise, all of which are available options in SPSS. In forward selection, variables are added one at a time until the addition of another variable accounts only for a small amount of variance. In backward selection, all variables are entered and then are deleted one at a time if they do not contribute significantly to the prediction of the outcome. Forward selection and backward deletion may not result in the same regression equation.[4] Stepwise is a combination of both forward selection and backward deletion in which variables are added one at a time and retained if they satisfy set statistical criteria but are deleted if they no longer contribute significantly to the model.[7]

In sequential multiple regression, which is also called hierarchical regression, the order of entering the explanatory variables is determined by the researcher using logical or theoretical factors, or by the strength of the correlation with the outcome variable. When each new variable is entered, the variance contributed by the variable, possible multicollinearity with other variables and the influence of the variable on the model are assessed. Variables can be entered one at a time or together in blocks and the significance of each variable, or each variable in the block, is assessed at each step. This method delivers a stable and reliable model and provides invaluable information about the inter-relationships between the explanatory variables.

Another method of entry in SPSS is remove, in which all variables in a block are removed in a single step.

7.3.3   *Sample size considerations*

For multiple regression, it is important to have an adequate sample size. A simple rule that has been suggested for predictive equations is that the minimum number of cases should be at least 100 or, for stepwise regression, that the number of cases should be at least $40 \times m$, where m is the number of variables in the model.[7] More precise methods for calculating sample size and power are available.[8] To avoid underestimating the sample size for regression, the sample size calculations should be based on the regression model itself and not on correlation coefficients.

It is important not to include too many explanatory variables in the model relative to the number of cases because this can inflate the R^2 value. When the sample size is very small, the R^2 value will be artificially inflated, the adjusted R^2 value will be reduced and the imprecise regression estimates may have no sensible interpretation. If the sample size is too small to support the number of explanatory variables being tested, the variables can be tested one at a time and only the most significant included in the final model. Alternatively, a new explanatory variable can be created that is a composite of the original variables, for example, BMI could be included instead of weight and height.

A larger sample size increases the precision around the estimates by reducing the standard errors and often increases the generalizability of the results. The sample size needs to be increased if a small effect size is anticipated, if the distribution of any of the variables is skewed or if there is substantial measurement error in any variable. All of these factors tend to reduce statistical power to demonstrate significant associations between the outcome and explanatory variables.

It is important to achieve a balance in the regression model with the number of explanatory variables and sample size, because even a small R value will become statistically significant when the sample size is very large. Thus, when the sample size is large it is prudent to be cautious about type I errors. When the final model is obtained, the clinical importance of estimates of effect size should be used to interpret the coefficients for each variable rather than reliance on P values.

7.3.4 Multicollinearity

Collinearity is a term that is used when two explanatory variables are significantly related to one another. The issue of collinearity is only important for the relationships between explanatory variables and naturally does not need to be considered in relationships between the explanatory variables and the outcome. Multicollinearity will occur in the regression model if two or more explanatory variables are significantly related to one other.

Regression is more robust to some degrees of multicollinearity than ANOVA but the smaller the sample size and the larger the number of variables in the model, the more problematic collinearity becomes. Important degrees of multicollinearity need to be reconciled because they can distort the regression coefficients and lead to a loss of precision, that is inflated standard errors of the beta coefficients, and thus to an unstable and unreliable model. In extreme cases of collinearity, the direction of effect, that is the sign, of a regression coefficient may change.

Correlations between explanatory variables cause logical as well as statistical problems. If one variable accounts for most of the variation in another explanatory variable, the logic of including both explanatory variables in the model needs to be considered since they are approximate measures of the same entity. The correlation (r) between explanatory variables in a regression model should not be greater than 0.70.[7] For this reason, the decision of which variables to include should be based on theoretical constructs rather than statistical considerations based on regression estimates. Variables that can be measured with reliability and with minimum measurement error are preferred, whereas measurements that are costly, invasive, unreliable or removed from the main causal pathway are less useful in predictive models.

The amount of mulitcollinearity in a model is estimated by the variance inflation factor (VIF), which is calculated as $1/(1 - R^2)$ where R^2 is the squared multiple correlation coefficient. In essence, VIF measures how much the variance of the regression coefficient has been inflated due to multicollinearity with other explanatory variables.[9] In regression models, P values rely on an estimate of variance around the regression

Table 7.3 Relation between R, tolerance
and variance inflation factor (VIF)

R	Tolerance	VIF
0.25	0.94	1.07
0.50	0.75	1.33
0.70	0.51	1.96
0.90	0.19	5.26
0.95	0.10	10.26

coefficients, which is proportional to the VIF and thus if the VIF is inflated, the P value may be unreliable. A VIF that is large, say greater than or equal to 4, is a sign of mulitcollinearity and the regression coefficients, their variances and their P values are likely to be unreliable

In SPSS, mulitcollinearity is estimated by tolerance, that is $1 - R^2$. Tolerance has an inverse relationship to VIF in that VIF $= 1/$tolerance. Tolerance values close to zero indicate mulitcollinearity.[9] In regression, tolerance values less than 0.2 are usually considered to indicate mulitcollinearity. The relation between R, tolerance and VIF is shown in Table 7.3. A tolerance value below 0.5, which corresponds with an R value above 0.7 is of concern.

Mulitcollinearity can be estimated from examining the standard errors and the tolerance values as described in the examples below, or multicollinearity statistics can be obtained in the *Statistics* options under the *Analyze → Regression → Linear* commands.

7.3.5   Multiple linear regression: Testing for group differences

Regression can be used to test whether the relation between the outcome and explanatory variables is the same across categorical groups, say males and females. Rather than split the data set and analyze the data from males and females separately, it is often more useful to incorporate gender as a binary explanatory variable in the regression model. This process maintains statistical power by maintaining sample size and has the advantage of providing an estimate of the size of the difference between the gender groups.

Binary variables are often included in a regression model in experimental studies in which a continuous outcome variable is adjusted for a continuous baseline variable before testing for a between-group difference.[10] In observational studies, a binary variable can be added to a regression model to compute the mean difference between two groups after adjusting for a covariate. It is simple to include a categorical variable in a regression model when the variable is binary, that is, has two levels only. Binary regression coefficients have a straight forward interpretation if the variable is coded 0 for the comparison group, for example, a factor that is absent or a reply of no, and 1 for the group of interest, for example, a factor that is present or a reply that is coded yes.

Research question

The spreadsheet **weights.sav** used previously in this chapter will be used to answer the following research questions.

Questions: Do length, gender or the number of siblings influence the weight of babies at one month of age? Does the length of babies by gender influence the weight of babies differently?

Variables: Outcome variable = weight (continuous)

Explanatory variables = length (continuous), gender (category, two levels) and parity (category, two levels)

In this model, length is included because it is an important predictor of weight. In effect, the regression model is used to adjust weight for differences in length between babies and then to test the null hypothesis that there is no difference in weight between groups defined by gender and parity.

The *Transform → Recode* commands shown in Box 1.9 can be used to recode gender into a new variable labelled gender2 with values 0 and 1, making an arbitrary decision to code male gender as the comparison group (i.e. male = 0, female = 1). Similarly, parity can be re-coded into a new variable, parity2 with the value 0 for singletons unchanged and with values of 1 or greater re-coded to 1 using the *Range* option from *1 through 3*. Once re-coded, values and labels for both variables need to be added in the Variable View screen and the numbers in each group verified as correct using the frequency commands shown in Box 1.7. It is important to always have systems in place to check for possible recoding errors and to document re-coded group numbers in any new variables.

In this chapter, regression equations are built using the sequential method. To add variables to the regression model in blocks, the commands shown in Box 7.8 can be used with the enter method and block option. Prior bivariate analysis using *t*-tests for gender and one-way ANOVA for parity (not shown) indicated that the association between gender and weight is stronger than the association between parity and weight. Therefore, gender is added in the model before parity. Using the sequential method, the statistics of the two models are easily compared, multicollinearity between variables can be identified and reasons for any inflation in standard errors and loss of precision become clear.

Box 7.8 SPSS commands to generate a regression model with a binary explanatory variable

SPSS Commands

weights.sav − IBM SPSS Statistics Data Editor
         Analyze → Regression → Linear
Linear Regression
         Highlight Weight, click into Dependent box
         Highlight Length, click into Independent(s) box
         Under Block 1 of 1, click Next
         Highlight Gender recoded, click into Independent(s) box in Block 2 of 2
         Method = Enter (default)
         Click Statistics

Linear Regression: Statistics
> *Select Estimates for Regression Coefficients (default) and tick Model fit (default) and R squared change, click Continue*
> *Click OK*

The Model Summary table indicates the strength of the predictive or explanatory variables in the regression model. The first model contains length and the second model contains length and gender. Because there are a different number of variables in the two models, the adjusted R square value is used when making direct comparisons between the models. The adjusted R square value can be used to assess whether the fit of the model improves with inclusion of the additional variable, that is, whether the amount of explained variation increases.

Model Summary

Model	R	R Square	Adjusted R square	Std. error of the estimate	Change statistics				
					R square change	F Change	df1	df2	Sig. F change
1	0.713[a]	0.509	0.508	0.42229	0.509	567.043	1	548	0.000
2	0.741[b]	0.549	0.548	0.40474	0.041	49.543	1	547	0.000

[a]Predictors: (constant), length (cm).
[b]Predictors: (constant), length (cm), gender re-coded.

By comparing the adjusted R square of Model 1 generated in Block 1 with the adjusted R square of Model 2 generated in Block 2, it is clear that adding gender improves the model fit because the adjusted R square increases from 0.508 to 0.548. This indicates that 54.8% of the variation is now explained. It is important to know whether the R square increases by a significant amount. The R Square Change and the Change Statistics indicates that in Model 1 with length only, R^2 changes from 0 to 0.509 and in Model 2 with gender re-coded included as a predictor, R^2 increases by 0.041. The corresponding P values shown in the column labelled Sig. F Change are less than 0.05 and are significant indicating the amount of variation accounted for by the model has significantly increased.

ANOVA[a]

Model		Sum of squares	df	Mean square	F	Sig.
1	Regression	101.119	1	101.119	567.043	0.000[b]
	Residual	97.723	548	0.178		
	Total	198.842	549			
2	Regression	109.235	2	54.617	333.407	0.000[c]
	Residual	89.607	547	0.164		
	Total	198.842	549			

[a]Dependent variable: weight (kg).
[b]Predictors: (constant), length (cm).
[c]Predictors: (constant), length (cm), gender re-coded.

In the ANOVA table, the regression mean square decreases from 101.119 in Model 1 to 54.617 in Model 2 when gender is added because more of the unexplained variation is now explained. With high F values, both models are clearly significant as expected.

In the Coefficients table, the standard error around the beta coefficient for length remains at 0.007 in both models indicating that the model is stable. An increase of more than 10% in a standard error indicates multicollinearity between the variables in the model and the variable being added.

Coefficients[a]

Model		Unstandardized coefficients		Standardized coefficients		
		B	Std. error	Beta	t	Sig.
1	(Constant)	−5.412	0.0411		−13.167	0.000
	Length (cm)	0.178	0.007	0.713	23.813	0.000
2	(Constant)	−4.563	0.412		−11.074	0.000
	Length (cm)	0.165	0.007	0.660	22.259	0.000
	Gender re-coded	−0.251	0.036	−0.209	−7.039	0.000

[a]Dependent variable: weight (kg).

Wiith two explanatory variables in the model, the regression line will be of the form of $y = a + b_1 x_1 + b_2 x_2$, where x_1 is length and x_2 is gender. Substituting the variables and the unstandardized coefficients from the Coefficients table, the equation for model is as follows:

$$\text{Weight} = -4.563 + (0.165 \times \text{Length}) - (0.251 \times \text{Gender})$$

Because males are coded zero, the final term in the equation is removed for males. The term for gender indicates that, after adjusting for length, females are 0.251 kg lighter than males. In effect this means that the y intercept is −4.563 for males and −4.814 (i.e. −4.563 − 0.251) for females. Thus, the lines for males and females are parallel but females have a lower y-axis intercept.

The unstandardized coefficients cannot be directly compared to assess their relative importance because they are in the original units of the measurements. However, the standardized coefficients indicate the relative importance of each variable in comparable standardized units (z scores). The Coefficients table shows that length with a standardized coefficient of 0.660 is a more significant predictor of weight than gender with a standardized coefficient of 0.209. As with an R value, the negative sign is an indication of the direction of effect only. The standardized coefficients give useful additional information because they show that although both predictors have the same P values, they are not of equal importance in predicting weight.

The Excluded Variables table shows the model with gender omitted. The 'Beta ln' is the standardized coefficient that would result if gender is included in the model and is identical to the standardized coefficient in the Coefficients table above. The partial correlation is the unique contribution of gender to predicting weight after the effect of length is removed and is an estimate of the relative importance of this predictive variable in isolation from length. The collinearity statistic tolerance is close to 1 indicating that the predictor variables are not closely related to one another and that the regression assumption of independence between predictive variables is not violated.

Excluded Variables[a]

Model	Beta In	t	Sig.	Partial correlation	Collinearity statistics Tolerance
1 Gender re-coded	−0.209[b]	−7.039	0.000	−0.288	0.936

[a]Dependent variable: weight (kg).
[b]Predictors in the model: (constant), length (cm).

7.3.6 *Plotting a regression line with one categorical explanatory variables*

To plot a regression equation, it is important to ascertain the range of the explanatory variable values because the line should never extend outside the absolute range of the data. To obtain the minimum and maximum values of length for males and females the SPSS commands *Analyze → Compare Means → Means* can be used with length as the dependent variable and gender2 as the independent variable, and *Options* clicked to request minimum and maximum values. This provides the information that the length of male babies ranges from 50 to 62 cm and that the length of female babies ranges from 48 to 60.5 cm.

Table 7.4 shows how an Excel spreadsheet can be used to compute the coordinates for the beginning and end of the regression line for each gender. The regression coefficients from the equation are entered in the first three columns, and the minimum and maximum values for length and indicators of gender are entered in the next two columns. The predicted weight is then calculated using the equation of the regression line and the calculation function in Excel.

Table 7.4   Excel spreadsheet to calculate regression line coordinates

Column 1 a	Column 2 b1	Column 3 b2	Column 4 length	Column 5 gender2	Column 6 predicted weight
−4.563	0.165	−0.251	50	0	3.687
−4.563	0.165	−0.251	62	0	5.667
−4.563	0.165	−0.251	48	1	3.106
−4.563	0.165	−0.251	60.5	1	5.169

The line coordinates from columns 4 and 6 can be copied and pasted into SigmaPlot to draw the graph using the commands shown in Box 7.9. The SigmaPlot spreadsheet should have the lower and upper coordinates for males in columns 1 and 2 and the lower and upper coordinates for females in columns 3 and 4 as follows:

Column 1	Column 2	Column 3	Column 4
50.0	3.69	48.0	3.11
62.0	5.67	60.5	5.17

Box 7.9 SigmaPlot commands to plot regression lines

SigmaPlot commands

Data 1*
  Click on Create Graph tab at top of the screen
  Click on Line in sub-menu
  Click on Simple Straight Line in Line Group
Create Graph – Data Format
  Data format = Highlight 'XY Pair', click Next
Create Graph – Select Data
  Highlight Column 1, click into Data for X
  Highlight Column 2, click into Data for Y
  Click Finish

The second line for females can be added using *Graph Page → Add Plot* and using the same command sequence shown in Box 7.9, except that the *Data for X* is column 3 and the *Data for Y* is column 4. The resulting graph can then be customized using the many options in *Graph Page*. The completed graph shown in Figure 7.5 is a method for presenting summary results in a way that shows the relationship between weight and length and the size of the difference between the genders.

7.3.7 Regression models with two explanatory categorical variables

Having established the relationship between weight, length and gender, the re-coded binary variable parity2 can be added to the model. Using the commands shown in Box 7.8, length and gender re-coded can be added as independent variables into Block 1 of 1 and parity re-coded (binary) as an independent variable into Block 2 of 2 to obtain the following output.

The Model Summary table shows that adding parity to the model improves the adjusted R square value only slightly from 0.548 in Model 1 to 0.556 in Model 2, and that is, 55.6% of the variation is now explained. However, the Change Statistics with P value less than 0.05 indicates that this small increase is significant.

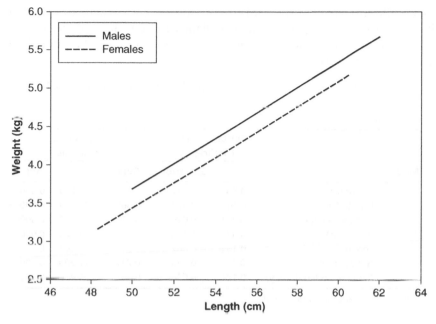

Figure 7.5 Equations for predicting weight at 1 month of age in term babies.

Regression

Model Summary

Model	R	R square	Adjusted R square	Std. error of the estimate	Change statistics				
					R square change	F change	df1	df2	Sig. F change
1	0.741[a]	0.549	0.548	0.40474	0.549	333.407	2	547	0.000
2	0.747[b]	0.559	0.556	0.40088	0.009	11.597	1	546	0.001

[a]Predictors: (constant), gender re-coded, length (cm).
[b]Predictors: (constant), gender re-coded, length (cm), parity re-coded (binary).

In the ANOVA table, the mean square decreases from 54.617 in Model 1 to 37.033 in Model 2 because more of the unexplained variation is now explained.

ANOVA[a]

Model		Sum of squares	df	Mean square	F	Sig.
1	Regression	109.235	2	54.617	333.407	0.000[b]
	Residual	89.607	547	0.164		
	Total	198.842	549			
2	Regression	111.098	3	37.033	230.443	0.000[c]
	Residual	87.744	546	0.161		
	Total	198.842	549			

[a]Dependent variable: weight (kg).
[b]Predictors: (constant), gender re-coded, length (cm).
[c]Predictors: (constant), gender re-coded, length (cm), parity re-coded (binary).

In the Coefficients table, the standard error for length remains at 0.007 in both models and the standard error for gender decreases slightly from 0.036 in Model 1 to 0.035 in Model 2 indicating that the model is stable. The unstandardized coefficients indicate that the equation for the regression model is now as follows:

$$\text{Weight} = -4.572 + (0.164 \times \text{Length}) - (0.255 \times \text{Gender}) + (0.124 \times \text{Parity})$$

Coefficients[a]

Model		Unstandardized coefficients		Standardized coefficients		
		B	Std. error	Beta	t	Sig.
1	(Constant)	−4.563	0.412		−11.074	0.000
	Length (cm)	0.165	0.007	0.660	22.259	0.000
	Gender re-coded	−0.251	0.036	−0.209	−7.039	0.000
2	(Constant)	−4.572	0.408		−11.203	0.000
	Length (cm)	0.164	0.007	0.655	22.262	0.000
	Gender re-coded	−0.255	0.035	−0.212	−7.200	0.000
	Parity re-coded (binary)	0.124	0.036	0.097	3.405	0.001

[a]Dependent variable: weight (kg).

When parity status is singleton, that is, parity equals zero, the final term of the regression equation will return a zero value and will therefore be removed for singleton babies. Therefore, the model indicates that, after adjusting for length and gender, babies who have siblings are on average 0.124 kg heavier than singleton babies.

The standardized coefficients in the Coefficients table show that length and gender are more significant predictors than parity in that their standardized coefficients are larger. These coefficients give a useful estimate of the size of effect of each variable when, as in this case, the P values are similar.

Excluded Variables[a]

Model		Beta in	t	Sig.	Partial correlation	Collinearity statistics Tolerance
1	Parity re-coded (binary)	0.097[b]	3.405	0.001	0.144	0.997

[a]Dependent variable: weight (kg).
[b]Predictors in the model: (constant), gender re-coded, length (cm).

The Excluded Variables table shows that tolerance remains high at 0.997 indicating that there is no collinearity between variables.

7.3.8   Plotting regression lines with two explanatory categorical variables

The regression lines plotted for a single binary explanatory variable are shown in Figure 7.5. To include the second binary explanatory variable of sibling status in the graph, two line coordinates are computed for each of the four groups, that is males

Table 7.5   Excel spreadsheet for calculating coordinates for regression lines with two binary explanatory variables

| | | | | | | | Column 8 |
| Column 1 | Column 2 | Column 3 | Column 4 | Column 5 | Column 6 | Column 7 | predicted |
a	b1	b2	b3	length	gender2	parity2	weight
-4.572	0.164	-0.255	0.124	50	0	0	3.63
-4.572	0.164	-0.255	0.124	62	0	0	5.60
-4.572	0.164	-0.255	0.124	49	1	0	3.21
-4.572	0.164	-0.255	0.124	58.5	1	0	4.77
-4.572	0.164	-0.255	0.124	50	0	1	3.75
-4.572	0.164	-0.255	0.124	62	0	1	5.72
-4.572	0.164	-0.255	0.124	48	1	1	3.17
-4.572	0.164	-0.255	0.124	60.5	1	1	5.22

with no siblings; males with one or more siblings; females with no siblings and females with one or more siblings. To obtain the minimum and maximum values for each of these groups, the data can be split by gender using the *Split File* command shown in Box 4.8 and then the SPSS commands *Analyze → Compare Means → Means* can be used with length as the dependent variable and parity2 as the independent variable and *Options* clicked to request minimum and maximum values.

Again, Excel can be used to calculate the regression coordinates using the regression equation and with an indicator for parity included in an additional column. The Excel spreadsheet from Table 7.5 and the commands from Box 7.9 can be used to plot the figure in SigmaPlot with additional lines included using *Add Plot* under *Graph Page.*

The coordinates from columns 5 and 8 can be copied and pasted into SigmaPlot and then split and rearranged to form the following spreadsheet of line coordinates.

Line 1 − X	Line 1 − Y	Line 2 − X	Line 2 − Y	Line 3 − X	Line 3 − Y	Line 4 − X	Line 4 − Y
50.0	3.63	49.0	3.21	50.0	3.75	48.0	3.17
62.0	5.60	58.5	4.77	62.0	5.72	60.5	5.22

The SigmaPlot commands shown in Box 7.9 but with *Multiple Straight Lines* selected under the *Line Group* sub-menu can be used to draw the four regression lines as shown in Figure 7.6. Plotting the lines is a useful method to indicate the size of the differences in weight between the four groups.

7.3.9   Including multi-level categorical variables

The previous model includes categorical variables with only two levels, that is, binary explanatory variables. A categorical explanatory variable with three or more levels can also be included in a regression model but first needs to be transformed into a series of

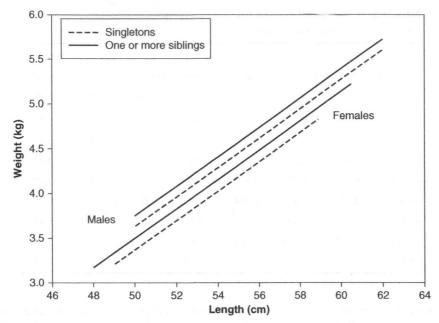

Figure 7.6 Regression lines by gender and parity status for predicting weight at 1 month of age in term babies.

binary variables. Simply adding a variable with three or more levels would produce a regression coefficient that indicates the effect for each level of the variable. If the effects for each level are unequal, the regression assumption that there is an equal (linear) effect across each level of the variable will be violated. Thus, multi-level categorical variables can be used only when there is a linearity of effect over the categories. This assumption of linearity is not required for ANOVA.

7.3.10 Dummy variables

When there are different effects across three or more levels of a variable, the problem of non-linearity can be resolved by creating dummy variables, which are also called indicator variables. It is not possible to include a dummy variable for each level of the variable because the dummy variables would lack independence and create multicollinearity. Therefore for k levels of a variable, there will be $k-1$ dummy variables, for example, for a variable with three levels, two dummy variables will be created. It is helpful in interpreting the results if each dummy variable has a binary coding of 0 or 1.

The variable parity1 with three levels from Chapter 5, that is parity coded as babies with 0, 1 or 2 or more siblings, can be recoded into dummy variables using *Transform → Recode into Different Variables.*

parityd1: Old Value = 1 → New Value = 1 (1 sibling)(same value as previously)
 Old Value: All other values → New Value = 0
parityd2: Old Value = 2 → New Value = 1 (2 or more siblings)
 Old Value: All other values → New Value = 0

Clearly a dummy variable for singletons is not required because if the values of parityd1 and parityd2 are both coded 0, the case is singleton. Dummy variables are invaluable for testing the effects of ordered groups that are likely to be different, for example, lung function in groups of non-smokers, ex-smokers and current smokers. It is essential that dummy variables are used when groups are non-ordered; for example, when marital status is categorized as single, married or divorced.

Using the SPSS commands shown in Box 7.8, length and gender2 can be added into the model as independent variables into Block 1 of 1 and the dummy variables parityd1 and parityd2 added in Block 2 of 2. Related dummy variables must always be included in a model together because they cannot be treated independently. If one dummy variable is significant in the model and a related dummy variable is not, they must both be left in the model together.

In the Model Summary table, the adjusted R square value shows that the addition of the dummy variables for parity improves the fit of the model only slightly from 0.548 to 0.556, that is, by 0.8%.

Model Summary

Model	R	R square	Adjusted R square	Std. error of the estimate	Change statistics				
					R square change	F change	df1	df2	Sig. F change
1	0.741[a]	0.549	0.548	0.40474	0.549	333.407	2	547	0.000
2	0.748[b]	0.559	0.556	0.40109	0.010	5.996	2	545	0.003

[a]Predictors: (constant), gender re-coded, length (cm).
[b]Predictors: (constant), gender re-coded, length (cm), dummy variable – parity = 1, dummy parity – parity ≥ 2.

In the Coefficients table, the P values for the unstandardized coefficients show that both dummy variables are significant predictors of weight with P values of 0.008 and 0.001, respectively. However, the low standardized coefficients and the small partial correlations in the Excluded Variables table show that the dummy variables contribute little to the model compared to length and gender.

Coefficients[a]

Model		Unstandardized coefficients		Standardized coefficients		
		B	Std. error	Beta	t	Sig.
1	(Constant)	−4.563	0.412		−11.074	0.000
	Length (cm)	0.165	0.007	0.660	22.259	0.000
	Gender re-coded	−0.251	0.036	−0.209	−7.039	0.000
2	(Constant)	−4.557	0.409		−11.144	0.000
	Length (cm)	0.164	0.007	0.654	22.182	0.000
	Gender re-coded	−0.255	0.035	−0.212	−7.216	0.000
	Dummy variable – parity = 1	0.111	0.042	0.088	2.678	0.008
	Dummy variable – parity ≥ 2	0.138	0.043	0.108	3.249	0.001

[a]Dependent variable: weight (kg).

Excluded variables[a]

Model		Beta In	t	Sig.	Partial correlation	Collinearity statistics tolerance
1	Dummy variable – parity = 1	0.034[b]	1.188	0.236	0.051	0.999
	Dummy parity – parity ≥ 2	0.063[b]	2.183	0.029	0.093	0.994

[a]Dependent variable: weight (kg).
[b]Predictors in the model: (constant), gender re-coded, length (cm).

Using the values in the Coefficients table, the regression equation is now as follows:

$$\text{Weight} = -4.557 + (0.164 \times \text{Length}) - (0.255 \times \text{Gender}) + (0.111 \times \text{Parityd1})$$
$$+ (0.138 \times \text{Parityd2})$$

Because of the binary coding used, the final two terms in the model are rendered zero for singletons because both dummy variables are coded zero. The coefficients for the final two terms indicate that after adjusting for length and gender, babies with one sibling are on average 0.111 kg heavier than singletons, and babies with two or more siblings are on average 0.138 kg heavier than singletons.

7.3.11 Multiple linear regression with two continuous variables and two categorical variables

Any combination of continuous and categorical explanatory variables can be included in a multiple linear regression model. The previous regression model with one continuous and two categorical variables, that is, length, gender and parity, can be further extended with the addition of second continuous explanatory variable, that is, head circumference.

Research question

Using the file **weights.sav,** the research question can be extended to examine whether head circumference contributes to the prediction of weight in 1 month-old babies after adjusting for length, gender and parity. The final predictive equation could be used to generate normal values for term babies, to calculate z scores for babies' weights, or to calculate per cent predicted weights.

Model Summary

Model	R	R square	Adjusted R square	Std. error of the estimate	Change statistics R square change	F change	df1	df2	Sig. F change
1	0.747[a]	0.559	0.556	0.40088	0.559	230.443	3	546	0.000
2	0.772[b]	0.596	0.593	0.38406	0.037	49.864	1	545	0.000

[a]Predictors: (constant), parity re-coded (binary), gender re-coded, length (cm).
[b]Predictors: (constant), parity re-coded (binary), gender re-coded, length (cm), head circumference (cm).

The regression model obtained previously can be built on to test the influence of the variable, head circumference. The model in which parity2 was included as a binary variable is used because including parity with three levels coded as dummy variables did not substantially improve the fit of the model. Using the SPSS commands shown in Box 7.8, length, gender2 and parity2 can be added in Block 1 of 1 and head circumference in Block 2 of 2 to generate the following output.

The Model Summary table shows that the adjusted R square increases slightly from 55.6 to 59.3% with the addition of head circumference. The Change Statistics indicates that the increase in R^2 from Model 1 to Model 2 is significant. In the Coefficients table, all predictors are significant and the standardized coefficients show that length contributes to the model to a greater degree than head circumference, but that head circumference makes a larger contribution than gender or parity.

Coefficients[a]

Model		Unstandardized coefficients		Standardized coefficients		
		B	Std. error	Beta	t	Sig.
1	(Constant)	4.572	0.408		-11.203	0.000
	Length (cm)	0.164	0.007	0.655	22.262	0.000
	Gender re-coded	-0.255	0.035	-0.212	-7.200	0.000
	Parity re-coded (binary)	0.124	0.036	0.097	3.405	0.001
2	(Constant)	6.890	0.511		-13.496	0.000
	Length (cm)	0.130	0.009	0.520	15.243	0.000
	Gender re-coded	-0.196	0.035	-0.163	-5.624	0.000
	Parity re-coded (binary)	0.093	0.035	0.073	2.638	0.009
	Head circumference (cm)	0.110	0.016	0.249	7.061	0.000

[a]Dependent variable: weight (kg).

However, the tolerance statistic in the Excluded Variables has fallen to 0.598 indicating some collinearity in the model. This is expected because the initial Pearson's correlations showed a significant association between length and head circumference with an r value of 0.598. As a result of the mutlicollinearity, the standard error for length has inflated from 0.007 in Model 1 to 0.009 in Model 2, a 29% increase. The benefit of explaining an extra 3.7% of the variation in length has to be balanced with this loss of precision.

Excluded Variables[a]

Model		Beta In	t	Sig.	Partial Correlation	Collinearity statistics Tolerance
1	Head circumference (cm)	0.249[b]	7.061	0.000	0.290	0.598

[a]Dependent variable: weight (kg).
[b]Predictors in the Model: (constant), parity re-coded (binary), gender re-coded, length (cm).

Deciding which variables to include in a model can be difficult. Head circumference is expected to vary with length as a result of common factors that influence body size and growth. In this situation, head circumference should be classified as an alternative outcome rather than an independent explanatory variable because it is on the same developmental pathway as length. Each model building situation will be different but it is important that the relationships between the variables and the purpose of building the model are always carefully considered.

7.4   Interactions

An interaction occurs when there is a multiplicative rather than additive relationship between two explanatory variables, that is, when the effect of one explanatory variable depends on the value of another variable. Interactions can occur between continuous and categorical variables. An additive effect of a binary variable was shown in Figure 7.5 where the lines for each gender had the same slopes so that they were parallel. If an interactive effect is present, the two lines would have different slopes and would cross over or intersect at some point.

To test for the presence of an interaction, the two variables are multiplied to create a cross-product term, which is included in the multiple regression model. In the following equation, the fourth term represents an interaction between length and gender. Also, once again, coding of binary variables as 0 and 1 is helpful for interpreting interactions. The last two terms in the model will be zero when gender is coded 0. When gender is coded as 1, the third term will add a fixed amount to the prediction of the outcome variable and the fourth interactive term will add an amount that increases as length increases, thereby causing the regression lines for each gender to increasingly diverge. The regression equation for a model with an interaction term would be as follows:

$$\text{Weight} = a + (b_1 \times \text{Length}) + (b_2 \times \text{Gender}) + (b_3 \times \text{Length} \times \text{Gender})$$

It is preferable to explore evidence that an interaction is present rather than testing for all possible interactions in the model. Testing for all interactions will almost certainly generate some spurious but significant P values.[11] Interactions naturally introduce mulitcollinearity into the model because the interaction term correlates with both of its derivatives. This will result in an unstable model, especially when the sample size is small. To avoid multicollinearity, the explanatory variables and their interaction can be centered before inclusion in the regression model,[7] which will be discussed later in this chapter.

7.4.1   Identifying interactions

Interactions between variables can be identified by plotting the dependent variable against the explanatory variable for each group within a factor. The regression plots can then be inspected to assess whether there is a different linear relationship across the groups. By using the SPSS *Split File* option with groups based in gender (see Box 4.8) and the commands shown in Box 7.7 and not requesting Confidence Intervals, the plots shown in Figures 7.7 and 7.8 can be obtained.

The regression equations for weight and length shown in Figure 7.7 indicate that the y intercept is different for males and females as expected from the former regression equations. When the values of the data points are a long way from zero, as in these plots,

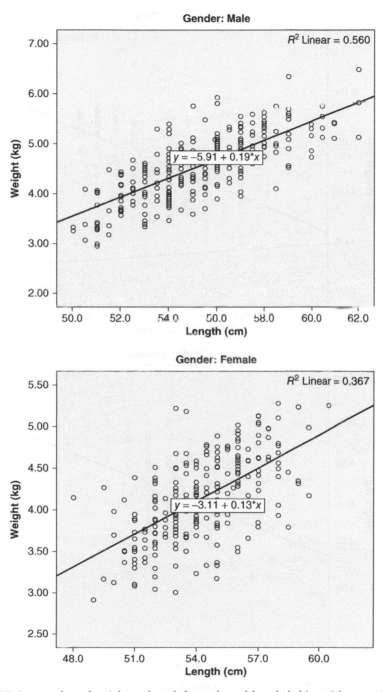

Figure 7.7 Scatter plots of weight on length for male and female babies with regression line.

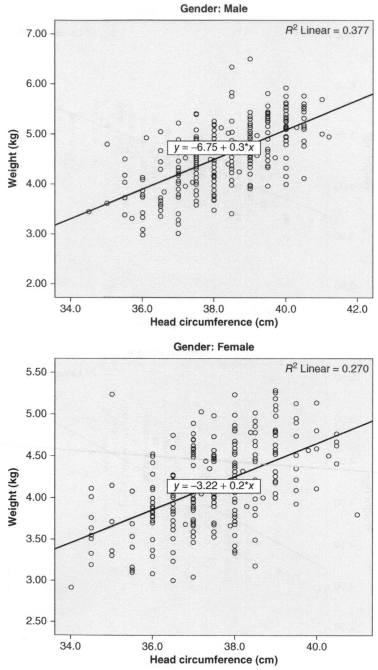

Figure 7.8 Scatter plots of weight on head circumference for male and female babies with regression line.

the y intercepts have no meaningful interpretation although they can indicate that the slopes are different. However, the slope of the line through the points is similar at 0.19 for males and 0.13 for females. This similarity of slopes suggests that there is no important interaction between length and gender in predicting weight. The graphs can be repeated to investigate a possible interaction between head circumference and gender.

The plots for weight and head circumference shown in Figure 7.8 indicate that the intercept is different between the genders at −6.75 for males and −3.22 for females. Moreover, the slope of 0.30 for males is 50% higher than the slope of 0.20 for females as shown by the different slopes of the regression lines through the plots. If plotted on the same figure, the two regression lines would intersect at some point indicating an interaction between head circumference and gender.

7.4.2 Including interactions in the model

The interaction term can be computed for inclusion in the model as shown in Box 7.10. In practice, head circumference would be omitted from the model because of its collinearity with length but it is included in this model solely for demonstrating the effect of an interaction term. The model is obtained using the commands shown in Box 7.8 and by adding length, gender2, parity2 and head circumference into Block 1 of 1 and the interaction term headxgen into Block 2 of 2.

Box 7.10 SPSS command to compute an interaction term

SPSS Commands

weights.sav – IBM SPSS Statistics Data Editor
      Transform → Compute Variable
Compute Variable
      Target Variable = headxgen
      Numeric Expression = Head circumference*Gender recoded
      Click OK

The Model Summary table shows that the interaction term only slightly improves the fit of the model by increasing the adjusted R square from 0.593 to 0.597. The Change Statistics columns indicate that this increase is significant.

Model Summary

Model	R	R square	Adjusted R square	Std. error of the estimate	R square change	F change	$df1$	$df2$	Sig. F change
					Change Statistics				
1	0.772[a]	0.596	0.593	0.38406	0.596	200.766	4	545	0.000
2	0.775[b]	0.601	0.597	0.38211	0.005	6.587	1	544	0.011

[a]Predictors: (constant), head circumference (cm), parity re-coded (binary), gender re-coded, length (cm).
[b]Predictors: (constant), head circumference (cm), parity re-coded (binary), gender re-coded, length (cm), head by gender interaction.

In the Coefficients table, the interaction term in Model 2 is significant with a P value of 0.011 and therefore must be included because it helps to describe the true relationship between weight, head circumference and gender. If an interaction term is included then both derivative variables, that is, head circumference and gender, must be retained in the model regardless of their statistical significance. Once an interaction is present, the coefficients for the derivative variables have no interpretation except that they form an integral part of the mathematical equation.

Coefficients[a]

Model		Unstandardized coefficients		Standardized coefficients		
		B	Std. error	Beta	t	Sig.
1	(Constant)	−6.890	0.511		−13.496	0.000
	Length (cm)	0.130	0.009	0.520	15.243	0.000
	Gender recoded	−0.196	0.035	−0.163	−5.624	0.000
	Parity recoded (binary)	0.093	0.035	0.073	2.638	0.009
	Head circumference (cm)	0.110	0.016	0.249	7.061	0.000
2	(Constant)	−8.086	0.689		−11.731	0.000
	Length (cm)	0.128	0.009	0.512	15.034	0.000
	Gender recoded	2.282	0.966	1.898	2.362	0.019
	Parity recoded (binary)	0.093	0.035	0.073	2.651	0.008
	Head circumference (cm)	0.144	0.020	0.326	7.063	0.000
	Head by gender interaction	−0.065	0.025	−2.040	−2.567	0.011

[a]Dependent variable: weight (kg).

The Coefficients table shows that inclusion of the interaction term inflates the standard error for head circumference from 0.016 in Model 1 to 0.02 in Model 2 and significantly inflates the standard error for gender from 0.035 to 0.966. These standard errors have inflated as a result of the collinearity with the interaction term and, as a result, the tolerance value in the Excluded Variables table is very low and unacceptable at 0.001, also a sign of mutlicollinearity. In addition, while the change in R square from Model 1 to Model 2 was significant, it is important to assess the clinical significance of this increase, in conjunction with a less precise model. This example highlights the trade-off between building a stable predictive model and deriving an equation that describes an interaction between variables. Multicollinearity caused by interactions can be removed by centering[12] which is described later in this chapter.

Excluded Variables[a]

Model		Beta In	t	Sig.	Partial Correlation	Collinearity Statistics Tolerance
1	Head by gender interaction	−2.040[b]	−2.567	.011	−.109	.001

[a]Dependent variable: weight (kg)
[b]Predictors in the model: (constant), head circumference (cm), parity re-coded (binary), gender re-coded, length (cm).

The final model with all variables and the interaction term included could be considered to be over-fitted. By including variables that explain little additional variation and by including the interaction term, the model not only becomes complex but the precision around the estimates is sacrificed and the regression assumptions of independence are violated. Head circumference should be omitted because of its relation with length and because it explains only a small additional amount of variation in weight. Thus, the interaction term is also omitted. The final model with only length, gender and parity is parsimonious. Once the final model is reached, the remaining regression assumptions should be confirmed.

7.5   Residuals

The residuals are the distances between each data point and the value predicted by the regression equation, that is, the variation about the regression line shown in Figure 7.2. The residual distances are converted to standardized residuals that are in units of standard deviations from the regression. Standardized residuals are assumed to have a normal or approximately normal distribution with a mean of zero and a standard deviation of 1

Given the characteristics of a normal distribution, it is expected that 5% of standardized residuals will be outside the area that lies between −1.96 and +1.96 standard deviations from the mean (see Figure 2.1). In addition, 1% of standardized residuals are expected to lie outside the area between −3 and +3 standard deviations from the mean.

As the sample size increases, there will be an increasing number of potential outliers. In this sample size of 550 babies, it is expected that five children will have a standardized residual that will be outside the area that lies between −3 and +3 standard deviations from the mean.

An assumption of regression is that the residuals are normally distributed. The residual for each case can be saved to a data column using the *Save* option and the plots of the residuals can be obtained while running the model as shown in Box 7.11. The normality of the residuals can then be inspected using *Analyze → Descriptive Statistics → Explore* as discussed in Chapter 2.

Box 7.11 SPSS commands to test the regression assumptions

SPSS Commands

weights.sav – IBM SPSS Statistics Data Editor
        Analyze → Regression → Linear
Linear Regression
        Highlight Weight, click into the Dependent box
        Highlight Length, Gender recoded, Parity recoded (binary), click into the
            Independent(s) box
        Click on Statistics
Linear Regression: Statistics
        Under Regression Coefficients, tick Estimates (default)
        Tick Model fit (default) and Collinearity diagnostics

> *Under Residuals, tick Casewise diagnostics – Outliers outside 3 standard deviations*
> *(default), click Continue*
> *Linear Regression*
> * Click Plots*
> *Linear Regression: Plots*
> * Under Scatter 1 of 1, highlight *ZPRED and click into X; highlight*
> *   *ZRESID and click into Y*
> * Under Standardized Residual Plots, tick Histogram and Normal probability plot*
> * Click Continue*
> *Linear Regression*
> * Click on Save*
> *Linear Regression: Save*
> * Under Predicted Values, tick Standardized*
> * Under Residuals, tick Standardized*
> * Under Distances, tick Mahalanobis, Cook's and Leverage values*
> * Click Continue*
> *Linear Regression*
> * Click OK*

The Coefficients table shows the variables in the model and the high-tolerance values confirm their lack of multicollinearity. The Casewise Diagnostics table shows the cases that are more than three standard deviations from the regression line. There is only one case that has a standardized residual that is more than three standard deviations from the regression, that is, the baby with a weight of 5.23 kg compared with a predicted value of 3.9783 kg and with a standardized residual of 3.122.

Regression

Coefficients[a]

Model		Unstandardized coefficients		Standardized coefficients			Collinearity statistics	
		B	Std. error	Beta	t	Sig.	Tolerance	VIF
1	(Constant)	−4.572	0.408		−11.203	0.000		
	Length (cm)	0.164	0.007	0.655	22.262	0.000	0.933	1.071
	Gender recoded	−0.255	0.035	−0.212	−7.200	0.000	0.935	1.069
	Parity recoded	0.124	0.036	0.097	3.405	0.001	0.997	1.003

[a]Dependent variable: weight (kg).

Casewise diagnostics[a]

Case number	Std. residual	Weight (kg)	Predicted value	Residual
404	3.122	5.23	3.9783	1.25169

[a]Dependent variable: weight (kg)

The Residuals Statistics table shows the minimum and maximum predicted values. The predicted values range from 3.159 to 5.707 kg and the unstandardized residuals range from 1.079 kg below the regression line to 1.252 kg above the regression line. This is the minimum and maximum distances of babies from the equation, which is the variation about the regression.

Residuals Statistics[a]

	Minimum	Maximum	Mean	Std. Deviation	N
Predicted value	3.1594	5.7069	4.3664	.44985	550
Std. predicted value	−2.683	2.980	0.000	1.000	550
Standard error of predicted value	0.027	0.060	0.034	0.006	550
Adjusted predicted value	3.1413	5.7047	4.3665	.44988	550
Residual	−1.07912	1.25169	0.00000	.39978	550
Std. residual	−2.692	3.122	0.000	.997	550
Stud. residual	−2.706	3.130	0.000	1.001	550
Deleted residual	−1.09043	1.25807	-.00008	.40276	550
Stud. deleted residual	−2.722	3.156	.000	1.003	550
Mahal. distance	1.469	11.372	2.995	1.529	550
Cook's distance	0.000	0.028	0.002	0.003	550
Centered leverage value	0.003	0.021	0.005	0.003	550

[a]Dependent variable: weight (kg).

The standardized predicted values and standardized residuals shown in the Residuals Statistics table are expressed in units of their standard deviation and have a mean of zero and a standard deviation of approximately or equal to 1, as expected when they are normally distributed.

The histogram and normal P–P plot shown in Figure 7.9 indicate that the distribution of the residuals deviates only slightly from a classically bell-shaped distribution.

The variance around the residuals can also be used to test whether the model violates the assumption of homoscedasticity, that is, equal variance over the length of the regression model. Residual plots are a good method for examining the spread of variance. The scatter plot in Figure 7.9 shows that there is an equal spread of residuals across the predicted values indicating that the model is homoscedastic.

7.6 Outliers and remote points

Outliers are data points that are more than three standard deviations from the regression line. Outliers in regression are identified in a similar manner to outliers in ANOVA. Univariate outliers should be identified before fitting a model but multivariate outliers, if present, are identified once the model of best fit is obtained. Outliers that cause a poor fit degrade the predictive value of the regression model; however, this has to be balanced with loss of generalizability if the points are omitted.

Multivariate outliers are data values that have an extreme value on a combination of explanatory variables and exert too much leverage and/or discrepancy (see Chapter 5). Data points with high leverage and low discrepancy have no effect on the regression line but tend to increase the R square value and reduce the standard errors. On the other hand, data points with low leverage and high discrepancy tend to influence the

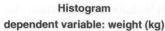

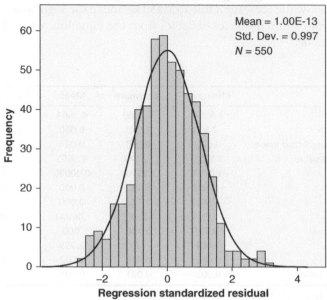

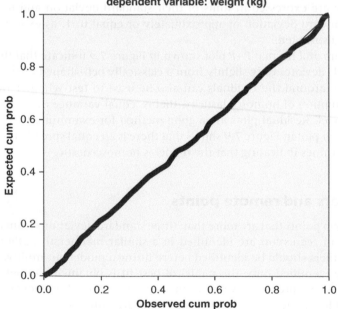

Figure 7.9 Histogram and plots of standardized residuals for regression on weight.

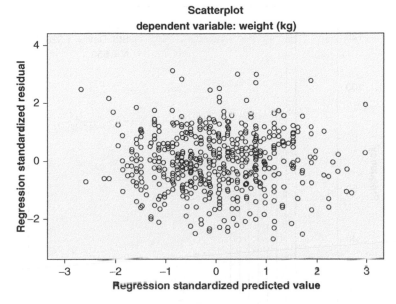

Figure 7.9 (*continued*)

intercept but not the slope of the regression or the R square value and tend to inflate the standard errors. Data points with both a high leverage and a high discrepancy influence the slope, the intercept and the R square value. Thus, a model that contains problematic data points with high leverage and/or high discrepancy values may not generalize well to the population.

Multivariate outliers can be identified using Cook's distances and leverage values as discussed in Chapter 5. The Residuals Statistics table shows that the largest Cook's distance is 0.028, which is below the critical value of 1, and the largest leverage value is 0.021, which is below the critical value of 0.05 indicating that there are no influential outliers in this model. In regression, Mahalanobis distances can also be inspected. Mahalanobis distances are evaluated using critical values of chi-square with degrees of freedom equal to the number of explanatory variables in the model. To adjust for the number of variables being tested, Mahalanobis distances are usually considered unacceptable at the $P < 0.001$ level, although the influence of any values with $P < 0.05$ should be examined.

To plot the Mahalanobis distances, which have been saved to a column at the end of the data sheet, the SPSS commands *Graphs → Histogram* can be used to obtain Figure 7.10. Any Mahalanobis distance that is greater than 16.266, that is, a chi-square value for $P < 0.001$ with three degrees of freedom (because there are three explanatory variables in the model), would be problematic. The graph shows that no Mahalanobis distances are larger than this. This is confirmed in the Residual Statistics table, which shows that the maximum Mahalanobis distance is 11.372.

If multivariate outliers are detected they can be deleted but it is not reasonable to remove troublesome data points simply to improve the fit of the model. In addition, when one extreme data point is removed another may take its place so it is important to

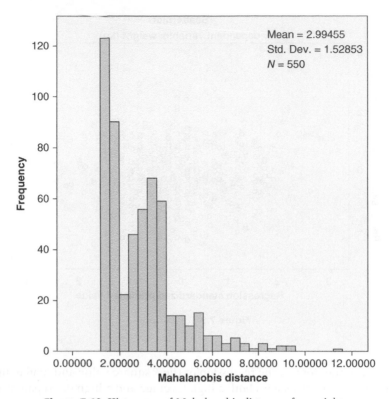

Figure 7.10 Histogram of Mahalanobis distances for weight.

recheck the data after deletion to ensure that there are no further multivariate outliers. Alternatively, the data can be transformed to reduce the influence of the multivariate outlier or the extreme data point can be re-coded to a less extreme value. However, a multivariate outlier depends on a combination of explanatory variables and therefore the scores would have to be adjusted for each variable. Any technique that is used to deal with multivariate outliers should be recorded in the study handbook and described in publications.

7.7 Validating the model

If the sample size is large enough, the model can be built using one-half of the data and then validated with the other half. If this is the purpose, the sample should be split randomly. Other selections of 60%–80% for building the model and 40–20% for validation can be used. A model built using one part of the data and validated using the other part of the data provides good evidence of stability and reliability. However, both models must have an adequate sample size and must conform to the assumptions for regression to minimize collinearity and maximize precision and stability.

7.8   Reporting a multiple linear regression

When reporting a multiple linear regression, a table is a concise and practical way to present the results. Information to include in a regression table are the unstandardized coefficients (95% CI) and corresponding standard errors, standardized beta coefficients, R^2 as a measure of a goodness of fit, the P values and the sample size.

In the research example, the most parsimonious model is the model with length, gender and parity as the significant predictive variables. With a hierarchical regression, this information should be reported at each step of the model as shown in Table 7.6. The R^2 for the initial model and the change in each step of the model in R^2 (represented by ΔR^2) is also reported. The 95% confidence intervals around the beta coefficients can be obtained by clicking on '*Statistics*' in the linear regression page and then ticking the option '*Confidence Intervals*' under the '*Regression Coefficients*' section. For gender, the beta coefficient shows the between-group difference after adjusting for length and parity. Similarly the beta coefficient for parity is the mean difference between babies with no siblings or one or more siblings after adjusting for length and gender.

In addition, information regarding how any outliers were dealt with, the method of entry used (e.g. stepwise) and for blockwise entry (or hierarchical), the reason why variables were selected to be entered into the model in that sequence should be reported. Also indicate whether the variables were tested for the presence of interactions and whether the model was validated.

Table 7.6   Reporting a hierarchical regression model with 3 explanatory variables

Predictor	*b* (95% CI)	SE B	β	*P* value
Step 1				
Intercept	−5.41 (−6.22, −4.61)	0.41		<0.0001
Length	0.18 (0.16, 0.19)	0.01	0.71	<0.0001
Step 2				
Intercept	−4.56 (−5.37, −3.75)	0.41		<0.0001
Length	0.17 (0.15, 0.18)	0.01	0.66	<0.0001
Gender[a]	−0.25 (−0.32, −0.18)	0.04	−0.21	<0.0001
Step 3				
Intercept	−4.57 (−5.37, −3.77)			
Length	0.16 (0.15, 0.18)		0.66	<0.0001
Gender[a]	−0.26 (−0.32, −0.19)		−0.21	<0.0001
Parity[b]	0.12 (0.05, 0.20)		0.10	0.001

Note. $R^2 = 0.71$ for step1; $\Delta R^2 = 0.04$ for step 2; $\Delta R^2 = 0.01$ for step 3.
[a] Coded 0 = male, 1 = female.
[b] Coded 0 = no siblings, 1 = 1 or more siblings.

7.9 Non-linear regression

If scatter plots suggest that there is a curved relationship between the explanatory and outcome variables, then a linear model may not be the best fit. Other non-linear models that may be more appropriate for describing the relationship can be examined using the SPSS commands shown in Box 7.12. Logarithmic, quadratic and exponential fits are the most common transformations used in medical research when data are skewed or when a relationship is not linear.

Box 7.12 SPSS commands for examining the equation that best fits data

SPSS Commands

weights.sav – IBM SPSS Statistics Data Editor
    Analyze → Regression → Curve Estimation
Curve Estimation
    Highlight Weight, click into Dependent(s) box
    Highlight Length, click into Independent Variable box
    Tick Include constant in equation (default) and Plot models (default)
    Under Models, tick Linear (default), Logarithmic, Quadratic and Exponential
    Click OK

In the Model Summary table, the Parameter Estimates for the Constant (the intercept) and the regression coefficients are reported. The equation of each model is as follows:

$$\text{Linear: } \text{Weight} = a + (b1 \times \text{Length})$$

$$\text{Logarithmic: } \text{Weight} = a + (b1 \times \log_e \text{Length})$$

$$\text{Quadratic: } \text{Weight} = a + (b_1 \times \text{Length}) + (b_2 \times \text{Length}^2)$$

$$\text{Exponential: } \text{Weight} = a + (b_1 \times e^{\text{length}})$$

Curve fit

Model Summary and Parameter Estimates
Dependent variable: weight (kg)

Equation	Model summary					Parameter estimates		
	R Square	F	df1	df2	Sig.	Constant	b1	b2
Linear	0.509	567.043	1	548	0.000	−5.412	0.178	
Logarithmic	0.508	566.399	1	548	0.000	−34.875	9.802	
Quadratic	0.509	283.034	2	547	0.000	−6.626	0.222	0.000
Exponential	0.503	555.229	1	548	0.000	0.458	0.041	

The independent variable is length (cm).

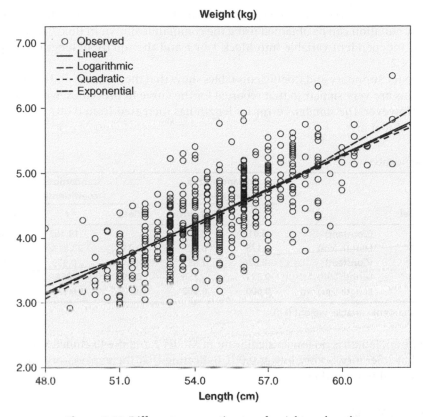

Figure 7.11 Different curve estimates of weight on length.

The R square values show that the linear and the quadratic models have the best fit with R square values of 0.509 closely followed by the logarithmic model with an R square of 0.508. The plots in Figure 7.11 show that the curves for the four models only deviate at the extremities of the data points, which are the regions in which prediction is less certain. Because the linear model is easier to communicate, in practice it would be the preferable model to use.

Model Summary

Model	R	R square	Adjusted R square	Std. error of the estimate	R square change	F change	$df1$	$df2$	Sig. F change
						Change statistics			
1	0.713[a]	0.509	0.508	0.42229	0.509	567.043	1	548	0.000
2	0.713[b]	0.509	0.507	0.42266	0.000	0.030	1	547	.863

[a]Predictors: (constant), length (cm).
[b]Predictors: (constant), length (cm), length squared.

If it was important to use the quadratic model, say to compare with other quadratic models in the literature, then the square of length can be computed as lensq using the

SPSS commands *Transform* → *Compute* using the formula lensq = length × length. The quadratic equation can be obtained using the commands shown in Box 7.8, with length added as independent variable into Block 1 of 1 and the square of length (lensq) into Block 2 of 2.

The Model Summary and Coefficients tables show that the R square and the regression coefficients are very similar to that reported for the curve fit procedure with a quadratic model. However, the standard error for length has increased from 0.007 in Model 1 to 0.256 in Model 2.

Coefficients[a]

Model		Unstandardized coefficients		Standardized coefficients		
		B	Std. error	Beta	t	Sig.
1	(Constant)	−5.412	0.411		−13.167	0.000
	Length (cm)	0.178	0.007	0.713	23.813	0.000
2	(Constant)	−6.626	7.053		−0.939	0.348
	Length (cm)	0.222	0.256	0.890	0.868	0.386
	Length squared	0.000	0.002	−0.177	−0.172	0.863

[a]Dependent variable: weight (kg).

In addition, length is no longer significant in Model 2 and the Excluded Variables table shows that tolerance is very low at 0.001 indicating that the explanatory variables are highly related to one other.

Excluded Variables[a]

Model		Beta In	t	Sig.	Partial Correlation	Collinearity Statistics Tolerance
1	Length squared	−0.177[b]	−0.172	0.863	−0.007	0..001

[a]Dependent variable: weight (kg).
[b]Predictors in the model: (constant), length (cm).

Collinearity can occur naturally when a quadratic term is included in a regression equation because the variable and its square are related. A scatter plot using the SPSS commands *Graphs* → *Legacy Dialogs* → *Scatter/Dot* → *Simple Scatter* to plot length squared against length demonstrates the direct relationship between the two variables as shown in Figure 7.12.

7.10   Centering

To avoid collinearity in quadratic equations, a mathematical solution of centering, that is, subtracting a constant from the data values, can be applied.[12] The constant that minimizes collinearity most effectively is the mean value of the variable. Using the following SPSS commands *Descriptive Statistics* → *Descriptives* shows that the mean of length is 54.841 cm. Using the commands *Transform* → *Compute* the mean value is used

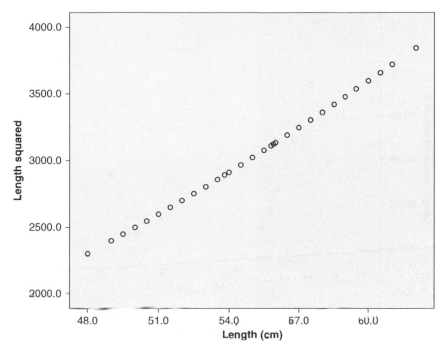

Figure 7.12 Scatter plot of length by length squared.

to compute a new variable for length centered (lencent) as 'length – 54.841' and then to compute another new variable, which is the square of lencent (lencntsq).

A scatter plot of length centered and its square in Figure 7.13 shows that the relationship is no longer linear simply because subtracting the mean value gives half of the values a negative value but then squaring all values returns a positive value again. The relation is thus U-shaped and no longer linear.

The regression can now be re-run using the commands shown in Box 7.8 but with length centered in Block 1 of 1 and its square in Block 2 of 2.

The Model Summary table shows that when length is centered, the adjusted R square value remains much the same from Model 1 to Model 2, with the Change Statistics also indicating no significant increase in the R value.

Model Summary

Model	R	R square	Adjusted R square	Std. error of the estimate	R square change	F change	$df1$	$df2$	Sig. F change
					Change statistics				
1	0.713[a]	0.509	0.508	0.42229	0.509	567.043	1	548	0.000
2	0.713[b]	0.509	0.507	0.42266	0.000	0.030	1	547	0.863

[a]Predictors: (constant), length centered.
[b]Predictors: (constant), length centered, length centered squared.

The Coefficients table shows the standard error for length is similar at 0.007 in Model 1 and 0.008 in Model 2. In addition, the unstandardized coefficients are now significant

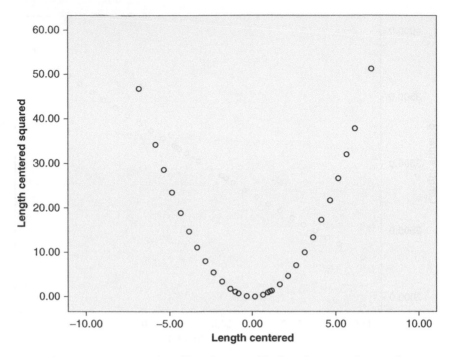

Figure 7.13 Scatter plot of length squared by length centered squared.

and the tolerance value is high at 0.973. The unstandardized coefficient for the square term is close to zero with a non-significant *P* value indicating its negligible contribution to the model. The equation for this regression model is as follows:

$$\text{Weight} = 4.369 + (0.179 \times (\text{Length} - 54.841) + (0.0001 \times (\text{Length} - 54.841)^2)$$

This centered model is a more stable quadratic model than the model given by the curve fit option and is therefore more reliable for predicting weight or for testing the effects of other factors on weight. However, length centered squared would not be included in the final regression model since it is not a significant predictor and is only reported here for illustrative purposes.

Coefficients[a]

Model		Unstandardized coefficients		Standardized coefficients		
		B	Std. error	Beta	t	Sig.
1	(Constant)	4.366	0.018		242.494	0.000
	Length centered	0.178	0.007	0.713	23.813	0.000
2	(Constant)	4.369	0.022		194.357	0.000
	Length centered	0.179	0.008	0.714	23.499	0.000
	Length centered squared	0.000	0.002	−0.005	−0.172	0.863

[a]Dependent variable: weight (kg).

The technique of centering can also be used to remove collinearity caused by interactions which are naturally related to their derivatives.[7]

Excluded Variables[a]

Model	Beta In	t	Sig.	Partial correlation	Collinearity statistics Tolerance
1 Length centered squared	−0.005[b]	−0.172	0.863	−0.007	0.973

[a]Dependent variable: weight (kg).
[b]Predictors in the model: (constant), length centered.

7.11   Notes for critical appraisal

When critically appraising a paper that reports simple or multiple linear regression analyses, the questions that should be asked are shown in Box 7.13.

Box 7.13 Questions to ask when critically appraising a regression analysis

The following questions should be asked when appraising published results from analyses in which regression has been used:
- Was the sample size large enough to justify using the model?
- Are the variables located on the correct axis, with the outcome on the y-axis and the explanatory variable on the x-axis?
- Were any repeated measures from the same participants treated as independent observations?
- Were all of the explanatory variables measured independently from the outcome variable?
- Have the explanatory variables been measured reliably?
- Is there any collinearity between the explanatory variables that could reduce the precision of the model?
- Are there any multivariate outliers that could influence the regression estimates?
- Is evidence presented that the residuals are normally distributed?
- Are there sufficient data at the extremities of the regression or should the prediction range be shortened?

References

1. Cohen, J. *Statistical power analysis for the behavioral sciences*, 2nd edn. Lawrence Erlbaum: NJ, 1988.
2. Peat J, Mellis C, Williams K, Xuan W. *Health science research: a handbook of quantitative methods*. Allen and Unwin: Crow's Nest, Sydney, 2001.
3. Simpson J, Berry G. Simple regression and correlation. In: Kerr C, Taylor R, Heard G, In: *Handbook of public health methods*. McGraw-Hill Companies Inc.: Roseville, Australia, 1998: 288–295.
4. Kachigan, SK. *Multivariate statistical analysis*, 2nd edn. Radius Press: New York, 1991.

5. Altman DG. *Practical statistics for medical research*. Chapman and Hall: London, 1991.

6. Stevens J. *Applied multivariate statistics for the social sciences*, 3rd edn. Lawrence Erlbaum Associates: Boston, MA, 1996.

7. Tabachnick BG, Fidell LS. *Using multivariate statistics*, 4th edn. Allyn and Bacon: Boston, MA, 2001.

8. Dupont WD, Plummer WD. Power and calculations for studies involving linear regression. *Control Clin Trials* 1998; **19**: 589–601.

9. Van Steen K, Curran D, Kramer J, Molenberghs G, Van Vreckem A, Bottomley A, Sylvester R. Multicollinearity in prognostic factor analyses using the EORTC QLQ-C30: identification and impact on model selection. *Stat Med* 2002; **21**: 3865–3884.

10. Vickers AJ, Altman DG. Analysing controlled trials with baseline and follow up measurements. *BMJ* 2001; **323**: 1123–1124.

11. Altman DG, Matthews JNS. Interaction 1: heterogeneity of effects. *BMJ* 1996; **313**: 486.

12. Kleinbaum DG, Kupper LL, Muller KE, Nizam A. *Applied regression analysis and other multivariable methods*. Duxbury Press: Pacific Grove, CA, 1998.

CHAPTER 8

Rates and proportions

When the methods of statistical inference were being developed in the first half of the twentieth century, calculations were done using pencil, paper, tables, slide rules and with luck a very expensive adding machine.[1]

MARTIN BLAND, STATISTICIAN

Objectives

The objectives of this chapter are to explain how to:
- use the correct summary statistics for rates and proportions
- present categorical baseline characteristics correctly
- crosstabulate categorical variables and obtain meaningful percentages
- conduct a test of chi-square and select the correct chi-square value
- plot percentages and interpret 95% confidence intervals
- manage cells with small numbers
- use trend tests for ordered exposure variables
- convert continuous variables with a non-normal distribution into categorical variables
- calculate the number needed to treat
- calculate significance and estimate effect size for paired categorical data
- calculate sample size requirements
- critically appraise the literature in which rates and proportions are reported

8.1 Summarizing categorical variables

Categorical variables are summarized using statistics called rates and proportions. A rate is a number used to express the frequency of a characteristic of interest in the population, such as 1 case per 10,000. In some cases, the rate is applied to a time period such as per annum. Frequencies can also be described using summary statistics such as a percentage, for example, 20% or a proportion, for example, 0.2. Rates, percentages and proportions are frequently used for summarizing information that is collected with forced choice response formats (e.g. tick box options) or Likert scales (e.g. disagree/neither agree or disagree/agree) on questionnaires.

Medical Statistics: A Guide to SPSS, Data Analysis and Critical Appraisal, Second Edition.
Belinda Barton and Jennifer Peat.
© 2014 John Wiley & Sons, Ltd. Published 2014 by John Wiley & Sons, Ltd.
Companion website: www.wiley.com/go/barton/medicalstatistics2e

Obtaining information about the distribution of the categorical variables in a study provides a good working knowledge of the characteristics of the sample. The spreadsheet **surgery.sav** contains data from a sample of 141 consecutive babies who were admitted to hospital to undergo surgery. The SPSS commands shown in Box 8.1 can be used to obtain frequencies and histograms for the categorical variables prematurity (1 = Premature; 2 = Term) and gender2 (1 = Male and 2 = Female). The frequencies for place of birth were obtained in Chapter 1.

Box 8.1 SPSS commands to obtain frequencies and histograms

SPSS Commands

surgery.sav – IBM SPSS Statistics Data Editor
   Analyze → Descriptive Statistics → Frequencies
Frequencies
   Highlight Prematurity and Gender recoded, click into Variable(s) box
   Click on Charts
Frequencies: Charts
   Chart Type: Tick Bar charts; Chart Values: Tick Frequencies (default) and click
   Continue
Frequencies
   Click Ok

Frequency table

Prematurity

		Frequency	Per cent	Valid per cent	Cumulative per cent
Valid	Premature	45	31.9	31.9	31.9
	Term	96	68.1	68.1	100.0
	Total	141	100.0	100.0	

Gender Recoded

		Frequency	Per cent	Valid per cent	Cumulative per cent
Valid	Male	82	58.2	58.2	58.2
	Female	59	41.8	41.8	100.0
	Total	141	100.0	100.0	

The valid per cent column in the first Frequency table indicates that 31.9% of babies in the sample were born prematurely and that 68.1% of babies in the sample were term births. The per cent and valid per cent columns are identical because all children in the sample have information of their birth status, that is, there are no missing data. In journal articles and scientific reports when the sample size is greater than 100, percentages such as these are reported with one decimal place only. When the sample size is less than 100, no decimal places are used. If the sample size was less than 20 participants, percentages would not be reported (see Chapter 1) although they are included on the SPSS output.

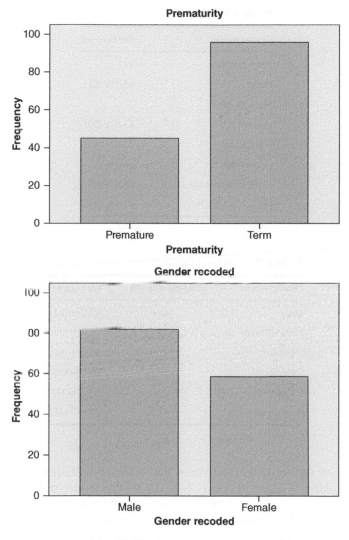

Figure 8.1 Number of babies by prematurity status and by gender.

The valid per cent column in the second Frequency table indicates that there are more males than females in the sample (58.2% vs 41.8%).

The bar charts shown in Figure 8.1 are helpful for comparing the frequencies visually and may be useful for a poster or a talk. However, these types of bar charts are not suitable for presenting sample characteristics in journal articles or other publications because accurate frequency information cannot be read from them and they are 'space hungry' for the relatively small amount of information provided.

8.2 Describing baseline characteristics

The baseline characteristics of the sample could be described as shown in Table 8.1 or Table 8.2. If the percentage of male children is included, it is not necessary to report

Table 8.1 Baseline characteristics

Characteristic	Per cent (n)
Total number	*141*
Male	58.2% (82)
Place of birth	
Local	63.8% (90)
Regional	23.4% (33)
Overseas	6.4% (9)
No information	6.4% (9)
Premature birth	31.9% (45)

Table 8.2 Baseline characteristics

Characteristic	Sample size (N)	Per cent (n)
Male	141	58.2% (82)
Place of birth	132	
Local		68.2% (90)
Regional		25.0% (33)
Overseas		6.8% (9)
Premature birth	141	31.9% (45)

the percentage of female children because this is the complement that can be easily calculated. Similarly, it is not necessary to include percentages of both term and premature birth since one can be calculated from the other. In some journals, observed numbers are not included in addition to percentages because the numbers can be calculated from the percentages and the total number of the sample. However, other journals request that the number of cases and the sample size, for example, 82/141, is reported in addition to percentages.

Although confidence intervals around percentage figures can be computed, these statistics are more appropriate for comparing rates in two or more different groups, as discussed later in this chapter, and not for describing the sample characteristics.

8.3   Incidence and prevalence

When describing frequencies, it is important to use the correct term. A common mistake is to describe prevalence as incidence, or vice versa, although these terms have different meanings and cannot be used interchangeably.

Incidence is a term used to describe the number of new cases with a condition divided by the population at risk. Prevalence is a term used to describe the total number of cases with a condition divided by the population at risk. The population at risk is the number of people during the specified time period who were susceptible to the condition. The prevalence of an illness in a specified period is the number of incident cases in that period plus the previous prevalent cases and minus any deaths or remissions.

Both incidence and prevalence are usually calculated for a defined time period; for example, for a 1-year or 5-year period. When the number of cases of a condition is measured at a specified point in time, the term 'point prevalence' is used. The terms incidence and prevalence should be used only when the sample is selected randomly from a population such as in a cross-sectional or cohort study. Obviously, the larger the sample size, the more accurately the estimates of incidence and prevalence will be measured.

When the sample has not been selected randomly from the population such as in some case-control or experimental studies, the terms percentage, proportion or frequency are more appropriate.

8.4 Chi-square tests

A chi-square test (denoted as χ^2) is used to assess whether the distribution of a categorical variable is significantly different between two or more groups. Tests of chi square are used to determine whether there is an association between two categorical variables. In health research, a test of chi-square is frequently used to assess whether disease (present/absent) is associated with exposure (yes/no). For example, a chi-square test could be used to examine whether the absence or presence of an illness is independent of whether a child was or was not immunized. Chi-square tests are appropriate for most study designs but the results are influenced by the sample size.

The data for chi-square tests are summarized using crosstabulations as shown in Table 8.3. These tables are sometimes called frequency or contingency tables. Table 8.3 is called a 2×2 table because each variable has two levels. Tables can have larger dimensions when either the exposure or the disease has more than two levels.

In a contingency table, one variable (usually the exposure) forms the rows and the other variable (usually the disease) forms the columns. For example, the exposure immunization (no, yes) would form the rows and the illness (present, absent) would form the columns. The four internal cells of the table show the counts for each of the disease/exposure groups; for example, cell 'a' shows the number who satisfy exposure present (immunized) and disease present (illness positive).

As in all analyses, it is important to identify which variable is the outcome variable and which variable is the explanatory variable. This is important for setting up the

Table 8.3 Crosstabulation for estimating chi-square

	Disease absent	Disease present	Total
Exposure absent	d	c	c + d
Exposure present	b	a	a + b
Total	b + d	a + c	Total

crosstabulation table to display the percentages that are appropriate for answering the research question. This can be achieved by either:

- entering the explanatory variable in the rows, the outcome in the columns and using row percentages, or
- entering the explanatory variable in the columns, the outcome in the rows and using column percentages.

A table set up in either of these ways will display the per cent of participants with the outcome of interest in each of the explanatory variable groups. In most study designs, the outcome is an illness or disease and the explanatory variable is an exposure or an experimental group. However, in case–control studies in which cases are selected on the basis of their disease status, the disease may be treated as the explanatory variable and the exposure as the outcome variable.

8.4.1 Assumptions

The assumptions for using a chi-square test are shown in Box 8.2.

Box 8.2 Assumptions for using chi-square tests

The assumptions that must be met when using a chi-square test are that:
- each observation must be independent
- each participant is represented in the table once only

A major assumption of chi-square tests is independence, that is, each participant must be represented in the analysis once only. Thus, if repeat data have been collected, for example, if data have been collected from hospital inpatients and some patients have been readmitted, a decision must be made about which data, for example, from the first admission or the last admission, are used in the analyses.

The expected frequency in each cell is an important concept in determining P values and deciding the validity of a chi-square test. The formula for calculating expected frequencies is given in Section 8.4.3. For each cell, a certain number of participants would be expected given the frequencies of each of the characteristics in the sample. When the expected frequency of cell is less than 5, the significance tests of the Pearson's chi-square distribution becomes inaccurate due to the small sample size. Thus, the Pearson's or continuity-corrected chi-square values should be used only when 80% of the expected cell frequencies exceed 5 and all expected cell frequencies exceed 1.

8.4.2 Which chi-square test and P value to report?

When a chi-square test is requested, most statistics programs provide a number of chi-square values on the output. The chi-square statistic that is conventionally used depends on both the sample size and the expected cell counts as shown in Table 8.4.

Table 8.4 Type and application of chi-square tests

Statistic	Application
Pearson's chi-square	Used when the sample size is very large, say over 1000
Continuity correction	Applied to 2 × 2 tables only and is an approximation to Pearson's for a smaller sample size, say less than 1000
Fisher's exact test	Must always be used when one or more cells in a 2 × 2 table have a small expected number of cases
Linear-by-linear	Used to test for a trend in the frequency of the outcome across an ordered exposure variable

However, these guidelines are quite conservative and if the result from a Fisher's exact test is available, it could be used in all situations because it is a gold standard test, whereas Pearson's chi-square and the continuity correction tests are approximations. Fisher's exact test is generally calculated for 2 × 2 tables and, depending on the program used, may also be produced for crosstabulations larger than 2 × 2.

In a 2 × 2 contingency table, the Pearson's chi square produces smaller P values than Fisher's exact and a type I error may occur.[2] A correction made to the calculation of Pearson's chi-square (Yates continuity correction) increases the P value. However, this correction tends to overestimate the P value and a type II error may occur.[2] Therefore, the Yates correction should generally not be applied except if the sample size is small. The linear-by-linear test is a trend test and is most appropriate in situations in which an ordered exposure variable has three or more categories and the outcome variable is binary.

When conducting a chi-square test in SPSS, the significance level is calculated using the 'asymptotic' method, which means that P values are calculated based on the assumption that the data has a large enough sample size to conform to a certain distribution. If the sample size is small or some cells have a low count, the 'exact' P values should be reported since the asymptotic P values will be unreliable. The exact calculation based on the exact distribution of the test statistics provides a reliable P value irrespective of the sample size or distribution of the data.

8.4.3 Calculating chi-square values

Chi-square values are calculated from the number of observed and expected frequencies (or counts) in each cell of the crosstabulation. The observed count is the actual count in the sample and is shown in each cell of the crosstabulation. The expected count is the expected value due by chance alone and is calculated for each cell as the:

$$\frac{\text{Row total} \times \text{Column total}}{\text{Grand total}}$$

For cell a in Table 8.3, the expected number is $((a + b) \times (a + c))/\text{Total}$

The chi-square statistic compares the observed count in each cell to the count which would be expected under the assumption of no association between the row and column classifications. The Pearson chi-square value is calculated by the following summation from all cells:

$$\text{Chi-squared value} = \frac{\sum (\text{Observed count} - \text{Expected count})^2}{\text{Expected count}}$$

The continuity corrected (Yates) chi-square is calculated in a similar way but with a correction made for a smaller sample size. The null hypothesis for a chi-square test is that there is no significant difference between the observed frequencies and expected frequencies. Obviously, if the observed and expected values are similar, then the chi-square value will be close to zero and therefore will not be significant. The larger the observed and expected values are from one another, the larger the chi-square value becomes and the more likely the P value will be significant.

Research question

The data set **surgery.sav** contains data from babies who were admitted to hospital for surgery. This sample was not selected randomly and therefore only percentages will apply and the terms incidence and prevalence cannot be used. However, chi-square tests are valid to assess whether there are any between-group differences in the proportion of babies with certain characteristics.

Question: Are males who are admitted for surgery more likely than females to have been born prematurely?

Null hypothesis: That the proportion of males in the premature group is equal to the proportion of females in the premature group.

Variables: Outcome variable = prematurity (categorical, two levels)
                    Explanatory variable = gender (categorical, two levels)

The command sequence to obtain a crosstabulation and chi-square test is shown in Box 8.3.

Box 8.3 SPSS commands to obtain a chi-square test

SPSS Commands

surgery.sav – IBM SPSS Statistics Data Editor
        Analyze → Descriptive Statistics → Crosstabs
Crosstabs
        Highlight Gender recoded and click into Row(s)
        Highlight Prematurity and click into Column(s)
        Click Statistics
Crosstabs: Statistics
        Tick Chi-square, click Continue
Crosstabs
        Click Cells
Crosstabs: Cell Display

> *Counts: tick Observed (default),*
> *Percentages: tick Row*
> *Noninteger Weights: tick Round cell count (default)*
> *Click Continue*
> *Crosstabs*
> *Click OK*

The Crosstabulation table shows that the two variables each have two levels to create a 2×2 table with four cells. The table shows that 40.2% of males in the sample were premature compared with 20.3% of females, that is, the rate of prematurity in the males is almost twice that in the females. In the Crosstabulation table, the smallest cell has an observed count of 12. The expected number for this cell is $59 \times 45/141$, or 18.83 as shown in the footnote of the Chi-Square Tests table.

Crosstabs

Gender Recoded * Prematurity Crosstabulation

| | | | Prematurity | | |
			Premature	Term	Total
Gender recoded	Male	Count	33	49	82
		% within gender recoded	40.2%	59.8%	100.0%
	Female	Count	12	47	59
		% within gender recoded	20.3%	79.7%	100.0%
Total		Count	45	96	141
		% within gender recoded	31.9%	68.1%	100.0%

Chi-Square Tests

	Value	df	Asymp. Sig. (2-sided)	Exact sig. (2-sided)	Exact sig. (1-sided)
Pearson Chi-square	6.256[a]	1	0.012		
Continuity correction[b]	5.374	1	0.020		
Likelihood ratio	6.464	1	0.011		
Fisher's exact test				.017	.009
Linear-by-linear association	6.212	1	0.013		
N of valid cases	141				

[a]0 cells (0.0%) have expected count less than 5. The minimum expected count is 18.83.
[b]Computed only for a 2×2 table.

In the Chi-Square Tests table, the third column's heading is 'Asymp. Sig. (two-sided)', which indicates the significance level for a two-sided test calculated asymptotically. In this example, the sample size is too small for the chi-square distribution to approximate the exact distribution of the Pearson statistic and so the Pearson chi-square value should not be reported. The continuity correction (Yates) results in a P value of 0.020, which is slightly higher than the P value of 0.017 for the Fisher's exact test. The Fisher's exact test would be reported in this study because the sample size is only 141 children.

This test is two-tailed and the corresponding value indicates that the difference in rates of prematurity between the genders is statistically significant at $P = 0.017$. This result can be reported as 'Fisher's exact test indicated that there was a significant difference in prematurity between males and females (40.2% vs 20.3%, $P = 0.02$)'.

8.4.4 Sample size requirements

Whether a difference in a rate between two groups is statistically significant is heavily influenced by the sample size. The larger the difference between the rates in two groups, the smaller the sample size required to show a statistically significant difference.

Table 8.5 shows the sample size needed in each group to detect a significant difference between two prevalence rates (power = 80%, $P < 0.05$).[3] The table shows that, in general, a large 30% difference between two groups in a 2×2 chi-square test will be statistically significant when the sample size is larger than 35 participants per group, a 20% difference will be statistically significant when the sample size is larger than 60 participants per group and a 10% difference will be statistically significant when the sample size is larger than 160 participants per group. Online programs such as GPower and StatsToDo which can be used for estimating more accurate sample size requirements for chi-square tests are listed in the Useful Websites section.

Table 8.5   Approximate sample size required per group to show that a difference in prevalence rates is statistically significant (power = 80%, $P < 0.05$, two-tailed) using a chi-square test

	Difference between two rates			
Lower rate	10%	20%	30%	40%
5%	160	60	35	25
10%	220	80	40	25
20%	320	100	45	30
30%	380	110	50	30
40%–50%	410	110	50	30

8.4.5 Confidence intervals

When between-group differences are compared, the summary percentages are best reported with 95% confidence intervals. It is useful to include the 95% confidence intervals when results are shown as figures because the degree of overlap between them provides an approximate significance of the differences between groups. The interpretation of the degree of overlap is discussed in Chapter 3 (also see Table 3.5).

Many statistics programs do not provide confidence intervals around frequency statistics. However, 95% confidence intervals can be easily computed using an Excel spreadsheet. The standard error around a proportion is calculated as $\sqrt{[p(1-p)/n]}$ where p is the proportion expressed as a decimal number and n is the number of cases in the group from which the proportion is calculated. The standard error (SE) around a proportion is rarely reported but is commonly converted into a 95% confidence interval which is $p \pm (SE \times 1.96)$.

An Excel spreadsheet in which the percentage is entered as its decimal equivalent in the first column and the number in the group is entered in the second column can be used to calculate confidence intervals as shown in Table 8.6.

The formula for the standard error is entered into the formula bar of Excel as sqrt $(p \times (1 - p)/n)$ and the formula for the width of the confidence interval is entered as $1.96 \times SE$. This width, which is the dimension of the 95% confidence interval that is entered into SigmaPlot to draw bar charts with error bars, can then be both subtracted and added to the proportion to calculate the 95% confidence interval values shown in the last two columns of Table 8.6.

The calculations are undertaken in proportions (decimal numbers) but are easily converted back to percentages by multiplying by 100, that is, by moving the decimal point two places to the right. Using the converted values, the result could be reported as 'the percentage of male babies born prematurely was 40.2% (95% CI 29.6–50.8%). This was significantly different than the percentage of female babies born prematurely which was 20.3% (95% CI 10.0–30.6%) $(P = 0.02)$'. The P value of 0.02 for this comparison is the rounded value derived from the P value of 0.017 in the Chi-Square Tests table.

Because the value of 'n' is integral in the denominator of the calculation of confidence intervals, the larger the sample size, the smaller the confidence will be, indicating greater precision in the result. Table 8.7 shows how the sample size influences the width of

Table 8.6   Excel spreadsheet to compute 95% confidence intervals around proportions

	Proportion	N	SE	Width	CI lower	CI upper
Male	0.402	82	0.054	0.106	0.296	0.508
Female	0.203	59	0.052	0.103	0.100	0.306

Table 8.7   Approximate sample size required to calculate 95% confidence intervals around a prevalence rate with the precision (width) shown (power = 80%, $P < 0.05$, two-tailed)

	Width of 95% confidence interval					
Prevalence	2%	3%	4%	5%	7.5%	10%
5%	460	200	110	70	35	35
10%	870	380	220	140	65	40
15%	1200	550	300	200	90	50
20%	1500	700	400	250	110	60
30%	2000	900	500	300	140	70
40%	2200	1000	600	380	160	90

95% confidence intervals.[3] The sample size required to calculate a rate with a 95% confidence interval of specified width is shown in Table 8.7. The precision depends on both the prevalence rate and the sample size. In general, a large sample size is required to reduce 95% confidence intervals below a width of 5%.

8.4.6   Creating a figure using SigmaPlot

The summary statistics from Table 8.6 can be entered into SigmaPlot by first using the commands *File → New* and then entering the percentages in column 1 and the width of the confidence interval, also converted to a percentage in column 2.

Column 1	Column 2
40.2	10.6
20.3	10.3

The SigmaPlot commands for plotting these summary statistics as a figure are shown in Box 8.4.

Box 8.4 SigmaPlot commands to draw simple histograms

SigmaPlot commands

Data 1*
        Click on Create Graph tab at top of the screen
        Click on Bar in sub-menu
        Click on Horizontal Bar - Error Bars in Bar Group
Create Graph – Error Bars
        Symbol Values = Worksheet Columns (default), click Next
Create Graph – Data Format
        Highlight Single X, click Next
Create Graph – Select Data
        Data for Bar = use drop box and select Column 1
        Data for Error = use drop box and select Column 2
        Click Finish

The graph can then be customized using the options under *Graph Page* to produce Figure 8.2 (see p.261). The lack of overlap between the confidence intervals is an approximate indication of a statistically significant difference between the two groups (see Table 3.5 for interpretation).

8.5   2 × 3 Chi-square tables

In addition to the common application of analyzing 2 × 2 tables, chi-square tests can also be used for larger tables, for example 2 × 3 tables, in which one variable has two levels and the other variable has three levels.

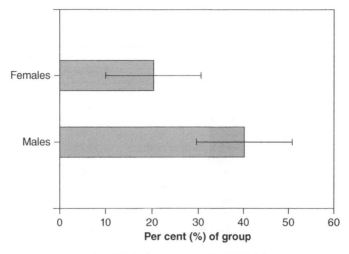

Figure 8.2 Per cent of male and female babies born prematurely.

Research question

Question: Are the babies born in regional centres (away from the hospital or overseas) more likely to be premature than babies born in local areas?

Null hypothesis: That the proportion of premature babies in the group born locally is not different to the proportion of premature babies in the groups born regionally or overseas.

Variables: Place of birth (categorical, three levels and) prematurity (categorical, two levels)

In this research question, there is no clear outcome or explanatory variable because both variables in the analysis are characteristics of the babies. This type of question is asked when it is important to know about the inter-relationships between variables in the data set. If prematurity has an important association with place of birth, this may need to be taken into account in multivariate analyses.

The SPSS commands shown in Box 8.3 can be used with place of birth recoded entered into the rows, prematurity entered into the columns and row percentages requested.

The row percentages in the Crosstabulation table show that there is a difference in the frequency of prematurity between babies born at different locations. The per cent of babies who are premature is 32.2% from local centres, 18.2% from regional centres and 55.6% from overseas centres. This difference in percentages fails to reach significance with a Pearson's chi-square value of 5.170 and a P value of 0.075. As mentioned previously, Pearson's chi-square may underestimate the P value when the sample size is small. For tables such as this that are larger than 2×2, an Exact chi-square test should be used when an expected count is low (see Section 8.7).

Crosstabs

Place of birth (recoded) * Prematurity Crosstabulation

				Prematurity		
				Premature	Term	Total
Place of birth (recoded)	Local	Count		29	61	90
		% within place of birth (recoded)		32.2%	67.8%	100.0%
	Regional	Count		6	27	33
		% within place of birth (recoded)		18.2%	81.8%	100.0%
	Overseas	Count		5	4	9
		% within place of birth (recoded)		55.6%	44.4%	100.0%
Total		Count		40	92	132
		% within place of birth (recoded)		30.3%	69.7%	100.0%

Chi-Square Tests

	Value	df	Asymp. sig. (two-sided)
Pearson chi-square	5.170[a]	2	0.075
Likelihood ratio	5.146	2	0.076
Linear-by-linear association	0.028	1	0.866
N of valid cases	132		

[a]1 cell (16.7%) has expected count less than 5. The minimum expected count is 2.73.

In the crosstabulation, the absolute difference in per cent of premature babies between regional and overseas centres is quite large at 55.6%−18.2% or 37.4%. The finding of a non-significant P value in the presence of this large between-group difference could be considered a type II error as a consequence of the small sample size. In this case, the sample size is too small to demonstrate statistical significance when a large difference of 37.4% exists. If the sample size had been larger, then the P value for the same between-group difference would be significant. Conversely, the difference between the groups may have been due to chance and a larger sample size might show a smaller between-group difference.

8.6 Cells with small numbers

A major problem with the previous analysis is the small numbers in some of the cells. There are only nine babies in the overseas group. The row percentages illustrate the problem that arises when some cells have small numbers. The five premature babies born overseas are 55.6% of their group because each baby is 1/9th or 11.1% of the group. When a group size is small, adding or losing a single case from a cell results in a large change in frequency statistics. Because there are some small group sizes, the footnote in the Chi-Square Tests table indicates that one cell in the table has an expected count less than five.

Using the formula shown previously (section 8.4.3), the expected number of premature babies referred from overseas is $9 \times 40/132$ or 2.73. This minimum expected cell count is printed in the footnote below the Chi-Square Tests table. If a table has less than five expected observations in more than 20% of cells, the assumptions for the chi-square test are not met. The warning message suggests that the P value of 0.075 is unreliable and probably an overestimate of significance.

Small cells cannot be avoided at times; for example, when a disease is rare. However, cells and groups with small numbers are a problem in all types of analyses because their summary statistics are often unstable and difficult to interpret. When calculating a chi-square statistic, most packages will give a warning message when the number of expected cases in a cell is low.

Pearson's chi-square tests may be valid when the number of observed counts in a cell is zero as long as the expected number is greater than 5 in 80% of the cells and greater than 1 in all cells. If expected numbers are less than this, then an exact chi-square based on alternative assumptions should be used.

8.7 Exact chi square test

An exact chi-square can be obtained for the 3×2 table above by clicking on the *Exact* button located in the top right hand corner of the *Crosstabs* dialogue box, and selecting *Monte Carlo*, entering 95% for *Confidence level* and *Number of samples* equal to 10,000 (default). The following table is obtained when the Monte Carlo method of computing the exact chi-square is requested. The Monte Carlo P value is based on a random sample of a probability distribution rather than a chi-square distribution which is an approximation. When the Monte Carlo option is selected, the P value will change slightly each time the test is run on the same data set because it is based on a random sample of probabilities.

Chi-Square Tests

| | Value | df | Asymp. sig. (2-sided) | Monte Carlo Sig. (2-sided) | | | Monte Carlo Sig. (1-sided) | | |
| | | | | | 95% Confidence interval | | | 95% Confidence interval | |
				Sig.	Lower bound	Upper bound	Sig.	Lower bound	Upper bound
Pearson Chi-square	5.170[a]	2	0.075	0.075[b]	0.070	0.081			
Likelihood ratio	5.146	2	0.076	0.100[b]	0.094	0.106			
Fisher's exact test	5.072			0.075[b]	0.070	0.081			
Linear-by-linear association	0.028[c]	1	0.866	0.879[b]	0.872	0.885	0.481[b]	0.472	0.491
N of valid cases	132								

[a] 1 cells (16.7%) have expected count less than 5. The minimum expected count is 2.73.
[b] Based on 10,000 sampled tables with starting seed 624387341.
[c] The standardized statistic is −0.168.

The Chi-Square Tests table shows that the asymptotic significance value of $P = 0.075$ is identical to the exact significance value obtained previously, that is, $P = 0.075$. The two-sided test should be used because the direction of effect could have been either way, that is, the proportion of premature babies could have been higher or lower in any of the groups.

An alternative to using exact methods is to merge the group with small cells with another group but only if the theory is valid. It is usually sensible to combine groups when there are less than 10 cases in a cell. Alternatively, the group can be omitted from the analyses although this will reduce the generalizability of the results.

8.8   Number of cells that can be tested

The number of viable cells for statistical analysis usually depends on sample size. As a rule of thumb, the maximum number of cells that can be tested using chi-square is the sample size divided by 10. Thus, a sample size of 160 could theoretically support 16 cells such as an 8×2 table, a 5×3 table or a 4×4 table. However, this relies on an even distribution of cases over the cells, which rarely occurs. In practice, the maximum number of cells is usually the sample size divided by 20. In this data set, this would be 141/20 or approximately seven cells which would support a 2×2 or 2×3 table. These tables would be viable as long as no cell size is particularly small.

The pathway for analyzing categorical variables when some cells have small numbers is shown in Figure 8.3.

Groups can be easily combined to increase cell size if the recoding is intuitive. However, if two or more unrelated groups need to be combined, they could be described with a generic label such as 'other' if neither group is more closely related to one of the other groups in the analysis. In the data set **surgery.sav**, it makes sense to combine the regional group with the overseas group because both are distinct from the local group. The SPSS commands to recode a variable into a different variable were shown in Box 1.9 in Chapter 1 and can be used to transform place2 with three levels into a binary variable called place3 (local, regional/overseas). To ensure that all output is self-documented, it is important to label each new variable in Variable View after re-coding and to verify the frequencies of place3 using the commands shown in Box 1.7.

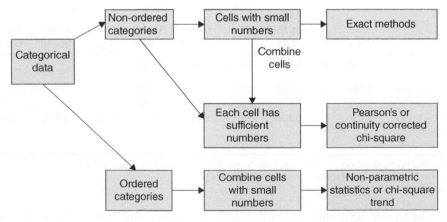

Figure 8.3 Pathway for analyzing categorical variables when some cells have small numbers.

Frequencies

Place of Birth (Binary)

		Frequency	Per cent	Valid per cent	Cumulative per cent
Valid	Local	90	63.8	68.2	68.2
	Regional or overseas	42	29.8	31.8	100.0
	Total	132	93.6	100.0	
Missing	System	9	6.4		
Total		141	100.0		

Having combined the small overseas group of nine children with the regional group of 33 children, the new combined group has 42 children. To answer the research question, the Crosstabulation table and tests of chi-square can be obtained by repeating the SPSS commands shown in Box 8.3 to compute a 2×2 table with the binary place of birth variable entered into the rows.

The Crosstabulation table shows that 32.2% of babies in the sample from the local area were premature compared to 26.2% of babies from regional centres or overseas. The Chi-Square Tests table shows Fisher's exact test *P* value of 0.546 which is not significant. This value, which is very different from the *P* value of 0.075 for the 3×2 table, is more robust because all cells have adequate sizes. With the small cells combined into larger cells, the footnote shows that no cell has an expected count less than five and thus the assumptions for chi-square are met.

Crosstabs

Place of Birth (Binary) * Prematurity Crosstabulation

		Prematurity		Total
		Premature	Term	
Place of birth Local	Count (binary) % within place of birth (binary)	29 32.2%	61 67.8%	90 100.0%
Regional or overseas	Count % within place of birth (binary)	11 26.2%	31 73.8%	42 100.0%
Total	Count % within place of birth (binary)	40 30.3%	92 69.7%	132 100.0%

Chi-Square Tests

	Value	df	Asymp. Sig. (2-sided)	Exact Sig. (2-sided)	Exact Sig. (1-sided)
Pearson Chi-square	0.493[a]	1	0.482		
Continuity correction[b]	0.249	1	0.618		
Likelihood ratio	0.501	1	0.479		
Fisher's exact test				0.546	0.312
Linear-by-linear association	0.490	1	0.484		
N of valid cases	132				

[a] 0 cells (0.0%) have expected count less than 5. The minimum expected count is 12.73.
[b] Computed only for a 2×2 table

Using the Excel spreadsheet created previously in Table 8.6, the percentages can be added as proportions and the confidence intervals calculated as shown in Table 8.8.

Table 8.8 Excel spreadsheet to compute confidence intervals around proportions

	Proportion	N	SE	Width	CI lower	CI upper
Local	0.322	90	0.049	0.097	0.225	0.419
Regional or overseas	0.262	42	0.068	0.133	0.129	0.395

8.9   Reporting chi-square tests and proportions

Generally, when reporting the results of chi-square test for publication, the chi-square value (if required), the total sample size, the P value and the degrees of freedom should be included. In addition, the odds ratio (as discussed in Chapter 9) can also be reported for 2×2 tables to indicate the size of the association between the two variables. In the example above, the results can be presented as 'Of the 132 babies, 29 of the 90 babies who were born locally were premature (32.2%) and 11 of the 42 were born regionally or overseas were premature (26.2%). A chi-square test indicated that there was no significant association between prematurity and place of birth $(P = 0.55)$'.

When presenting crosstabulated information of the effects of explanatory factors for a report, journal article or presentation, it is usual to present the results in tables with the outcome variable presented in the columns and the risk factors or explanatory variables presented in the rows as shown in Table 8.9.

The chi-square analyses show that the number of males and females referred for surgery is significantly different but that the per cent of premature babies from regional or overseas areas is not significantly different from the per cent of premature babies in the group born locally. The results of these analyses could be presented as shown in Table 8.9.

Table 8.9 Factors associated with prematurity in 141 children attending hospital for surgery

Risk factor	Per cent premature and 95% CI	P value
Male	40.2% (29.6, 50.8)	0.02
Female	20.3% (10.0, 30.6)	
Born in local area	32.2% (22.5, 41.9)	0.55
Born in regional area or overseas	26.2% (12.9, 39.5)	

The overlap of the 95% confidence intervals in this table is consistent with the P values and shows that there is only a minor overlap of 95% confidence intervals between genders but a large overlap of 95% confidence intervals between regions.

8.9.1   Differences in percentages

When comparing proportions between two groups, it can be useful to express the size of the absolute difference in proportions between the groups. A 95% confidence interval around this difference is valuable in interpreting the significance of the difference

Table 8.10 Excel spreadsheet to compute confidence intervals around a difference in proportions

	p_1	n_1	p_2	n_2	$1-p_1$	$1-p_2$	Difference	SE	Width	CI lower	CI upper
Gender	0.402	82	0.203	59	0.598	0.797	0.199	0.075	0.148	0.051	0.347
Place	0.322	90	0.262	42	0.678	0.738	0.06	0.084	0.164	−0.104	0.224

Note: p — proportion

Table 8.11 Risk factor for prematurity in 141 children attending for surgery

Risk factor	Per cent premature	Difference and 95% confidence interval	P value
Male	40.2%	19.9% (5.1, 34.7)	0.02
Female	20.3%		
Born locally	32.2%	6.0% (−10.4, 22.4)	0.55
Born regionally/overseas	26.2%		

because if the interval does not cross the line of no difference (zero value) then the difference between groups is statistically significant.

The Excel spreadsheet shown in Table 8.10 can be used to calculate the differences in proportions, the standard error around the differences and the width of the confidence intervals. The difference in proportions is calculated as $p_1 - p_2$ and the standard error of the difference as $\sqrt{((p_1 \times (1 - p_1)/n_1) + (p_2 \times (1 - p_2)/n_2))}$, where p_1 is the proportion and n_1 is the number of cases in one group and p_2 is the proportion and n_2 is the number of cases in the other group. The width of the confidence interval is calculated as before as $SE \times 1.96$.

The results from the above analyses can be presented as shown in Table 8.11 as an alternative to the presentation shown in Table 8.9. In Table 8.9, the precision in both groups could be compared but Table 8.11 shows the absolute difference between the groups. This type of presentation is useful, for example, when comparing percentages between two groups that were studied in different time periods and the outcome of interest is the change over time.

The 95% confidence interval for the difference between genders does not contain the zero value of no difference as expected because the P value is significant. On the other hand, the confidence interval for the difference between places of birth contains the zero value indicating there is little difference between groups and that the P value is not significant.

8.10 Large contingency tables

Small crosstabulations such as 2×2 tables are relatively straightforward to interpret but when using larger crosstabulations, such as 2×3 tables, it can be difficult to interpret the

P value without further sub-analyses, as shown when answering the following research question.

Research question

Question: Are babies who are born prematurely more likely to require different types of surgical procedures than term babies?

Null hypothesis: That the proportion of babies who require each type of surgical procedure in the group born prematurely is the same as in the group of term babies.

Variables: Outcome variable = procedure performed (categorical, three levels)
Explanatory variable = prematurity (categorical, two levels)

In situations such as this where the table is 3×2 because the outcome has three levels, both the row and column cell percentages can be used to provide useful summary statistics for between-group comparisons. The commands shown in Box 8.3 can be used with prematurity as the explanatory variable entered in the rows and procedure performed as the outcome variable in the columns. In addition, the column percentages can be obtained by clicking on *Cells* in the *Crosstabs* dialog box and ticking *Column* under *Percentages*.

Crosstabs

Prematurity * Procedure Performed Crosstabulation

			Procedure performed			
			Abdominal	Cardiac	Other	Total
Prematurity	Premature	Count	9	23	13	45
		% within prematurity	20.0%	51.1%	28.9%	100.0%
		% within procedure performed	17.0%	41.1%	40.6%	31.9%
	Term	Count	44	33	19	96
		% within prematurity	45.8%	34.4%	19.8%	100.0%
		% within procedure performed	83.0%	58.9%	59.4%	68.1%
Total		Count	53	56	32	141
		% within prematurity	37.6%	39.7%	22.7%	100.0%
		% within procedure performed	100.0%	100.0%	100.0%	100.0%

Chi-Square Tests

	Value	*Df*	Asymp. sig. (two-sided)
Pearson chi-square	8.718[a]	2	0.013
Likelihood ratio	9.237	2	0.010
Linear-by-linear association	6.392	1	0.011
N of valid cases	141		

[a]0 cell (0.0%) has expected count less than 5. The minimum expected count is 10.21.

The row percentages in the Crosstabulation table show that fewer of the premature babies required abdominal procedures than the term babies (20.0% vs 45.8%) and that more of the premature babies had cardiac procedures than the term babies (51.1% vs 34.4%). In addition, more of the premature babies than the term babies had other procedures (28.9% vs 19.8%). Since the contingency table is now larger than 2×2, the Fisher's exact test is not produced and the Pearson's chi-square test is used. The significance of these differences from the Chi-Square Tests table is $P = 0.013$. However, this P value does not indicate the specific between-group comparisons that are significantly different from one another. In practice, the P value indicates that there is a significant difference in percentages within the table but does not indicate which groups are significantly different from one another. In this situation where there is no ordered explanatory variable, the linear by linear association has no interpretation.

The column percentages shown in the Crosstabulation table can be used to interpret the 2×2 comparisons. These percentages show that rates of surgery types in premature babies are abdominal vs cardiac surgery 17.0% vs 41.1%, abdominal vs other surgery 17.0% vs 40.6% and cardiac vs other surgery 41.1% vs 40.6%. To obtain P values for these comparisons, the *Data → Select Cases → If condition is satisfied* option can be used to select two groups at a time and compute three separate 2×2 tables. For the three comparisons above, this provides P values of 0.011, 0.031 and 1.0, respectively.

The original P value from the 2×3 table was significant because the rate of prematurity was significantly lower in the abdominal surgery group compared to both the cardiac and other surgery groups. However, there was no significant difference between the cardiac vs other surgery group. This process of making multiple comparisons increases the chance of a type I error, that is, finding a significant difference when one does not exist. A preferable method is to compute confidence intervals as shown in the Excel spreadsheet in Table 8.6 and then examine the degree of overlap. The computed intervals are shown in Table 8.12.

The rates and their confidence intervals can then be plotted using SigmaPlot as shown in Box 8.5. The data sheet has the proportions and confidence interval widths converted into percentages for the premature babies in columns 1 and 2 and for the term babies in columns 3 and 4 as follows:

Column 1	Column 2	Column 3	Column 4
17.0	10.1	83.0	10.1
41.1	12.9	58.9	12.9
40.6	17.0	59.4	17.0

Table 8.12   Excel spreadsheet to compute confidence intervals around proportions

	Proportion	N	SE	Width	CI lower	CI upper
Abdominal-premature	0.17	53	0.052	0.101	0.069	0.271
Cardiac-premature	0.411	56	0.066	0.129	0.282	0.540
Other-premature	0.406	32	0.087	0.170	0.236	0.576
Abdominal-term	0.83	53	0.052	0.101	0.729	0.931
Cardiac-term	0.589	56	0.066	0.129	0.460	0.718
Other-term	0.594	32	0.087	0.170	0.424	0.764

Box 8.5 SigmaPlot commands for plotting multiple bars

SigmaPlot Commands

Data 1*

   Click on Create Graph tab at top of the screen
   Click on Bar in sub-menu
   Click on Grouped Horizontal Bar - Error Bars in Bar Group

Create Graph - Style

   Highlight Grouped Error Bars, click Next

Create Graph – Error Bars

   Symbol Values = Worksheet Columns (default), click Next

Create Graph – Data Format

   Highlight Many X, click Next

Create Graph – Select Data

   Data for Set 1 = used drop box and select Column 1
   Data for Error 1 = used drop box and select Column 2
   Data for Set 2 = used drop box and select Column 3
   Data for Error 2 = used drop box and select Column 4
   Click Finish

Figure 8.4 shows clearly that the 95% confidence intervals of the bars for the per cent of the abdominal surgery group who are term or premature babies do not overlap either of the other groups and therefore the percentages are significantly different as described by the P values. The per cent of premature babies in the cardiac surgery and other procedure groups are almost identical as described by the P value of 1.0 (see p.269).

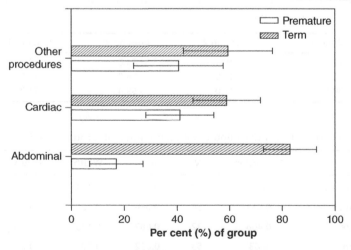

Figure 8.4 Percentage of surgical procedures in premature and term babies.

8.11   Categorizing continuous variables

In addition to 2×2 and 2×3 tables, chi-square tests can also be used to analyze tables of larger dimensions as shown in the following research question. However, the same assumptions apply and the sample size should be sufficient so that small cells with few expected counts are not created.

Research question

Question:	Do babies who have a cardiac procedure stay in hospital longer than babies who have other procedures?
Null hypothesis:	That length of stay is not different between children who undergo different procedures.
Variables:	Outcome variable = length of stay (categorized into quintiles)
	Explanatory variable = procedure performed (categorical, three levels)

In the data set, length of stay is a right skewed continuous variable (see Chapter 2). As an alternative to using rank-based non-parametric tests, it is often useful to divide non-normally distributed variables such as this into categories. Box 8.6 shows the SPSS commands that can be used to divide length of stay into quintiles, that is, five groups. The sample is divided with four cutpoints to give five roughly equal sized groups.

Box 8.6 SPSS commands to categorize variables

SPSS Commands

surgery.sav – IBM SPSS Statistics Data Editor
      Transform → Visual Binning
Visual Binning
      Highlight Length of stay and click into Variables to Bin box
      Click Continue
      Enter new variable name LOSquintiles into Binned Variable box
      Change variable label Length of Stay (Binned) to Length of stay quintiles
      Click on Make Cutpoints
Make Cutpoints
      Tick Equal Percentiles Based on Scanned Cases
      Number of Cutpoints: enter 4
      Tick Apply
Visual Binning
      Click on Make Labels to automatically label the new variable with cutpoint ranges
      Tick OK

Information about the sample size of each quintile and the range of values in each quintile band can be obtained using the following SPSS commands *Analyze → Descriptive Statistics → Frequencies* to obtain the following output:

Length of stay quintiles

		Frequency	Per cent	Valid per cent	Cumulative per cent
Valid	≤19	30	21.3	22.7	22.7
	20–22	24	17.0	18.2	40.9
	23–30	26	18.4	19.7	60.6
	31–44	26	18.4	19.7	80.3
	45+	26	18.4	19.7	100.0
	Total	132	93.6	100.0	
Missing	System	9	6.4		
Total		141	100.0		

In the length of stay quintiles table, it can be seen that the length of stay in hospital for 24 babies was between 20 and 22 days long. The ranges are important for describing the quintile values when reporting the results. The number of cases in some quintiles is unequal because there are some ties in the data.

Procedure performed * Length of stay quintiles Crosstabulation

			Length of stay quintiles					
			≤19	20–22	23–30	31–44	45+	Total
Procedure performed	Abdominal	Count	5	8	15	11	9	48
		% within procedure performed	10.4%	16.7%	31.3%	22.9%	18.8%	100.0%
	Cardiac	Count	15	13	7	12	6	53
		% within procedure performed	28.3%	24.5%	13.2%	22.6%	11.3%	100.0%
	Other	Count	10	3	4	3	11	31
		% within procedure performed	32.3%	9.7%	12.9%	9.7%	35.5%	100.0%
Total		Count	30	24	26	26	26	132
		% within procedure performed	22.7%	18.2%	19.7%	19.7%	19.7%	100.0%

Chi-Square Tests

	Value	df	Asymp. Sig. (2-sided)
Pearson chi-square	20.643[a]	8	0.008
Likelihood ratio	21.086	8	0.007
Linear-by-linear association	0.595	1	0.440
N of valid cases	132		

[a] 0 cells (0.0%) have expected count less than 5. The minimum expected count is 5.64.

The SPSS commands for obtaining crosstabulations shown in Box 8.3 can now be used to answer the research question. In the crosstabulation, the procedure performed is entered into the rows as explanatory variable and length of stay quintiles are entered in the columns as the outcome variable. The *row percentages* are selected in *Cells*.

It is very difficult to interpret large tables such as this 3×5 table. The crosstabulation has 15 cells, each with fewer than 20 observed cases. Although some cells have only two or three cases, the Chi-Square Tests footnote shows that no cells have an expected number less than 5, so that the analysis and the P value are valid. Although the P value is significant at $P = 0.008$, no clear trends are apparent in the table. If the cardiac and abdominal patients are compared, the abdominal group has fewer babies in the lowest quintile and the cardiac group has slightly fewer babies in the highest quintile. In the group of babies who had other procedures, most babies are either in the lowest or in the highest quintiles of length of stay. Thus, the P value is difficult to interpret without any further sub-group analyses and the interpretation of the statistical significance of the results is difficult to communicate. Again, in such a large table, the linear-by-linear statistic has no interpretation and should not be used. A solution to removing small cells for this research question would be to divide length of stay into two groups only, perhaps above and below the median value or above and below a clinically important threshold, and to examine the per cent of babies in each procedure group who have long or short stays.

8.12   Chi-square trend test for ordered variables

Chi-square trend test, which in SPSS is called a linear-by-linear association, is suitable when the exposure variable can be categorized into ordered groups, such as quintiles for length of stay, and the outcome variable is binary. The linear-by-linear statistic then indicates whether there is a trend for the outcome to increase or decrease as the exposure increases.

Research question

Question: Is there a trend for babies who stay longer in hospital to have a higher infection rate?

Null hypothesis: That infection rates do not change with length of stay.

Variables: Outcome variable = infection (categorical, two levels)
                     Explanatory/exposure variable = length of stay (categorized into quintiles, ordered)

In this research question, it makes sense to test whether there is a trend for the per cent of babies with infection to increase significantly with an increase in length of stay. The SPSS commands shown in Box 8.3 can be used with length of stay quintiles in the rows, infection in the columns and the row percentages requested.

The Crosstabulation table shows that the per cent of children with infection increases with length of stay quintile, from 23.3% in the lowest length of stay quintile group to

57.7% in the highest quintile group. The Pearson chi-square indicates that there is a significant difference in percentages between some groups in the table with $P = 0.033$. From this, it can be inferred that the lowest rate of infection in the bottom quintile is significantly different from the highest rate in the top quintile but not that any other rates are significantly different from one other. More usefully, the linear-by-linear association indicates that there is a significant trend for infection to increase with increasing length of stay at $P = 0.002$.

Length of stay quintiles * Infection Crosstabulation

			Infection		Total
			No	Yes	
Length of stay quintiles	≤19	Count	23	7	30
		% within Length of stay quintiles	76.7%	23.3%	100.0%
	20–22	Count	17	7	24
		% within Length of stay quintiles	70.8%	29.2%	100.0%
	23–30	Count	17	9	26
		% within Length of stay quintiles	65.4%	34.6%	100.0%
	31–44	Count	12	14	26
		% within Length of stay quintiles	46.2%	53.8%	100.0%
	45+	Count	11	15	26
		% within Length of stay quintiles	42.3%	57.7%	100.0%
Total		Count	80	52	132
		% within Length of stay quintiles	60.6%	39.4%	100.0%

Chi-Square Tests

	Value	df	Asymp. Sig. (2-sided)
Pearson chi-square	10.462[a]	4	.033
Likelihood ratio	10.578	4	.032
Linear-by-linear association	9.769	1	.002
N of valid cases	132		

[a] 0 cells (0.0%) have expected count less than 5. The minimum expected count is 9.45.

8.12.1   Reporting the results

When presenting the effects of an ordered exposure variable on several outcomes in a scientific table, the exposure groups are best shown in the columns and the outcomes in the rows. Using this layout the per cent of babies in each exposure group can be compared across a line of the table. The data from the Crosstabulation table above can be presented as shown in Table 8.13. If other outcomes associated with length of stay were also investigated, further rows could be added to the table.

Table 8.13   Rates of infection by length of stay

Range (days)	Length of stay in quintiles					P value	P value for trend
	1 **0–19**	**2** **20–22**	**3** **23–30**	**4** **31–44**	**5** **45–244**		
Number in group	30	24	26	26	26		
Percentage with infection	23.3%	29.2%	34.6%	53.8%	57.7%	0.033	0.002

To obtain a graphical indication of the magnitude of the trend across the data, a clustered bar chart can be requested using the SPSS commands shown in Box 8.7. If the number of cases in each group is unequal, as in this data set, then percentages rather than numbers must be selected in the *Bars Represent* option so that the height of each bar is standardized for the different numbers in each group and can be directly compared.

Box 8.7 SPSS commands to obtain a clustered bar chart

SPSS Commands

surgery.sav – IBM SPSS Statistics Data Editor
 Graphs → Legacy Dialogs → Bar
Bar Charts
 Click Clustered, tick Summaries for groups of cases (default), click Define
Define Clustered Bar: Summaries for Groups of Cases
 Bars Represent: Tick % of cases
 Highlight Infection and click into Category Axis
 Highlight Length of stay quintiles and click into Define Clusters by
 Click OK

In Figure 8.5, the group of bars on the left hand side of the graph shows the decrease in the per cent of babies who did not have infection across length of stay quintiles. The group of bars on the right hand side shows the complement of the data, that is, the increase across quintiles of the per cent of babies who did have infection. A way of presenting the data to answer the research question would be to draw a bar chart of the per cent of children with infection only as shown on the right hand side of Figure 8.5. This type of chart can be drawn in SigmaPlot using the commands shown in Box 8.4 with a vertical bar chart without error bars rather than a horizontal bar chart selected. Using the SigmaPlot commands *Analysis → Regression Wizard with the option Linear under the equation category Polynomial* will provide a trend line across the bars as shown as in Figure 8.6.

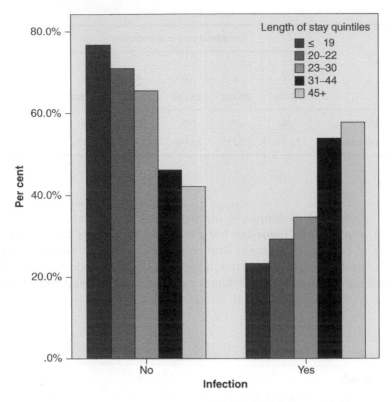

Figure 8.5 Length of stay quintiles for babies by infection status.

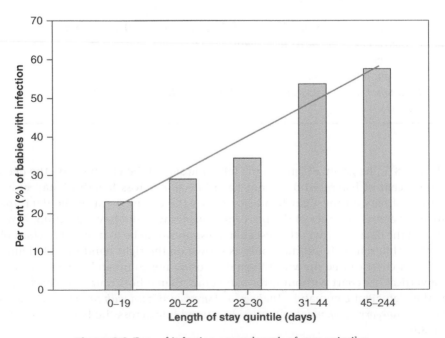

Figure 8.6 Rate of infection across length of stay quintiles.

8.13   Number needed to treat (NNT)

In interpreting the results from clinical trials, clinicians are often interested in how many patients need to be administered a treatment to prevent one adverse event. An adverse event is any unfavourable or undesirable effect that an individual experiences during the clinical trial (or period of observation) which may or may not be associated with the treatment. This statistic, which is called number needed to treat (NNT), can be calculated from clinical studies in which the effectiveness of an intervention is compared in two groups; for example, a standard treatment group and a new treatment group. For 2×2 crosstabulations, a chi-square test is used to indicate significance between the groups, or a difference in proportions is used to indicate whether the new treatment group has a significantly lower rate of adverse events than the standard treatment group. However, in clinical situations, these statistics, which describe the general differences between two groups, may not be the major results of interest. In a clinical setting, the statistic NNT provides a number that can be directly applied to individual patients and may therefore be more informative.

To calculate NNT, two categorical variables each with two levels are required in order to compute a 2×2 crosstabulation. One variable must indicate the presence or absence of the adverse event; for example, an outcome such as death or disability, and the other variable must indicate group status (exposure), for example, whether patients are in the intervention or control group.

Research example

The file **therapy.sav** contains data for 200 patients, half of whom were randomized to receive standard therapy and half of whom were randomized to receive a new therapy. The two outcomes that have been collected are the presence or absence of stroke and the presence or absence of disability. Each outcome variable is a binary yes/no response. Using the commands shown in Box 8.3, the following 2×2 tables for each outcome can be obtained. To calculate NNT, the outcome is entered as the rows, the treatment group is entered in the columns and column percentages are requested. In the cross-tabulation stroke is entered in row and treatment group is entered in column in the Crosstabs commands.

Crosstabs

Stroke * Treatment Group Crosstabulation

			Treatment group		Total
			New therapy	Standard treatment	
Stroke	No complications	Count	85	79	164
		% within treatment group	85.0%	79.0%	82.0%
	Stroke	Count	15	21	36
		% within treatment group	15.0%	21.0%	18.0%
Total		Count	100	100	200
		% within treatment group	100.0%	100.0%	100.0%

Chi-Square Tests

	Value	df	Asymp. sig. (two-sided)	Exact sig. (two-sided)	Exact sig. (one-sided)
Pearson chi-square	1.220[a]	1	0.269		
Continuity correction[b]	0.847	1	0.357		
Likelihood ratio	1.224	1	0.269		
Fisher's exact test				0.358	0.179
Linear-by-linear association	1.213	1	0.271		
N of valid cases	200				

[a]0 cell (0.0%) has expected count less than 5. The minimum expected count is 18.00.
[b]Computed only for a 2×2 table.

The first Crosstabulation table shows that the rate of stroke is 15% in the new treatment group compared to 21.0% in the standard treatment group. The Chi-Square Tests table shows the Fisher's exact test chi-square value of $P = 0.358$ which indicates that this difference in rates is not statistically significant. However, the statistical significance of between-group rates, which depends largely on sample size, may not be of primary interest in a clinical setting.

8.13.1   Calculating NNT

From the table, NNT is calculated from the absolute risk reduction (ARR), which is simply the difference in the per cent of patients with the outcome of interest between the groups. From the Crosstabulation table for stroke:

$$ARR = 21.0\% - 15.0\% = 6.0\%$$

then converted to a proportion, which in decimal format is 0.06, and the reciprocal is taken to obtain NNT:

$$NNT = 1/ARR = 1/0.06 = 16.67$$

Obviously, NNT is always rounded to the nearest whole number. This indicates that 17 people will need to receive the new treatment to prevent one extra person from having a stroke.

Crosstabs

Disability * Treatment Group Crosstabulation

			Treatment group		
			New therapy	Standard treatment	Total
Disability	No disability	Count	82	68	150
		% within treatment group	82.0%	68.0%	75.0%
	Disability	Count	18	32	50
		% within treatment group	18.0%	32.0%	25.0%
Total		Count	100	100	200
		% within treatment group	100.0%	100.0%	100.0%

Chi-Square Tests

	Value	df	Asymp. sig. (two-sided)	Exact sig. (two-sided)	Exact sig. (one-sided)
Pearson chi-square	5.227[a]	1	0.022		
Continuity correction[b]	4.507	1	0.034		
Likelihood ratio	5.281	1	0.022		
Fisher's exact test				0.033	0.017
Linear-by-linear association	5.201	1	0.023		
N of valid cases	200				

[a]0 cell (0.0%) has expected count less than 5. The minimum expected count is 25.00.
[b]Computed only for a 2×2 table.

The second Crosstabulation table shows that the rate of disability is 18% in the new treatment group compared to 32.0% in the standard treatment group. The Fisher's exact test chi-square value with $P = 0.033$ shows that this new treatment achieves a significant change in the rate of disability. The calculation of NNT is as follows:

$$ARR = 32.0\% - 18.0\% = 14.0\%$$

$$NNT = 1/ARR = 1/0.14 = 7.14$$

This indicates that seven people will need to receive the new treatment to prevent one extra person having a major disability. The larger the difference between groups as shown by a larger ARR, the fewer the number of patients who need to receive the treatment to prevent the occurrence of one additional adverse event. Methods for calculating confidence intervals for NNT, which must be a positive number, are reported in the literature.[4]

Occasionally in clinical trials there may be no adverse events in one group. If the *Crosstabs* procedure is repeated again, with the variable indicating survival (death) entered as the outcome in the rows, the shown table is produced.

Crosstabs

Death * Treatment Group Crosstabulation

			Treatment group		
			New therapy	Standard treatment	Total
Death	Survived	Count	100	92	192
		% within treatment group	100.0%	92.0%	96.0%
	Died	Count	0	8	8
		% within treatment group	0.0%	8.0%	4.0%
Total		Count	100	100	200
		% within treatment group	100.0%	100.0%	100.0%

Chi-Square Tests

	Value	df	Asymp. sig. (two-sided)	Exact sig. (two-sided)	Exact sig. (one-sided)
Pearson chi-square	8.333[a]	1	0.004		
Continuity correction[b]	6.380	1	0.012		
Likelihood ratio	11.424	1	0.001		
Fisher's exact test				0.007	0.003
Linear-by-linear association	8.292	1	0.004		
N of valid cases	200				

[a] Two cells (50.0%) have expected count less than 5. The minimum expected count is 4.00.
[b] Computed only for a 2×2 table.

The Crosstabulation shows that death occurs in 8% of the standard treatment group compared to 0% in the new treatment group. The Fisher's exact test chi-square value with $P = 0.007$ indicates that this a significant association between survival and type of treatment received. When no adverse events occur in a group, as for deaths in the new treatment group this does not mean that no deaths will ever occur in patients who receive the new treatment. One way to estimate the proportion of patients in this group who might die is to calculate the upper end of the confidence interval around the zero percentage. To compute a confidence interval around a percentage that is less than 1% requires exact methods based on a binomial distribution. However, a rough estimate of the upper 95% confidence interval around a zero percentage is $3/n$ where n is the number of participants in the group. From the Crosstabulation table, the upper 95% confidence interval around no deaths in the new therapy group would then be $3/100$, or 3%. This is an approximate calculation only and may yield a conservative estimate. The true binomial interval is 3.6%. For more accurate estimates, a binomial confidence calculator is available at StatPages (see Useful Websites).

8.13.2 How to report NNT

When reporting NNT, it is usual to show the rates of the events in the two treatment groups in addition to the P value from the chi-square tests. Table 8.14 shows how the results can be reported.

Table 8.14 Reporting the results from an experimental study of treatment effects

Outcome	New therapy	Standard treatment	NNT	P value
N	100	100		
Stroke	15%	21%	17	0.36
Disability	18%	32%	7	0.03
Death	0%	8%	13	0.01

8.14   Paired categorical variables: McNemar's chi-square test

Paired categorical measurements taken from the same participants on two occasions or categorical data collected in matched case-control studies must be analyzed using tests for repeated data.

The measurements collected in these types of study designs are not independent and therefore chi-square tests cannot be used because the assumptions would be violated. In this situation, McNemar's test is used to assess whether there is a significant change in proportions over time for paired data or whether there is a significant difference in proportions between matched cases and controls. In this type of analysis, the outcome of interest is the within-person changes (or within-pair differences) and there are no explanatory variables. McNemar's test can be used when the outcome variable has a binary response such as 'yes' and 'no'. McNemar's test is calculated by examining the number of the responses that are concordant for positive (yes on both occasions) and negative (no on both occasions), and the number of disconcordant pairs (yes and no, or no and yes).

The assumptions for using a paired McNemar's test are shown in Box 8.8.

Box 8.8 Assumptions for a paired McNemar's test

For a paired McNemar's test the following assumptions must be met:
- the outcome variable is binary
- each participant is represented in the table once only
- the difference between the paired proportions is the outcome of interest

---

Research question

The file **health-camp.sav** contains the data from 86 children who attended a camp to learn how to self-manage their illness. The children were asked whether they knew how to manage their illness appropriately (yes/no) and whether they knew when to use their rescue medication appropriately (yes/no) at both the start and completion of the camp. In this example, McNemar's test can be used to determine if the children's responses before the camp is equal to their responses after the camp.

Question: Did attendance at the camp increase the number of children who knew how to manage their illness appropriately?

Null hypothesis: That there was no change in children's knowledge of illness management between the beginning and completion of the health camp.

Variables: Appropriate knowledge (categorical, binary) at the beginning and completion of the camp.

In this research question the explanatory variable is time, which is built into the analysis, and knowledge at both Time 1 and Time 2 are the outcome variables. The relationship between the measurements is summarized using a paired 2×2 contingency table and McNemar's test can be obtained using the commands shown in Box 8.9.

Box 8.9 SPSS commands to obtain McNemar's test

SPSS Commands

health-camp.sav – IBM SPSS Statistics Data Editor
>   *Analyze → Descriptive Statistics → Crosstabs*

Crosstabs
>   *Highlight Knowledge-Time1 and click into Row(s)*
>   *Highlight Knowledge-Time2 and click into Column(s)*
>   *Click on Statistics*

Crosstabs: Statistics
>   *Tick McNemar, click Continue*

Crosstabs
>   *Click on Cells*

Crosstabs: Cell Display
>   *Counts: tick Observed (default)*
>   *Percentages: tick Total*
>   *Noninteger Weights: tick Round cell count (default)*
>   *Click Continue*

Crosstabs
>   *Click OK*

In the Crosstabulation table, the total column and total row cells indicate that 34.9% of children had appropriate knowledge at the beginning of the camp (Yes at Time 1) and 61.6% at the end of the camp (Yes at Time 2). More importantly, the internal cells of the table show that 31.4% of children did not have appropriate knowledge on both occasions and 27.9% did have appropriate knowledge on both occasions. The percentages also show that 33.7% of children improved their knowledge (i.e. went from No at Time 1 to Yes at Time 2) and only 7.0% of children reduced their knowledge (i.e. went from Yes at Time 1 to No at Time 2).

Crosstabs

Knowledge-Time 1 * Knowledge-Time 2 Crosstabulation

			Knowledge-Time 2		Total
			No	Yes	
Knowledge-Time 1	No	Count	27	29	56
		% of total	31.4%	33.7%	65.1%
	Yes	Count	6	24	30
		% of total	7.0%	27.9%	34.9%
Total		Count	33	53	86
		% of total	38.4%	61.6%	100.0%

Chi-Square Tests

	Value	Exact Sig. (two-sided)
McNemar test		0.000[a]
N of valid cases	86	

[a]Binomial distribution used.

The Chi-Square Tests table shows a McNemar P value of <0.0001 indicating that children's knowledge of the management of their illness significantly changed after attending the camp. The percentages from the crosstabulation indicate that their knowledge improved.

When reporting paired information, summary statistics that reflect how many children improved their knowledge compared to how many children reduced their knowledge are used. This difference in proportions with its 95% confidence interval can be calculated using Excel.

In computing these statistics from the Crosstabulation table, the concordant cells are not used and only the information from the discordant cells is of interest as shown in Table 8.15. In Table 8.15, the two concordant cells (a and d) show the number of children who did or did not have appropriate knowledge at both the beginning and end of the camp. The two discordant cells (b and c) show the number of children who changed their knowledge status in either direction between the two occasions.

Table 8.15 Presentation of data showing discordant cells

	No at end of camp		Yes at end of camp	Total
No at beginning of camp	27		29	56
		a b		
		c d		
Yes at beginning of camp	6		24	30
Total	33		53	n 86

8.14.1 Calculating the change in proportion

The counts in the discordant cells are used in calculating the change as a proportion and the SE of difference from the cell counts as follows:

$$\text{Difference in proportions} = \frac{(b-c)}{n}$$

$$\text{SE of difference} = \frac{1}{n} \times \sqrt{b+c- \left(\frac{(b-c)^2}{n} \right)}$$

For large sample sizes, the 95% confidence interval around the difference in proportions is calculated as $1.96 \times \text{SE}$. These statistics can be computed using the discordant

Table 8.16   Excel spreadsheet to compute differences for paired data

	p_2 Yes-Time 2	p_1 Yes-Time 1	Total N	Difference	SE	95% CI width	CI lower	CI upper
Knowledge	0.616	0.349	86	0.267	0.062	0.122	0.145	0.390

Note: p = proportion

cell counts in an Excel spreadsheet as shown in Table 8.16 and the proportions for appropriate knowledge at the beginning of the camp (Yes at Time 1) and end of the camp (Yes at Time 2). The table shows that the increase in knowledge converted back to a percentage is 26.7% (95% CI 14.5, 39.0). The 95% confidence interval does not cross the zero line of no difference which reflects the finding that the change in proportions is statistically significant.

Research question

A second outcome that was measured in the study was whether children knew when to use their rescue medication appropriately. The SPSS commands shown in Box 8.9 can be used to obtain a McNemar's test for this outcome by entering medication-time 1 into the rows and medication-time 2 into the columns of the crosstabulation. Again, only the total percentages are requested.

In the Crosstabulation table, the percentages in the discordant cells indicate a small increase in knowledge of 15.1% to 12.8% or 2.3%. The Chi-Square Tests table shows that this difference is not significant with a P value of 0.839.

Crosstabs

Medication-Time 1 * Medication-Time 2 Crosstabulation

			Medication-Time 2		
			No	Yes	Total
Medication-Time 1	No	Count	17	13	30
		% of total	19.8%	15.1%	34.9%
	Yes	Count	11	45	56
		% of total	12.8%	52.3%	65.1%
Total		Count	28	58	86
		% of total	32.6%	67.4%	100.0%

Chi-Square Tests		
	Value	Exact sig. (two-sided)
McNemar test		0.839[a]
N of valid cases	86	

[a]Binomial distribution used.

The Excel spreadsheet shown in Table 8.16 can be used to obtain the paired difference and its 95% confidence interval as proportions as shown in Table 8.17. The increase in knowledge is 2.3% (95% CI −8.8%, 13.5%). The 95% confidence interval crosses the

Table 8.17   Excel spreadsheet to compute differences for paired data

	p_2 Yes- Time 2	p_1 Yes- Time 1	Total *N*	Difference	SE	95% CI width	CI lower	CI upper
Medication	0.674	0.651	86	0.023	0.057	0.112	−0.088	0.135

Note: p = proportion

zero line of no difference reflecting the finding that the change in proportions is not statistically significant.

8.14.2   *Reporting the results of paired data*

The analyses show that the number of children who knew how to manage their illness significantly changed after camp, with almost one third of the group reporting increased knowledge after attending the camp. The number of children who knew when to use their rescue medication slightly changed but not significantly on completion of the camp. These results could be presented as shown in Table 8.18. By reporting the per cent of children with knowledge on both occasions, the per cent increase and the *P* value, all information that is relevant to interpreting the findings is included.

Table 8.18   Changes in knowledge of management and medication use in 86 children following camp attendance

	Knowledge prior	Knowledge on completion	% increase and 95% CI	*P* value
Management	34.9%	61.6%	26.7% (14.5, 39.0)	<0.0001
Medication use	65.1%	67.4%	2.3% (−8.8, 13.5)	0.84

8.15   Notes for critical appraisal

There are many ways in which crosstabulations can be used and chi-square values can be computed. The *P* values often depend on the sample size and can be biased by cells with only a small number of expected counts. When critically appraising an article that presents categorical data analyzed using univariate statistics or crosstabulations, it is important to ask the questions shown in Box 8.10.

Box 8.10 Questions for critical appraisal

The following questions should be asked when appraising published results from analyses in which crosstabulations are used:
- Has any participant been included in an analysis more than once?
- Have the correct terms to describe rates or proportions been used?
- Is the correct chi-square value presented?

- Could any small cells have biased the *P* value?
- Are percentages reported so that the size of the difference is clear?
- Have 95% confidence intervals for percentages been reported?
- If two groups are being compared, is the difference between them shown?
- If the exposure variable is ordered, is a trend statistic reported?
- Is it clear how any 'missing data' have influenced the results?
- Are the most important findings reported as a figure?
- If the results of a trial to test an intervention are being reported, is NNT presented?
- If the data are paired, has a paired statistical test been used?

References

1. Bland M. *An introduction to medical statistics*, 2nd edn. Oxford University Press: Oxford, UK, 1996.
2. Field A. *Discovering statistics using IBM SPSS Statistics*, 4th edn. Sage: London, 2013.
3. Peat J, Mellis C, Williams K, Xuan W. *Health science research: a handbook of quantitative methods*. Allen and Unwin: Crow's Nest, Sydney, 2001.
4. Altman DG. Confidence intervals for number needed to treat. *BMJ* 1998; **317**: 1309–1312.

CHAPTER 9
Risk statistics

Clinicians have a good intuitive understanding of risk and even of a ratio of risks. Gamblers have a good intuitive understanding of odds. No one (with the possible exception of certain statisticians) intuitively understands a ratio of odds.[1,2]

Objectives

The objectives of this chapter are to explain how to:
- decide whether odds ratio or relative risk is the appropriate statistic to use
- use logistic regression to compute adjusted odds ratios
- report and plot unadjusted and adjusted odds ratios
- change risk estimates to protection and vice versa
- calculate 95% confidence intervals around estimates of risk
- critically appraise the literature in which estimates of risk are reported

9.1 Risk statistics

Chi-square tests indicate whether two binary variables such as an exposure and an outcome measurement are independent or are significantly related to each other. However, apart from the *P* value, chi-square tests do not provide a statistic for describing the strength of the relationship. Two risk statistics that are useful for measuring the magnitude of the association between two binary variables measured in a 2×2 table are the odds ratio and the relative risk. Both of these statistics are estimates of risk and, as such, describe the probability that people who are exposed to a certain factor will have a disease compared to people who are not exposed to the same factor.

The odds ratio is the odds of the outcome occurring in one group divided by the odds of the outcome occurring in another group. Relative risk is the ratio of the probability of the outcome occurring in one group (i.e. exposed) to the probability of the outcome occurring in another group (i.e. non-exposed). The choice of using an odds ratio or a relative risk depends on both the study design and whether bivariate or multivariate analyses are required.

Medical Statistics: A Guide to SPSS, Data Analysis and Critical Appraisal, Second Edition.
Belinda Barton and Jennifer Peat.
© 2014 John Wiley & Sons, Ltd. Published 2014 by John Wiley & Sons, Ltd.
Companion website: www.wiley.com/go/barton/medicalstatistics2e

9.2 Study design

Both odds ratio and relative risk are widely used in epidemiological and clinical research to describe the risk of people having a disease (or an outcome) in the presence of an exposure, which may be an environmental factor, a treatment or any other type of explanatory factor. Odds ratios have the advantage that they can be used in any study design, including experimental and case–control studies in which the proportion of cases is unlikely to be representative of the proportion in the population. Thus, odds ratio are commonly used to measure the effect size. In addition, direct comparisons of effect can be made between different study designs and odds ratios from different studies can be compared and combined, and are often used to report the results of systematic reviews and meta-analyses. Odds ratios can be adjusted for the effects of other related exposures in multivariate analyses in which case the summary estimates are called 'adjusted' odds ratios, which are discussed later in this chapter.

The relative risk statistic relies on the probability of the outcome in the sample being the same as the probability of the outcome in the population. Therefore, relative risk can be calculated when the sample has been selected randomly or when a representative sample has been enrolled. Random samples are often enrolled in cross-sectional studies, some cohort studies and clinical trials. As such, relative risk is commonly calculated in these types of studies and when only bivariate analyses are required. In non-random samples, the probability of outcome will be altered by the selection criteria and therefore the relative risk will not represent the population risk. Thus, relative risk should only be calculated from a sample that has the same characteristics as the population from which it is drawn and in which the proportion of people with the outcome represents the population prevalence rate of the disease.

Odds ratios should not be used to estimate the relative risk. The odds ratio will always overestimate the effect when interpreted as a relative risk and the degree of overestimation will increase as the effect becomes larger.[3] Only when the outcome of interest is low (<10%) does the odds ratio approximate to the risk ratio.[3]

9.3 Odds ratio

The odds ratio is the odds of a person having a disease if exposed to the risk factor divided by the odds of a person having a disease if not exposed to the risk factor. Conversely, an odds ratio can be interpreted as the odds of a person having been exposed to a factor when having the disease compared to the odds of a person having been exposed to a factor when not having the disease. This converse interpretation is useful for case–control studies in which participants are selected on the basis of their disease status and their exposures are measured. In this type of study, the odds ratio is interpreted as the odds that a case has been exposed to the risk factor of interest compared to the odds that a control has been exposed.

9.3.1 Assumptions

The assumptions for using odds ratio are exactly the same as the assumptions for using chi-square tests shown in Box 8.2 in Chapter 8.

Table 9.1 Table to measure the relation between a disease and an exposure

	Disease present	Disease absent	Total
Exposure present	a	b	$a+b$
Exposure absent	c	d	$c+d$
Total	$a+c$	$b+d$	N

9.3.2 Calculating odds ratio

The way in which tables to calculate risk statistics are classically set up in the clinical epidemiology textbooks is shown in Table 9.1.

The odds ratio is a ratio of the probability of an event occurring to the probability of an event not occurring.[4] The odds ratio is calculated by comparing the odds of an event in one group (e.g. exposure present) to the odds of the same event in another group (e.g. exposure absent). From Table 9.1, the odds of the disease in the exposed group compared to the odds of the disease in the non-exposed group can be calculated as shown below. This calculation shows why an odds ratio is sometimes called a ratio of cross-products.

$$\text{Odds ratio (OR)} = \frac{(a/b)}{(c/d)} = \frac{(a \times d)}{(b \times c)}$$

9.3.3 Coding

A problem arises in calculating odds ratio and relative risk using some statistical packages because the format of the table that is required to compute the correct statistics is different from the format used in clinical epidemiology textbooks. To use SPSS to compute these risk statistics, the variables need to be coded as shown in Table 9.2.

Table 9.2 Possible coding of variables to compute risk

Code	Alternate code	Condition	Interpretation
1	0	Disease absent	Outcome negative
2	1	Disease present	Outcome positive
1	0	Exposure absent	Risk factor negative
2	1	Exposure present	Risk factor positive

This will invert the table shown in Table 9.1 but as shown later in this chapter, this will allow the odds ratio to be read directly from the SPSS output generated in both the *Analyze → Frequencies Crosstabs* and the *Analyze → Regression → Binary Logistic* menus.

If the reverse notation is used as in Table 9.1, the odds ratio and relative risk statistics printed by SPSS have to be inverted to obtain the correct direction of effect. The options are to either:

i. code the data as shown in Table 9.2 and in Table 8.3, which inverts the location of cells in Table 9.1 but not the statistics or

ii. code the data as shown in Table 9.1 which inverts the statistics but not the table.

In this chapter, the first option is used so that the layout of the tables is as shown in Table 8.3.

9.3.4   Interpreting the odds ratio

Both odds ratio and relative risk are invaluable statistics for describing the magnitude of the relationship between the exposure and the outcome variables because they provide a size of effect that adds to the information provided by the chi-square value. A chi-square test indicates whether the difference in the proportion of participants with and without disease in the exposure present and exposure absent groups is statistically significant, but an odds ratio quantifies the relative size of the difference between the groups.

Odds ratio is a less valuable statistic than relative risk because it represents the odds of disease, which is not as intuitive as the relative risk. Although the odds ratio is not the easiest of statistics to explain or understand, it is widely used for describing an association between an exposure and a disease because it can be calculated from studies of any design, including cross-sectional, cohort studies, case–control studies and experimental trials as shown in Table 9.3.

Odds ratio has the advantage that it can be used to make direct comparisons of results from studies of different designs and, for this reason, odds ratios are often used in meta-analyses. The odds ratio and the relative risk are always in the same direction of risk or protection. However, the odds ratio does not give a good approximation of the relative risk when the exposure and/or the disease are relatively common.[5] The odds ratio is always larger than relative risk and therefore generally overestimates the true association between variables.

The calculation of the odds ratio from the data shown in Table 9.4 is as follows:

$$\text{Odds ratio} = (a/b)/(c/d)$$
$$= (40/25)/(60/75)$$
$$= (8/5)/(4/5)$$
$$= 2.0$$

Table 9.3   Study type and statistics available

Type of study	Odds ratio	Relative risk
Cross-sectional	Yes	Yes
Cohort	Yes	Sometimes
Case–control	Yes	No
Clinical trial	Yes	Sometimes

Table 9.4   2 × 2 crosstabulation of disease and exposure

	Disease absent	Disease present	Total
Exposure absent	75	60	135
	d	c	
	b	a	
Exposure present	25	40	65
Total	100	100	200

When an odds ratio equals 1.0 then the odds that people with and without the disease have been exposed is equal and the exposure presents no difference in risk. An odds ratio of 2.0 can be interpreted as the odds that an exposed person has the disease present are twice that of the odds that a non-exposed person has the disease present. That is, if a person who is exposed to a risk factor and a person who is not exposed to the same risk factor are compared, a gambler would break even by betting 2:1 that the person who had been exposed would have the disease. However, this interpretation is not intuitive for most researchers and clinicians.

An odds ratio calculated in this way from a 2 × 2 table is called an unadjusted odds ratio because it is not adjusted for the effects of possible confounders. Odds ratios calculated using logistic regression are called 'adjusted odds ratios' because they are adjusted for the effects of the other variables in the model.

The size of odds ratio that is important is often debated and in considering this the clinical importance of the outcome and the number of people exposed need to be taken into account. An odds ratio above 2.0 is usually important. However, a smaller odds ratio between 1.0 and 2.0 can have public health importance if a large number of people are exposed to the factor of interest. For example, approximately 25% of the 5 million children aged between 1 and 14 years living in Australasia have a mother who smokes. The odds ratio for children to wheeze if exposed to environmental tobacco smoke is 1.3, which is close to 1.0. On the basis of this odds ratio and the high exposure rate, a conservative estimate is that 320 000 children have symptoms of wheeze as a result of being exposed, which amounts to an important public health problem.[6] If only 5% of children were exposed or if the outcome was more trivial, the public health impact would be less important.

Research question

The spreadsheet **asthma.sav** contains data from a random cross-sectional sample of 2464 children aged 8 to 10 years in which the exposure of allergy to housedust mites (HDM), the exposure to respiratory infection in early life, the characteristic gender and the presence of the disease (asthma) were measured in all children.

Question:	Are HDM allergy, early infection or gender independent risk factors for asthma in this sample of children?
Null hypothesis:	That HDM allergy, respiratory infection in early life and gender are not independent risk factors for asthma.
Variables:	Outcome variable = Diagnosed asthma (categorical, two levels)
	Explanatory variables (risk factors) = allergy to HDM (categorical, two levels), early infection (categorical, two levels) and gender (categorical, two levels).

The SPSS commands shown in Box 9.1 can be used to obtain the crosstabulations for the three risk factors and their risk statistics. In calculating risk, the risk factors are entered in the rows, the outcome in the columns and the row percentages are requested. Each explanatory variable is crosstabulated separately with the outcome variable so three different crosstabulation tables are produced.

Box 9.1 SPSS commands to obtain risk statistics

SPSS Commands

asthma.sav –IBM SPSS Statistics Data Editor
> *Analyze → Descriptive Statistics → Crosstabs*

Crosstabs
> *Highlight Allergy to HDM, Early infection, and Gender and click into Row(s)*
> *Highlight Diagnosed asthma and click into Column(s)*
> *Click Statistics*

Crosstabs: Statistics
> *Tick Chi-square, tick Risk, Click Continue*

Crosstabs
> *Click Cells*

Crosstabs: Cell Display
> *Counts: tick Observed (default)*
> *Percentages: tick Row*
> *Noninteger Weights: tick Round cell count (default), click Continue*

Crosstabs
> *Click OK*

Crosstabs

Allergy to HDM * Diagnosed asthma Crosstabulation

			Diagnosed asthma		
			No	Yes	Total
Allergy to HDM	No	Count	1414	125	1539
		% within allergy to HDM	91.9%	8.1%	100.0%
	Yes	Count	529	396	925
		% within allergy to HDM	57.2%	42.8%	100.0%
Total		Count	1943	521	2464
		% within allergy to HDM	78.9%	21.1%	100.0%

The Crosstabulation table for allergy to HDM and asthma shows that in the group of children who did not have HDM allergy 8.1% had been diagnosed with asthma and in the group of children who did have HDM allergy 42.8% had been diagnosed with asthma.

The Pearson's chi-square value in the Chi-Square Tests table is used to assess significance because the sample size is in excess of 1000. The P value is highly significant at $P < 0.0001$ indicating that the frequency of HDM allergy is significantly different between the two groups and there is an association between HDM allergy and asthma. The odds ratio can be calculated from the crosstabulation table as (396/529)/(125/1414), which is 8.468. This is shown in the Risk Estimate table, which also gives the 95% confidence interval.

Chi-Square Tests

	Value	df	Asymp. sig. (two-sided)	Exact sig. (two-sided)	Exact sig. (one-sided)
Pearson chi-square	416.951[a]	1	0.000		
Continuity correction[b]	414.874	1	0.000		
Likelihood ratio	411.844	1	0.000		
Fisher's exact test				0.000	0.000
Linear-by-linear association	416.782	1	0.000		
N of valid cases	2464				

[a]0 cell (0.0%) has expected count less than 5. The minimum expected count is 195.59.
[b]Computed only for a 2×2 table.

In the Risk Estimate table the odds ratio for the association between a diagnosis of asthma and HDM allergy is large at 8.468 (95% CI 6.765–10.60) reflecting the large difference in percentages of outcome given exposure and thus a strong relation between the two variables in this sample of children. The 95% confidence interval does not contain the value of 1.0, which represents no difference in risk, and therefore is consistent with an odds ratio that is statistically significant.

The cohort statistics reported below the odds ratio can also be used to generate relative risk, which is explained later in this chapter.

Risk Estimate

	Value	95% confidence interval Lower	Upper
Odds ratio for allergy to HDM (no/yes)	8.468	6.765	10.600
For cohort diagnosed asthma = no	1.607	1.516	1.702
For cohort diagnosed asthma = yes	0.190	0.158	0.228
N of valid cases	2464		

The Crosstabulation table for early infection and asthma shows that of the children diagnosed with asthma, 19.7% did not have a respiratory infection in early life compared with 27.5% of the group who did have an early respiratory infection. Although the difference in percentages in this table (27.5% vs 19.7%) is not as large as for HDM allergy, the Pearson's chi-square value in the Chi-Square Tests table shows that this difference is similarly highly significant at $P < 0.0001$.

Crosstabs

Early infection * Diagnosed asthma Crosstabulation

			No	Yes	Total
Early infection	No	Count	1622	399	2021
		% within early infection	80.3%	19.7%	100.0%
	Yes	Count	321	122	443
		% within early infection	72.5%	27.5%	100.0%
Total		Count	1943	521	2464
		% within early infection	78.9%	21.1%	100.0%

Chi-Square Tests

	Value	df	Asymp. sig. (two-sided)	Exact sig. (two-sided)	Exact sig. (one-sided)
Pearson chi-square	13.247[a]	1	0.000		
Continuity correction[b]	12.784	1	0.000		
Likelihood ratio	12.599	1	0.000		
Fisher's exact test				0.000	0.000
Linear-by-linear association	13.242	1	0.000		
N of valid cases	2464				

[a]0 cell (0.0%) has expected count less than 5. The minimum expected count is 93.67.
[b]Computed only for a 2×2 table.

However, the Risk Estimate table shows that the odds ratio for the association between a diagnosis of asthma and an early respiratory infection is much lower than for HDM allergy at 1.545 (95% CI 1.221–1.955). Again, the statistical significance of the odds ratio is reflected in the 95% confidence interval, which does not contain the value of 1.0, which represents no difference in risk.

Risk Estimate

	Value	95% Confidence interval	
		Lower	Upper
Odds ratio for early infection (no/yes)	1.545	1.221	1.955
For cohort diagnosed asthma = no	1.108	1.042	1.178
For cohort diagnosed asthma = yes	0.717	0.602	0.854
N of valid cases	2464		

For gender, the Crosstabulation table shows that 18.8% of females had a diagnosis of asthma compared with 23.4% of males. At $P = 0.005$, the Pearson's chi-square value in the Chi-Square Tests table is less significant than for the other two variables. In the Risk Estimate table, the odds ratio of 1.319 is also smaller (95% CI 1.085–1.602), reflecting the smaller difference in proportions in diagnosed asthma between the two gender groups.

Crosstabs

Gender * Diagnosed asthma Crosstabulation

| | | | Diagnosed asthma | | |
			No	Yes	Total
Gender	Female	Count	965	223	1188
		% within gender	81.2%	18.8%	100.0%
	Male	Count	978	298	1276
		% within gender	76.6%	23.4%	100.0%
Total		Count	1943	521	2464
		% within gender	78.9%	21.1%	100.0%

Chi-Square Tests

	Value	df	Asymp. sig. (two-sided)	Exact sig. (two-sided)	Exact sig. (one-sided)
Pearson chi-square	7.751[a]	1	0.005		
Continuity correction[b]	7.478	1	0.006		
Likelihood ratio	7.778	1	0.005		
Fisher's exact test				0.006	0.003
Linear-by-linear association	7.747	1	0.005		
N of valid cases	2464				

[a]0 cell (0.0%) has expected count less than 5. The minimum expected count is 251.20.
[b]Computed only for a 2 × 2 table.

Risk Estimate

| | Value | 95% Confidence interval | |
		Lower	Upper
Odds ratio for gender (female/male)	1.319	1.085	1.602
For cohort diagnosed asthma = no	1.060	1.017	1.104
For cohort diagnosed asthma = yes	0.804	0.689	0.938
N of valid cases	2464		

9.3.5   Reporting odds ratios

The results from these tables can be presented as shown in Table 9.5. When reporting an odds ratio or relative risk, the per cent of cases with the outcome in the two comparison groups of interest are included. It is often useful to rank explanatory variables in order of the magnitude of risk.

Odds ratios larger than 1.0 are reported with only one decimal place because the precision of 1/100th or 1/1000th of an estimate of risk is not required. The decision of whether to include a column with the chi-square values is optional since the only interpretation of the chi-square value is the *P* value. From the table, it is easy to see how the odds ratio describes the strength of the associations between variables in a way that is not discriminated by the *P* values.

Table 9.5 Unadjusted associations between risk factors and diagnosed asthma in a random sample of 2464 children aged 8–10 years

Risk factor (exposure)	% diagnosed asthma in exposed group	% diagnosed asthma in non-exposed group	Unadjusted odds ratio and 95% CI	Chi-square	P value
Allergy to HDM	42.8%	8.1%	8.5 (6.8, 10.6)	417.0	<0.0001
Early infection	27.5%	19.7%	1.5 (1.2, 2.0)	13.2	<0.0001
Gender	23.4%	18.8%	1.3 (1.1, 1.6)	7.8	0.005

9.4 Protective odds ratios

An odds ratio greater than 1.0 indicates that the risk of disease in the exposed group is greater than the risk in the non-exposed group. If the odds ratio is less than 1.0, then the risk of disease in the exposed group is less than the risk in the non-exposed group.

Whether odds ratios represent risk or protection largely depends on the way in which the variables are coded. For example, having HDM allergy is a strong risk factor for diagnosed asthma in the study sample but if the coding had been reversed with not having HDM allergy coded as 2, then not having HDM allergy would be a strong protective factor. For ease of interpretation, comparison and communication, it is usually better to present all odds ratios in the direction of risk rather than presenting some odds ratios as risk and some as protection.

To illustrate this, the commands shown in Box 1.9 in Chapter 1 can be used to reverse the coding of HDM allergy from 2 = exposure to 1 = exposure and from 1 = no exposure to 2 = no exposure. In this example, the new variable is called hdm2 and its values have been added in Variable View before conducting any analyses. The SPSS commands shown in Box 9.1 can then be used with allergy to HDM re-coded as the row variable, diagnosed asthma as the column variable and the row percentages requested.

Crosstabs

Allergy to HDM – Re-coded * Diagnosed Asthma Crosstabulation

			Diagnosed asthma		Total
			No	Yes	
Allergy to HDM – re-coded	Allergy	Count	529	396	925
		% within allergy to HDM – re-coded	57.2%	42.8%	100.0%
	No Allergy	Count	1414	125	1539
		% within allergy to HDM – re-coded	91.9%	8.1%	100.0%
Total		Count	1943	521	2464
		% within allergy to HDM – re-coded	78.9%	21.1%	100.0%

Chi-Square Tests

	Value	df	Asymp. sig. (two-sided)	Exact sig. (two-sided)	Exact sig. (one-sided)
Pearson chi-square	416.951[a]	1	0.000		
Continuity correction[b]	414.874	1	0.000		
Likelihood ratio	411.844	1	0.000		
Fisher's exact test				0.000	0.000
Linear-by-linear association	416.782	1	0.000		
N of valid cases	2464				

[a]0 cell (0.0%) has expected count less than 5. The minimum expected count is 195.59.
[b]Computed only for a 2×2 table.

Risk Estimate

	Value	95% Confidence interval	
		Lower	Upper
Odds ratio for allergy to HDM – re-coded (allergy/no allergy)	0.118	0.094	0.148
For cohort diagnosed asthma = no	0.622	0.588	0.659
For cohort diagnosed asthma = yes	5.271	4.386	6.334
N of valid cases	2464		

The per cent of children with diagnosed asthma in the exposed and unexposed groups and the P value are obviously exactly the same as before. The only difference in the Crosstabulation table is that the rows have been interchanged. The odds ratio is now a protective factor of 0.118 (95% 0.094–0.148) rather than a risk factor of 8.468 (95% CI 6.765–10.60) as it was in the first analysis.

9.4.1   Changing the direction of risk statistics

Summary statistics of odds ratio can easily be changed from protection to risk or vice versa by calculating the reciprocal value, that is

$$\text{odds ratio (risk)} = 1/\text{odds ratio (protection)}$$

$$= 1/0.118$$

$$= 8.474$$

When recalculated, the upper confidence interval becomes the lower confidence interval and vice versa.

Figure 9.1 shows an odds ratio expressed as a risk factor or as a protective factor. The x-axis is a logarithmic scale because odds ratios are derived from logarithmic values. In Figure 9.1, the dotted line passing through 1 indicates the line of no effect, that is, no difference in risk. When a factor is coded as risk or protection, the effect size is the same because on a logarithmic scale the odds ratios are symmetrical on either side of the line of unity.

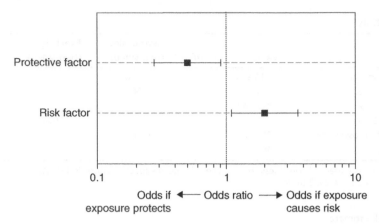

Figure 9.1 Effect of an exposure on a disease shown as both a protective factor and as a risk factor.

Ways in which the direction of risk can be changed during the analysis are to recode the dependent variable so that the category for which risk is of interest is coded with a higher number than the reference category. Alternatively, when running a binary logistic regression, the reference category can be changed under '*Categorical, Change Contrast*'.

9.5   Adjusted odds ratios

A problem with odds ratios calculated from 2×2 crosstabulations is that some explanatory factors may be related to one another. If cases with one factor present also tend to have another factor present, the effects of both factors will be included in each odds ratio. Thus, each odd ratio will be artificially inflated with the effect of the associated exposure; that is, confounding will be present. Logistic regression is used to calculate the effects of risk factors as independent odds ratios with the effects of other confounders removed. These odds ratios are called adjusted odds ratios.

Figure 9.2 shows the percentage of cases with disease in each of three exposure groups. In group 1, participants had no exposure, in group 2 participants had exposure to factor I and in group 3 participants had exposure to factor I and factor II. If an unadjusted odds ratio were used to calculate the risk of disease in the presence of exposure to factor I, then in a bivariate analysis, groups 2 and 3 would be combined and compared with group 1. The effect of including cases also exposed to factor II would inflate the estimate of risk because their rate of disease is higher than for cases exposed to factor 1. Logistic regression is used to mathematically separate out the independent risk associated with exposure to factor I or to factor II.

9.5.1   *Binary logistic regression*

Binary logistic regression is not really a regression analysis in the classic sense of the term but is a mathematical method to measure the effects of explanatory variables (or risk factors) on a binary outcome variable while adjusting for inter-relationships between them.

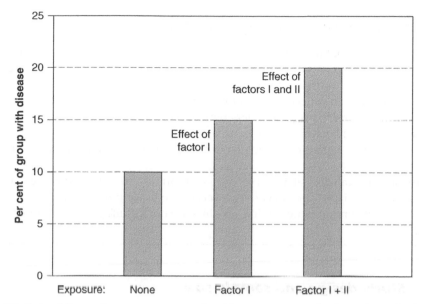

Figure 9.2 Rate of disease in group not exposed and in groups exposed to factor I or to both factors I and II.

In binary logistic regression, the variables that affect the probability of the outcome are measured as odds ratios, which are called adjusted odds ratios.

Logistic regression is primarily used to determine which explanatory variables independently predict the outcome, when the outcome is a binary variable.[7] The outcome variable could be a condition or a disease; for example, the presence or absence of asthma, or the occurrence or absence of a heart attack. In linear regression, the values of the outcome variables are predicted form one or more explanatory variables (see Chapter 7). In logistic regression, since the outcome is binary, the probability of the outcome occurring is calculated based on the given values of the explanatory variables. Logistic regression is similar to the linear regression in that a regression equation can be used to predict the probability of an outcome occurring. However, the logistic regression equation is expressed in logarithmic terms (or logits) and therefore regression coefficients must be converted to be interpreted.

Although the explanatory variables or predictors in the model can be continuous or categorical variables, logistic regression is best suited to measure the effects of exposures or explanatory variables that are binary variables. Continuous variables can be included but logistic regression will produce an estimate of risk for each unit of measurement. Thus, the assumption that the risk effect is linear over each unit of the variable must be met and the relationship should not be curved or have a threshold value over which the effect occurs. In addition, interactions between explanatory variables can be included.

9.5.2 Assumptions of logistic regression

The assumptions for using logistic regression are shown in Box 9.2. The assumptions for the chi-square test as shown in Box 8.2 in Chapter 8 must also be met.

Box 9.2 Assumptions for using logistic regression

The assumptions that must be met when using logistic regression are as follows:
- the sample is representative of the population to which inference will be made
- the sample size is sufficient to support the model
- the data have been collected in a period when the relationship between the outcome and the explanatory variable/s remains constant
- all important explanatory variables are included
- the explanatory variables do not have a high degree of collinearity with one another
- if an ordered categorical variable or a continuous variable is included as an explanatory variable, the effect over levels of the factor must be linear
- alternate outcome and intervening variables are not included as explanatory variables

9.5.3 Study design and sample size

Logistic regression is most suitable for studies with a large randomly selected sample such as cross-sectional or cohort studies but is also appropriate for use in studies with a non-random population such as case–control and experimental studies. Logistic regression is not suitable for matched or paired data or for repeated measures because the measurements are not independent – in these situations, conditional logistic regression is used. In addition, variables that are alternative outcome variables because they are on the same pathway of development as the outcome variable must not be included as independent risk factors.

A large sample size is usually required to support a reliable binary logistic regression model because a cell is generated for each unit of the variable. The data are divided into a multi-dimension array of cells in exactly the same way as for factorial ANOVA shown in Table 5.6 but the outcome variable is also included in the array. If three variables each with two levels are included in the analysis, for example, an outcome and two explanatory variables, the number of cells in the model will be $2 \times 2 \times 2$, or eight cells. As with chi-square analyses, a general rule of thumb is that the number of cases in any one cell should be at least 10. When there are empty cells or cells with a small number of cases, estimates of risk can become unstable and unreliable. Thus, it is important to have an adequate sample size to support the analysis.

9.5.4 Model building

Although SPSS provides automatic forward and backward stepwise processes for building multivariate models, it is more informative to build a logistic regression model using the same sequential method described for multiple regression in Chapter 7. Using this method, variables are added to the model one at a time in order of the magnitude of the chi-square association, starting with the largest estimate. At each step, changes to the model can be examined to assess multicollinearity and instability in the model.

If an a priori decision is made to include known confounders, these can be entered first into the logistic regression and the model built up from there. Alternatively, confounders can be entered at the end of the model building sequence and only retained in the model if they change the size of the coefficients of the variables already in the model by more than 10%.

At each step of adding a variable to the model, it is important to compare the *P* values, the standard errors and the odds ratios in the model from Block 1 of 1 with the values from the second model in Block 2 of 2. A standard error that increases by an important amount, say by more than 10% when another variable is added to the model, is an indication that the model has become less precise. In this situation, the model is less stable as a result of two or more variables having some degree of multicollinearity and thus sharing variation. The effect of shared variation is to inflate the standard errors. If this occurs, then one of the variables must be removed. If the standard error decreases, the model has become more precise. This indicates that the variable added to the model is a good predictor of the outcome and explains some of the variance. As with any multivariate model, the decision of which variable to remove or maintain is based on biological plausibility for the effect and decisions about the variables that can be measured with most accuracy. A commonly used criterion for retaining variables in a model is a *P* value < 0.1.[8]

Occasionally in logistic regression, complete separation can occur where the outcome variable can be perfectly predicted by one or more explanatory variables. For example, this may occur when predicting an age-related disease (e.g. Alzheimer's) and the explanatory variable is age coded in categories (e.g. $1 = 25-40$ years, $2 = 41-55$ years and $3 = 56-70$ years). All people with the disease are 56 years and older and all people aged less than 56 do not have the disease. Therefore, age group 3 predicts the presence of the disease and the age groups of 1 and 2 predict the absence of the disease. Here, the outcome groups (presence or absence of a disease) can be separated by the explanatory variable. Complete separation results in large standard errors as a result of overfitting the regression model.[9]

9.5.5   *Assessing the model and predictors*

In logistic regression, to test the goodness of fit of the model to the data, Cox and Snell *R* square and Nagelkerke *R* square can be examined. The Cox and Snell *R* square is similar to the multiple correlation coefficient in linear regression and measures the strength of the association. This coefficient which takes sample size into consideration is based on log likelihoods and cannot reach its maximum value of 1.[8] The Nagelkerke *R* square is a modification of the Cox and Snell so that a value of 1 can be obtained. Consequently, the Nagelkerke *R* square is generally higher than Cox's and has values that range between 0 and 1.

To evaluate the contribution of an explanatory variable to the model, the Wald statistic can be used. This statistic has a chi-square distribution and is the result of dividing the *B* value by its standard error and then squaring the result. This value is used to calculate the significance (*P*) value for each factor in the model. In logistic regression, the constant is used in the prediction of probabilities but does not have a practical interpretation. It should be noted that when the absolute value of the *B* coefficient is large, the standard error increases which results in the Wald statistic being underestimated.[9] Consequently, the occurrence of Type II errors is increased. In this case, other methods such as a sequential method of entering variables should be used to assess the contribution of the variable to the model.

Research question

The risk factors for asthma in the research question can now be examined in a multivariate model by building a logistic regression using the SPSS commands shown in Box 9.3. On the basis of the magnitude of the chi square values, the variable allergy to HDM will be entered first, then early infection and finally gender.

Box 9.3 SPSS commands to build a logistic regression model

SPSS Commands

asthma.sav –IBM SPSS Statistics Data Editor
    Analyze → Regression → Binary Logistic
Logistic Regression
    Highlight Diagnosed asthma and click into Dependent
    Highlight Allergy to HDM and click into Covariates
    Method = Enter (default)
    Under Block 1 of 1, click Next
    Highlight Early infection and click into Covariates under Block 2 of 2
    Method = Enter (default)
    Click on Options
Logistic regression: Options
    Under Statistics and Plots, tick CI for exp(B):95%
    Tick Include constant in model (default)
    Click Continue
Logistic Regression
    Click OK

The Omnibus Tests of Model Coefficients reports the chi-square value for the overall model, as well as the change from the previous model and the corresponding significance level. In this model, the comparison model is no predictors, with only the constant (intercept) included. The level of block is significant ($P < 0.001$), indicating that the model has improved significantly by including the variable, allergy to HDM.

Logistic regression

Omnibus Tests of Model Coefficients

		Chi-square	df	Sig.
Step 1	Step	411.844	1	0.000
	Block	411.844	1	0.000
	Model	411.844	1	0.000

In the Model Summary table, the Nagelkerke R square indicates that 23.9% of the variation in diagnosed asthma is explained by HDM allergy. The Variables in the Equation table shows the model coefficients but the interpretation of the coefficients is different to those obtained in linear regression. The B estimate for HDM allergy of 2.136 is the odds ratio in units of natural logarithms, that is, to the base e. A positive coefficient indicates that the predicted odds increase as the explanatory variable increases. A negative coefficient indicates that the predicted odds decrease as the explanatory variable increases. The standard error of this estimate in log units is 0.115. When adding further variables to the model, it is important that this standard error does not inflate by more than 10%. The actual odds ratio of 8.468 is shown as the anti-log (or exponential, e^b) of the B estimate in the column labelled Exp(B). This value indicates the changes in odds associated with a unit increase in the explanatory variable and when there is only one explanatory variable in the model is the same as the estimate from the 2×2 crosstabulation.

Model Summary

Step	−2 Log likelihood	Cox & Snell R square	Nagelkerke R square
1	2130.337[a]	0.154	0.239

[a] Estimation terminated at iteration number 5 because parameter estimates changed by less than 0.001.

Variables in the Equation

		B	S.E.	Wald	df	Sig.	Exp(B)	95% C.I.for EXP(B) Lower	Upper
Step 1[a]	hdm	2.136	0.115	347.771	1	0.000	8.468	6.765	10.600
	Constant	−4.562	0.198	530.349	1	0.000	0.010		

[a] Variable(s) entered on step 1: hdm.

The Omnibus Tests of Model Coefficients table indicates the change in the chi-square value from the previous model and whether this change is significant. The P value is of 0.022 is significant and indicates that the fit of the model to the data has significantly improved by including infection as an explanatory variable.

Omnibus Tests of Model Coefficients

		Chi-square	df	Sig.
Step 1	Step	5.275	1	0.022
	Block	5.275	1	0.022
	Model	417.119	2	0.000

The Model Summary table from Block 2 shows that the Nagelkerke R square has increased slightly from 0.239 to 0.242 and the odds ratio for HDM allergy has decreased slightly from 8.467 to 8.360. Importantly, the standard error for HDM allergy has remained unchanged at 0.115 indicating that the model is stable. The odds ratio for infection, which is the exponential of the beta coefficient (B) 0.307, that is 1.360, is significant at $P = 0.02$. This estimate of risk is reduced compared to the unadjusted odds ratio of 1.545 obtained from the 2×2 table because the effect of confounding is removed.

Model Summary

Step	−2 Log likelihood	Cox & Snell R Square	Nagelkerke R Square
1	2125.062[a]	0.156	0.242

[a]Estimation terminated at iteration number 5 because parameter estimates changed by less than 0.001.

Variables in the Equation

		B	S.E.	Wald	df	Sig.	Exp(B)	95% C.I.for EXP(B) Lower	Upper
Step 1[a]	Hdm	2.123	0.115	342.608	1	.000	8.360	6.677	10.468
	Infect	0.307	0.133	5.369	1	.020	1.360	1.049	1.764
	Constant	−4.911	0.252	380.375	1	.000	.007		

[a]Variable(s) entered on step 1: infect.

The effect of gender can be added to the model using the commands shown in Box 9.3 by entering the variables allergy to HDM and early infection for the stable model in Block 1 of 1 and entering gender in Block 2 of 2.

Logistic regression

Omnibus Tests of Model Coefficients

		Chi-square	df	Sig.
Step 1	Step	0.274	1	0.600
	Block	0.274	1	0.600
	Model	417.393	3	0.000

Model Summary

Step	−2 Log likelihood	Cox & Snell R Square	Nagelkerke R Square
1	2124.788[a]	0.156	0.242

[a]Estimation terminated at iteration number 5 because parameter estimates changed by less than 0.001.

Variables in the Equation

		B	S.E.	Wald	df	Sig.	Exp(B)	95% C.I.for EXP(B) Lower	Upper
Step 1[a]	hdm	2.118	0.115	338.103	1	0.000	8.313	6.633	10.419
	infect	0.302	0.133	5.155	1	0.023	1.353	1.042	1.756
	gender	0.058	0.110	0.274	1	0.600	1.059	0.854	1.314
	Constant	−4.985	0.289	297.409	1	0.000	0.007		

[a]Variable(s) entered on step 1: gender.

The Omnibus Tests of Model Coefficients table shows that the chi-square value has slightly changed, which is not significant indicating that adding gender to the model did not improve the fit of the model. The addition of gender does not change the R square statistics in the Model Summary table and hardly changes the odds ratio for HDM allergy in the Variables in the Equation table. The odds ratio for HDM allergy falls slightly from 8.360 to 8.313 and there is no change in the standard error of 0.115. The odds ratio for infection falls slightly from 1.360 to 1.353, again with no change in the standard error of 0.133. Gender which was a significant risk factor in the unadjusted analysis at $P = 0.005$ is no longer a significant predictor with $P = 0.60$. The unadjusted odds ratio for gender was 1.319 in bivariate analyses compared to the adjusted value which is now 1.059.

The reduction in this odds ratio suggests that there is a degree of confounding between gender and HDM allergy or infection. The extent of the confounding can be investigated using the SPSS commands in Box 8.3 in Chapter 8 with allergy to HDM and early infection entered in the rows, gender entered in the columns and column percentages requested to produce the following output.

Crosstabs

Allergy to HDM * Gender Crosstabulation

			Gender		Total
			Female	Male	
Allergy to HDM	No	Count	805	734	1539
		% within gender	67.8%	57.5%	62.5%
	Yes	Count	383	542	925
		% within gender	32.2%	42.5%	37.5%
Total		Count	1188	1276	2464
		% within gender	100.0%	100.0%	100.0%

Chi-Square Tests

	Value	df	Asymp. sig. (two-sided)	Exact sig. (two-sided)	Exact sig. (one-sided)
Pearson chi-square	27.499[a]	1	0.000		
Continuity correction[b]	27.064	1	0.000		
Likelihood ratio	27.600	1	0.000		
Fisher's exact test				0.000	0.000
Linear-by-linear association	27.487	1	0.000		
N of valid cases	2464				

[a]0 cell (0.0%) has expected count less than 5. The minimum expected count is 445.98.
[b]Computed only for a 2 × 2 table.

Crosstabs

Early infection * Gender Crosstabulation

			Gender		Total
			Female	Male	
Early infection	No	Count	1016	1005	2021
		% within gender	85.5%	78.8%	82.0%
	Yes	Count	172	271	443
		% within gender	14.5%	21.2%	18.0%
Total		Count	1188	1276	2464
		% within gender	100.0%	100.0%	100.0%

Chi-Square Tests

	Value	df	Asymp. sig. (two-sided)	Exact sig. (two-sided)	Exact sig. (one-sided)
Pearson chi-square	19.065[a]	1	0.000		
Continuity correction[b]	18.610	1	0.000		
Likelihood ratio	19.228	1	0.000		
Fisher's exact test				0.000	0.000
Linear-by-linear association	19.058	1	0.000		
N of valid cases	2464				

[a]0 cell (0.0%) has expected count less than 5. The minimum expected count is 213.59.
[b]Computed only for a 2×2 table.

9.5.6   Interpretation of confounding effects

The P values for the Pearson chi-square tests indicate that allergy to HDM and early respiratory infection are both significantly related to gender. Examination of the Crosstabulation tables shows that males have a higher percentage of allergy and early respiratory infections compared to females. Thus, gender was a risk factor in the unadjusted estimates because of confounding between gender and the other two risk factors. The logistic regression shows that once the effects of confounding are removed, gender is no longer a significant independent risk factor for diagnosed asthma.

The interpretation of this model is that boys have a higher rate of diagnosed asthma because they have a higher rate of allergy to HDM and a higher rate of early respiratory infection than girls, and not because they are male per se. Separating out the confounding and identifying the independent effects of risk factors makes an invaluable contribution towards identifying pathways to disease.

9.5.7   Reporting adjusted odds ratios

When reporting odds ratios from any type of study design, the percentages from which they are derived must also be reported so that the level of exposure can be used to interpret the findings. In this research question, the data were derived from a cross-sectional study and thus it is important to report the proportion of children who had asthma in the groups that were exposed or not exposed to the risk factors of interest as shown in Table 9.6. In a case–control study, it would be important to report the per cent of participants in the case and control groups who were exposed to the factors of interest. It is also important to report the unadjusted and adjusted values so that the importance of confounding factors is clear. The adjusted odds ratios from the binary logistic regression are smaller but provide an estimate that is not biased by confounding.

Odds ratios are multiplicative. Table 9.6 shows that the odds ratio for the association between childhood asthma and allergy to HDM is 8.3. However, the odds ratio for children to have diagnosed asthma if they are exposed to both allergy to HDM and to

Table 9.6   Unadjusted and adjusted risk factors for children to have asthma

Risk factor	Exposed % with asthma	Non-exposed % with asthma	Unadjusted odds ratio (95% CI)	Adjusted odds ratio (95% CI)	P value
HDM allergy	42.8%	8.1%	8.5 (6.8, 10.6)	8.3 (6.6, 10.4)	<0.0001
Early infection	27.5%	19.7%	1.5 (1.2, 2.0)	1.4 (1.0, 1.8)	0.02
Gender	23.4%	18.8%	1.4 (1.1, 1.6)	1.1 (0.9, 1.3)	0.60

an early respiratory infection compared to the odds they are not exposed to either risk factor is 8.3×1.4 or 11.6.

9.5.8   Plotting the results in a figure

The lower and upper endpoints of the 95% confidence intervals have different widths as a result of being computed in logarithmic units; therefore, they need to be overlaid as separate plots when using SigmaPlot as shown in Box 9.4. The estimates of odds ratios and confidence interval widths can be entered into SigmaPlot worksheet with the odds ratio in column 1, the lower endpoint of the 95% confidence interval in column 2 and the upper endpoint in column 3 as follows:

Column 1	Column 2	Column 3
8.314	1.678	2.102
1.353	0.310	0.403
1.060	0.206	0.255

The graph can then be plotted using the commands shown in Box 9.4.

Box 9.4 SigmaPlot commands to plot odds ratios

SigmaPlot Commands

Data 1*
       Click on Create Graph tab at top of the screen
       Click on Scatter in sub-menu
       Click on Simple Scatter - Horizontal Error Bars in Scatter Group
Create Graph – Error Bars
       Symbol Values = Worksheet Columns (default), click Next
Create Graph – Data Format
       Data Format = Highlight Many X, click Next

Create Graph – Select Data
    Data for Bar = use drop box and select Column 1
    Data for Error = use drop box and select Column 2
    Click Finish

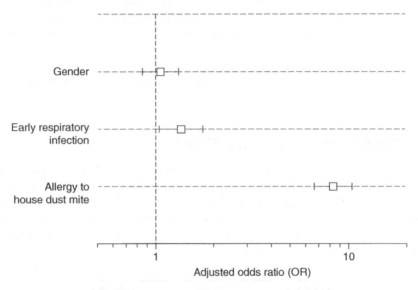

Figure 9.3 Independent risk factors for diagnosed asthma in children.

The sequence is then repeated in *Graph Page → Add Plot* with column 1 again as the data for the bar and column 3 as the data for the error. Once this basic graph is obtained, the labels, symbols, axes, ticks and labels can be customized under the *Graph Page* options menus to obtain Figure 9.3. The *x*-axis needs to be a logarithmic base 10 scale, the first plot should have negative error bars only and the second plot should have positive error bars only. The errors bars can be changed by clicking on a bar and altering the attributes in the *Page Objects* box on the right hand side of the screen.

Figure 9.3 shows the relative importance of the odds ratios. Early infection and allergy to HDM are significant risk factors which are reflected by their 95% confidence intervals not crossing the line of no effect (unity). For gender, the odds ratio is close to unity and the confidence intervals lie on either side of the line of unity indicating a possible effect from protection to risk, which is therefore ambiguous.

9.6   Relative risk

Relative risk is calculated as the ratio of the probability of the outcome occurring in the exposed group compared to the probability of the outcome occurring in the non-exposed group. Relative risk can only be used when the sample is randomly selected from the population and cannot be used in other studies, such as case–control studies or some clinical trials, in which the percentage of the sample with the disease is determined by the sampling method.

9.6.1   Assumptions

The assumptions for using relative risk are the same as for odds ratio (see Section 9.3.1).

9.6.2   Calculating relative risk

Relative risk is calculated as the ratio of the probability of the outcome occurring in the exposed group compared to the probability of the outcome occurring in the non-exposed group and is calculated as follows using the coding displayed in Table 9.1:

$$\text{Relative risk (RR)} = \frac{a/(a+b)}{c/(c+d)}$$

If the summary data shown in Table 9.4 had been collected from a random sample the relative risk would be calculated as follows, with the recoding of data cells for SPSS:

$$\text{Relative risk} = \frac{d/(d+c)}{b/(b+a)}$$

$$= (40/40 + 25)/(60/60 + 75)$$

$$= 0.62/0.44$$

$$= 1.4$$

Thus, the risk estimates are calculated by dividing the per cent of disease positive cases in one row by the per cent of disease positive cases in the other row. The calculation shows how the odds ratio of 2.0 calculated previously with the same data can overestimate the relative risk of 1.4.

9.6.3   Interpreting the relative risk

The advantage of calculating the relative risk is that it is has an intuitive interpretation. A relative risk of 2 indicates that the prevalence of the outcome (present) in the exposed group is twice as high as the prevalence of the outcome (present) in the non-exposed group. That is, people in the exposed group are two times more likely than people in the non-exposed group to have the disease, indicating that the exposure confers a risk for disease. A relative risk of 0.5 would indicate that the prevalence of the outcome (present) in the exposed group is half of the prevalence of the outcome (present) in the non-exposed group, that is, the exposure confers protection against disease. A relative risk of 1 indicates equal risk in the two exposure groups and therefore that the outcome is not related to the exposure.

9.6.4   Requesting relative risk statistics using SPSS

In requesting risk statistics in conjunction with a 2×2 table in SPSS, three estimates are shown in the Risk Estimate table. The first set of statistics is the odds ratio and the next two sets of estimates are labelled 'For cohort = No' and 'For cohort = Yes'. If the 2×2

table is set up appropriately, one of these two statistics is the relative risk. If the 2×2 table is not set up appropriately, relative risk has to be computed from the risk estimates.

For obtaining relative risk in SPSS, the crosstabulation table needs to be set up with the outcome in the columns, the risk factor in the rows and the row percentages requested. If a table is constructed in this way, then either of the following two options can be used.

Option 1

The risk factor but not the outcome has to be re-coded with the exposure present (yes) coded as 1 and the exposure absent (no) coded as 2.

On the spreadsheet **asthma.sav,** allergy to HDM has been recoded in this way into the variable HDM2. This coding is exactly opposite to the coding needed to easily interpret the output from logistic and linear regressions. This coding scheme will 'invert' the crosstabulation table so that the positive exposure is shown on the top row and no exposure is shown on the row below. This table with HDM allergy recoded, which was shown previously, is shown again below. The relative risk can then be calculated as the row percentage for positive outcome divided by the row percentage for negative outcome, that is, 42.8/8.1 or 5.28. This statistic is given in the line 'For cohort = Yes', with a negligible difference from the calculated value resulting from rounding of decimal places.

Crosstabs

Allergy to HDM – Re-coded * Diagnosed Asthma Crosstabulation

			Diagnosed asthma		Total
			No	Yes	
Allergy to HDM – re-coded	Allergy	Count	529	396	925
		% within allergy to HDM – re-coded	57.2%	42.8%	100.0%
	No allergy	Count	1414	125	1539
		% within allergy to HDM – re-coded	91.9%	8.1%	100.0%
Total		Count	1943	521	2464
		% within allergy to HDM – re-coded	78.9%	21.1%	100.0%

Risk Estimate

	Value	95% confidence interval	
		Lower	Upper
Odds ratio for HDM allergy – re-coded (allergy/no allergy)	0.118	0.094	0.148
For cohort diagnosed asthma = no	0.622	0.588	0.659
For cohort diagnosed asthma = yes	5.271	4.386	6.334
N of valid cases	2464		

In the Risk Estimate table, 'For cohort diagnosed asthma = yes' shows the relative risk for children to have diagnosed asthma in the presence of HDM allergy is 5.271 (95% CI 4.386, 6.334). As with odds ratio, only the number of decimal places that infer precision that can be interpreted is reported so the risk estimates from this table would be reported as a relative risk of 5.3 (95% CI 4.4, 6.3).

Option 2

If the risk factor for exposure is maintained as coded as 1 for exposure absent (no) and 2 for exposure present (yes), then the table that was obtained previously is shown again below.

Crosstabs

Allergy to HDM * Diagnosed Asthma Crosstabulation

			Diagnosed asthma		Total
			No	Yes	
Allergy to HDM	No	Count	1414	125	1539
		% within allergy to HDM	91.9%	8.1%	100.0%
	Yes	Count	529	396	925
		% within allergy to HDM	57.2%	42.8%	100.0%
Total		Count	1943	521	2464
		% within allergy to HDM	78.9%	21.1%	100.0%

Risk Estimate

	Value	95% confidence interval	
		Lower	Upper
Odds ratio for allergy to HDM (no/yes)	8.468	6.765	10.600
For cohort diagnosed asthma = no	1.607	1.516	1.702
For cohort diagnosed asthma = yes	0.190	0.158	0.228
N of valid cases	2464		

In this case, the relative risk shown in the table is calculated as 8.1/42.8, or 0.190 and is in the direction of protection. The estimate in the direction of risk and the 95% confidence interval can be computed as the reciprocal of the estimates given for 'For cohort diagnosed asthma = yes' as follows:

$$1/0.190 = 5.263$$

$$1/0.158 = 6.329$$

$$1/0.228 = 4.386$$

Thus, the relative risk for children to have asthma in the presence of HDM allergy is 5.3 (95% CI 4.4, 6.3), which is identical to using the first option.

For both options, the estimate 'For cohort . . . = no' is the relative risk of children having diagnosed asthma in the group that is not exposed to the risk factor of interest. This statistic is rarely used.

9.7   Number needed to be exposed for one additional person to be harmed (NNEH)

In epidemiological studies in which the influence of an exposure is described by an odds ratio, inclusion of the statistic 'number needed to be exposed for one additional person to be harmed' (NNEH) can be a useful statistic that applies to a person rather than to a sample. As such, this statistic provides the number of people who need to be exposed to the risk factor of interest to cause harm to one additional person.

As with calculating NNT in Chapter 8, NNEH is calculated from a 2×2 table in which both the outcome and the exposure are coded as binary variables. The statistic NNEH can be easily calculated from a 2×2 crosstabulation in which the outcome is entered in the rows, the exposure is entered in the columns and the column percentages are requested. The statistic NNEH is then calculated from the absolute risk increase (ARI), which is simply the difference in the proportion of participants with the outcome of interest in the exposed and unexposed groups. From the tables for asthma and HDM allergy:

$$ARI = 0.43 - 0.08 = 0.35$$

$$NNEH = 1/ARI = 1/0.35 = 2.9$$

This indicates that for every three children with allergy to HDM, one additional child will be diagnosed with asthma. NNEH is only reported to whole numbers.

For early infection,

$$ARI = 0.275 - 0.197 = 0.078$$

$$NNEH = 1/ARR = 1/0.078 = 12.8$$

This indicates that for every 13 children who have respiratory infection in early life, one additional child will be diagnosed with asthma. Obviously, the larger the odds ratio, the fewer the number of people who need to be exposed to cause harm.

9.8   Notes for critical appraisal

When critically appraising an article that reports risk statistics, it is important to ask the questions shown in Box 9.5.

Box 9.5 Questions to ask when critically appraising the literature in which risk statistics are presented

The following questions should be asked of studies that report risk statistics:
- If relative risk is reported, was the sample randomly selected?
- Have the proportions of disease in the exposed and non-exposed groups been reported in addition to the odds ratio or relative risk?
- Is it difficult to compare estimates if some of the factors are presented as risk factors and others as protective factors?

- Are confidence intervals presented for all estimates of odds ratio or relative risk?
- Can all of the variables in the model be classified as independent exposure factors or have alternative outcomes and intervening variables also been included?
- What type of method was used to build the logistic regression model and was collinearity between variables tested?

References

1. Sackett DL. Down with odds ratios! *Evid Based Med* 1996; **1**: 164–166.
2. Sinclair JC, Bracken MB. Clinically useful measures of effect in binary analyses of randomized trials. *J Clin Epidemiol* 1994; **47**: 881–889.
3. Katz, KA. The (relative) risks of using odds ratios. *Arch Dermatol* 2006; **142**: 761–764.
4. Bland JM, Altman DG. The odds ratio. *BMJ* 2000; **320**: 1468.1
5. Deeks J. When can odds ratios mislead. *BMJ* 1998; **317**: 1155–1156.
6. Peat JK. Can asthma be prevented? Evidence from epidemiological studies in children in Australia and New Zealand in the last decade. *Clin Exp Allergy* 1998; **28**: 261–265.
7. Wright RE. Logistic regression. In: *Reading and understanding multivariate statistics*, Grimm LG, Yarnold PR (editors). American Psychological Association: Washington, USA, 1995: 217–244.
8. Hosmer DW, Lemeshow S. *Applied logistic regression*. Wiley: New York, 2000.
9. Tabachnick BG, Fidell LS. *Using multivariate statistics*, 4th edn. Allyn and Bacon: Boston, MA, 2001.

CHAPTER 10

Tests of reliability and agreement

Truth cannot be defined or tested by agreement with 'the world'; for not only do truths differ for different worlds but the nature of agreement between a world apart from it is notoriously nebulous.
NELSON GOODMAN, PHILOSOPHER

Objectives

The objectives of the chapter are to explain how to:

- measure the reliability and agreement of categorical information, for example information collected by questionnaires
- measure the reliability and agreement of continuous measurements
- calculate the sample size needed to measure reliability
- critically appraise the literature that reports tests of reliability and agreement

---

10.1 Reliability and agreement

In research studies, it is important that the outcome measures used are reliable and accurate. This is especially important when the results are used to guide clinical practice and develop or change current treatment practice. In this, measures should have a high degree of reproducibility, that is, the results between repeated administrations by either the same raters (also called observers) or at different time points under the same conditions are very similar.

Measures of reliability and agreement are both used to assess reproducibility. It is important to distinguish between the terms 'reliability' and 'agreement', since they are often used interchangeably. The different types of reliability and agreement are shown in Table 10.1.

10.1.1 Reliability

Reliability is used to measure the ratio of the variability between the same participants (e.g. by different raters or at different times) to the total variability of all participants in the sample.[1] Therefore, reliability describes the ability of a measure to distinguish

---

Medical Statistics: A Guide to SPSS, Data Analysis and Critical Appraisal, Second Edition.
Belinda Barton and Jennifer Peat.
© 2014 John Wiley & Sons, Ltd. Published 2014 by John Wiley & Sons, Ltd.
Companion website: www.wiley.com/go/barton/medicalstatistics2e

Table 10.1   Definitions of reliability and agreement

Statistic	Measurement
Agreement	The degree to which scores are similar or different.
Reliability	The ability of the measure to differentiate between participants.
Intra-rater (or intra-observer) agreement	The degree to which responses of 2 or more different raters are concordant under the same or similar conditions.
Inter-rater (inter-observer) reliability	The degree to which responses of 2 or more different raters are able to differentiate between participants under the same or similar conditions.
Test–retest reliability (or intra-rater reliability)	The degree to which the measure is able to differentiate between participants under repeated administration of the measure under the same or similar conditions. The characteristic being measured in the participant should not change during that time.

between participants despite the measurement error. In this, the measurement error is related to the variability between participants.[2] The reliability of a measure can be measured as given below:

$$\text{Reliability} = \frac{\text{Variation between participants}}{\text{Variation between participants} + \text{measurement error}}$$

For a measure to be reliable, the measurement error should be small relative to the variability between participants, so that participants can accurately be distinguished. Clearly, if the scores for two participants are far apart, that is, there is wide between participant variation, the ability of the measure to distinguish between them will not be influenced by a measurement error which is small in comparison. However, if the scores are close together, the measurement error will influence the ability to distinguish between them and the reliability of the measure will be low. Because reliability statistics are calculated from the between participant variation, one of their features is that they are influenced by the heterogeneity of the study sample.[2] For a measure to be reliable, the measurement error should be small relative to the variability between participants, so that participants can accurately be distinguished.

The statistics that are used to describe reliability and agreement and which are discussed in this chapter are shown in Table 10.2.

Table 10.2   Statistics used to describe reliability and agreement

	Reliability	Agreement
Categorical measurements	Kappa	Per cent in agreement
Continuous measurements	ICC	Measurement error
	Cronbach's alpha	Error range
		Differences versus means plot
		Limits of agreement

ICC = intra-class correlations; SEM = standard error of measurement

10.1.2 *Agreement*

Agreement is the degree to which scores are similar or different when two or more measurements are taken from the same participants on different occasions. For example, if a measurement was taken from the same group of participants on two occasions under the same conditions (e.g. 1 week apart), statistics of agreement would be used to determine how close or how different the two measurements are. Test–retest reliability is a measure of agreement. With agreement, the measurement error is of interest and the variability within and between participants is not of interest. When the measurement error is large, small changes in the measurements between the two occasions will not be detected.[2]

10.1.3 *Study design*

Studies that are designed to assess reliability or agreement must be conducted in a setting in which they do not produce a false impression of the accuracy of the measurement. Box 10.1 shows the assumptions under which the reliability and/or agreement of categorical measurements and continuous measurements are tested. All of the assumptions relate to the study design.

Box 10.1 Assumptions for measuring reliability and/or agreement

The following methods must be incorporated into the study design:
- The method of administration and the conditions must be identical on each occasion.
- At the second administration, both the participant and the raters must be blinded to prior measurement values.
- The time to the second administration should be short enough so that the (i) severity of the condition has not changed since the first administration; (ii) no new treatment or intervention has been implemented between measurements; and (iii) there has been no significant change that could bias the second administration (e.g. patient's health has improved or deteriorated).
- If a questionnaire is being tested, the time between administrations must be long enough for participants to have forgotten their previous responses.
- The setting in which reliability or agreement is established must be the same as the setting in which the questionnaire or measurement will be used.
- Each participant has the same number of measurements and participants are selected to represent the entire range of measurements that can be encountered.

If a measure such as a questionnaire is to be used in a community setting, then reliability has to be established in a similar community setting and not for example in a clinic setting where the patients form a well-defined sub-sample of a population. Patients who frequently answer questions about their illness may have well-rehearsed responses to questions and may provide an artificial estimate of reliability when compared to people in the general population who rarely consider aspects of an illness or condition that they do not have.

Questionnaires are widely used in research studies to obtain information about personal characteristics, illnesses and exposure to environmental factors. For a questionnaire to be a useful research tool, the responses to questions must not have a substantial amount of measurement error. To measure test–retest reliability, the questionnaire is given to the same people on two separate occasions. Alternatively, if a questionnaire is designed to be administered by a clinician or researcher, it is administered on different occasions by different raters. An important concept is that the condition that the questionnaire is designed to measure must not have changed in the period between administrations and the time period must be long enough for the participants to have little recollection of their previous responses.

10.2   Kappa statistic

In clinical research, it is important to accurately identify the presence or absence of a disease or condition. This process may involve clinicians interpreting findings from physical examinations or imaging techniques such as X-rays. For example, a physician and a radiologist may independently review a series of patients' digital chest X-rays to determine the presence or absence of tuberculosis. To assess the degree of concordance between the two clinicians' ratings, the per cent agreement between the raters could be reported (e.g. 50% of raters responded 'yes' on both occasions). However, this percentage could be misleading since it does not take into account the level of concordance between the two raters that may occur by chance. The kappa statistic can be used to assess the concordance of responses for two or more raters after taking account of chance agreement. Kappa is an estimate of the proportion in agreement between raters in excess of the agreement that would occur by chance.

This statistic can be used to measure reliability between raters or between administrations for both binary and nominal scales.[3] The interpretation of kappa values is shown in Table 10.3.[4] When the observed proportion in agreement is less than that expected

Table 10.3   Kappa value and corresponding level of agreement[4]

Kappa value	Interpretation
<0.00	Poor
0.00–0.20	Slight agreement
0.21–0.40	Fair agreement
0.41–0.60	Moderate agreement
0.61–0.80	Substantial agreement
0.81–1.00	Almost perfect agreement

by chance, kappa will have a negative value indicating no agreement. A kappa value that equals 0 indicates that the observed agreement is equal to the chance agreement.

There are different types of kappa statistics. For data with three or more possible responses or for ordered categorical data, weighted kappa should be used so that the responses that are further away from concordance are more heavily weighted than those close to concordance. SPSS does not provide estimates of weighted kappa and therefore more specialized software is required. In SPSS, Cohen's kappa is calculated which is suitable when there are two raters. The assumptions for Cohen's kappa are that participants or items to be rated are independent, and also that the raters and categories are independent. Kappa values are influenced by the prevalence of the condition or disease being rated which is demonstrated in the research question below.

10.2.1 Sample size

Before undertaking a study of reliability, the minimum sample size required to detect a significant kappa value can be calculated. With two observers rating a binary variable or a questionnaire administered on two occasions, the null hypothesis is that the kappa value equals zero (two-tailed). For a significance level of 0.05 and power of 80%, the sample size required to detect a significant kappa value of 0.40 is 50. A sample size of 32 is required for a kappa value of 0.5; 22 for a kappa value of 0.6; 17 for a kappa value of 0.7; 13 for a kappa value of 0.8; and 10 for a kappa value of 0.9.[5]

Research question

The file **questionnaires.sav** contains the data of three questions which required a 'yes' or 'no' response. The questions were administered on two occasions to the same 50 people at an interval of 3 weeks. The research aim was to measure the test–retest reliability of the questions.

Question: Do the questions have a high level of test-retest reliability?

Null hypothesis: The proportion in agreement is no greater than that expected by chance (i.e. kappa value = 0).

Variables: Questions (nominal) and time (ordinal)

It is important to establish how reliable questions are because questions that are prone to a significant amount of random error or bias do not make good outcome or explanatory variables. The SPSS commands shown in Box 10.2 can be used to obtain a kappa statistic.

This command sequence can then be repeated to obtain the following tables and statistics for questions 2 and 3 of the questionnaire.

From the Crosstabulation table for question 1, the per cent in agreement is estimated from the per cent who are concordant, which is shown on the diagonal of the table in the No at Time 1-No at Time 2 and Yes at Time 1-Yes at Time 2 cells. Thus, the per cent in agreement is 40% + 22%, or 62%, which is 0.62 as a proportion. The kappa value is low at 0.252 indicating only fair agreement after chance is taken into account. Kappa is always lower than the proportion in agreement. The Symmetric Measures table shows that the *P* value of 0.048 is just significant indicating that the level of agreement is different from that expected by chance. Since the level of significance is two-tailed, the *P* value does not indicate whether the agreement is worse or better than chance. However, agreement worse than that expected by chance rarely occurs in clinical contexts.

Box 10.2 SPSS commands to measure reliability

SPSS Commands

questionnaires.sav – IBM SPSS Statistics Data Editor
      Analyze → Descriptive Statistics → Crosstabs
Crosstabs
      Highlight Question 1-time 1 and click into Row(s)
      Highlight Question1-time 2 and click into Column(s)
      Click on Statistics
Crosstabs: Statistics
      Tick Kappa, tick Continue
Crosstabs
      Click on Cells
Crosstabs: Cell Display
      Counts: tick Observed (default)
      Percentages: tick Total
      Noninteger Weights: tick Round cell counts (default), Click Continue
Crosstabs
      Click OK

Crosstabs

Question 1 – Time 1 * Question 1 – Time 2 crosstabulation

			Question 1 – time 2		
			No	Yes	Total
Question 1 – time 1	No	Count	20	15	35
		Percentage of total	40.0	30.0	70.0
	Yes	Count	4	11	15
		Percentage of total	8.0	22.0	30.0
Total		Count	24	26	50
		Percentage of total	48.0	52.0	100.0

Symmetric measures

	Value	Asymp. std. error[a]	Approx. t^{b}	Approx. sig.
Measure of agreement kappa	0.252	0.123	1.977	0.048
N of valid cases	50			

[a]Not assuming the null hypothesis.
[b]Using the asymptotic standard error assuming the null hypothesis.

It should be noted that the *P* value is not a good indication of reliability because its interpretation is that the kappa value is significantly different from zero. Measurements taken from the same people on two occasions are closely related by nature and thus the *P* value is expected to indicate some degree of agreement. The standard error is also reported and can be used to calculate a confidence interval around kappa.

In the Crosstabulation table for question 2, the per cent in agreement is 68% + 10%, which is 78% or 0.78 as a proportion, and kappa is higher than in the first table (Question 1) at 0.337.

Crosstabs

Question 2 – Time 1 * Question 2 – Time 2 crosstabulation

			Question 2 – time 2		Total
			No	Yes	
Question 2 – time 1	No	Count	34	5	39
		Percentage of total	68.0	10.0	78.0
	Yes	Count	6	5	11
		Percentage of total	12.0	10.0	22.0
Total		Count	40	10	50
		Percentage of total	80.0	20.0	100.0

Symmetric measures

	Value	Asymp. std. error[a]	Approx. t^b	Approx. sig.
Measure of agreement kappa	0.337	0.159	2.390	0.017
N of valid cases	50			

[a]Not assuming the null hypothesis.
[b]Using the asymptotic standard error assuming the null hypothesis.

In the Crosstabulation table for question 3, although the per cent in agreement is 34% + 44%, which is also 78% or 0.78 as a proportion, kappa is higher than that for Question 2 at 0.556 and the *P* value increases in significance from 0.017 to <0.001. Thus, kappa varies for the same proportion in agreement. With a higher per cent of 'Yes' replies (56% for question 3 compared with 22% for question 2), kappa increases from the fair to moderate range.

Crosstabs

Question 3 – Time 1 * Question 3 – Time 2 crosstabulation

			Question 3 – time 2		Total
			No	Yes	
Question 3 – time 1	No	Count	17	5	22
		Percentage of total	34.0	10.0	44.0
	Yes	Count	6	22	28
		Percentage of total	12.0	44.0	56.0
Total		Count	23	27	50
		Percentage of total	46.0	54.0	100.0

Symmetric measures

	Value	Asymp. std. error[a]	Approx. t^b	Approx. sig.
Measure of agreement kappa	0.556	0.118	3.933	0.000
N of valid cases	50			

[a]Not assuming the null hypothesis.
[b]Using the asymptotic standard error assuming the null hypothesis.

A feature of kappa is that the value increases as the proportion of 'No' and 'Yes' responses become more equal and when the proportion in agreement remains the same. This feature is a major barrier to comparing kappa values across measurements or between different studies. For this reason, the value of kappa, the percentage of positive responses and the per cent in agreement must all be reported to help assess reliability and agreement.

10.2.2   Reporting kappa results

Information about the test–retest reliability of the three questions can be reported as shown in Table 10.4. The kappa value, the per cent in agreement and the *P* value should be reported. It is difficult to say which question is the most reliable and has the least non-systematic bias because all three questions have a different percentage of positive responses and therefore the kappa values cannot be compared. However, both questions 2 and 3 have a higher per cent in agreement than question 1. The differences in percentages of positive responses suggest that the three questions are measuring different entities.

Table 10.4   Test–retest reliability for three questions administered to 50 people at a 3 week interval

	Percentage of positive responses at time 1	Percentage of positive responses at time 2	Proportion in agreement	Kappa 95% CI	P
Question 1	30%	52%	0.62	0.25 (0.01, 0.49)	0.05
Question 2	22%	20%	0.78	0.34 (0.03, 0.65)	0.02
Question 3	56%	54%	0.78	0.56 (0.32, 0.79)	<0.001

10.3   Reliability of continuous measurements

Continuous measurements must also have a high degree of reliability to be useful as a research tool. A measure is reliable if it produces the same value under all possible situations, that is, with different raters, in different settings and at different times. A measurement that has poor reliability will not be accurate at measuring the construct that it has been designed to measure and will also be unstable over repeated administrations, that is have poor test–retest reliability.

Variations in continuous measurements can result from inconsistent measurement practices, from equipment variations or from ways in which results are read or interpreted. These sources can be measured as within-rater (intra-rater) variation, between-rater (inter-rater) variation, or within-participant variation (see Table 10.1). Variations that result from the ways in which researchers administer, read, or interpret tests are within-rater or between-rater variations. Variations that arise from patient compliance factors or from biological changes are within-participant variations. To quantify these measurement errors, the same measurement is taken from the same participants on two occasions, or from the same participants by two or more raters, and the results are compared.

10.4 Intra-class correlation

The intra-class correlation coefficient (ICC) can be used to describe the relative extent to which two continuous measurements taken by different raters or two measurements taken by the same rater on different occasions are reliable. ICCs are frequently used to assess inter-rater reliability for ordinal, interval, and ratio scales where there are two or more raters.

ICC values range from 0 to 1. ICC is calculated as a ratio of the between participant variance to the 'between and within' participant variance. If each participant has the same score on two occasions (i.e. perfect concordance between measurements), there would be no within-participant variation and all of the variation would be due to differences between participants so that the ICC would equal 1. A high value of ICC of 0.95 indicates that 95% of the variance in the measurement is due to the true variance between the participants. The remaining 5% of the variance is due to measurement error or the variance within the participants or between the raters.

The advantage of ICC is that, unlike Pearson's correlation coefficient, a value of unity is only obtained when the two measurements are identical to one another. The ICC is a relative measure whose magnitude depends on both the amount of variability in the sample and the differences between repeated measurements. As such, the ICC is a measure of the proportion of 'true' variance in the sample. However, because ICC depends on the range of values in a sample, it may not be comparable between studies. A disadvantage of ICC is that the same instrument may be judged reliable or unreliable depending on the population in which it is assessed.

10.4.1 Different types of intra-class correlation

There are three classes of the ICC which relate to the study design[6]:

1. One-way random (ICC (1)) is used when raters are selected at random. That is, there are different raters and not the same raters are used for all participants. Also different raters may be used at different sites, however this is uncommon. This ICC does not separate the effects of rater and participant variation and will always be the lowest of the ICC values.
2. Two-way random (ICC (2)) is used when the same raters rate each case. Raters in the sample are considered a random sample from a population of raters. When there are the same raters for each participant, ICC (2), which controls for raters effects is used. This is the model most frequently encountered in clinical research when the same raters carry out measurements on all of the participants. The value of ICC (2) will always be larger than for ICC (1) because it models two effects – the effect of the rater and of the participant.

3. Two-way mixed (ICC (3)) is used when the same raters rate each participant in the study and only the raters are of interest. This is uncommon because the raters usually represent an unlimited number of people who could make the observations. The ICC estimate only applies the raters in the study and hence findings cannot be generalized. This value will be larger than ICC (1) and ICC (2).

10.4.2   Intra-class correlation notation

The notation that is used to describe the different formulas to calculate ICC is shown in Table 10.5. The number '1' is added to the ICC when it relates to the reliability of single raters and 'k' is added when the ICC relates to the mean of the raters (where k is the number of raters). The value for 'single measures' statistic is an index of reliability for typical single raters, which is the most common situation in clinical research. The 'average measures' statistic is an index of reliability for different raters averaged together for example when the measurements are a mean of the measurements obtained by different raters.

For ICC $(2,k)$ and ICC $(3,k)$, there is an option to use 'consistency' or 'absolute agreement'. Consistency is used when a systematic difference between raters is not of interest. To determine how well a measurement assesses the true value of a participant, the option 'absolute agreement' is used.

Table 10.5   ICC notation and corresponding SPSS classification

ICC class	SPSS nomenclature
ICC (1,1)	One-way random, single measures
ICC (1,k)	One-way random, average measures
ICC (2,1)	Two-way random, single measures
ICC (2,k)	Two-way random, average measures
ICC (3,1)	Two-way mixed, single measures
ICC (3,k)	Two-way mixed, average measures

Research question

The file **observer-weights.sav** contains data from 32 babies who had their weight measured by two nurses who had no knowledge of each other's measurements.

Question: Do measurements of babies' weights have a high degree of reliability?

Null hypothesis: The ICC value equals 0 indicating random concordance.

The SPSS commands to obtain ICC are shown in Box 10.3.

Box 10.3 SPSS commands to measure reliability

SPSS Commands

observer-weights.sav – IBM SPSS Statistics Data Editor
        Analyze → Scale → Reliability Analysis
Reliability Analysis
        Highlight Weight–observer 1 and Weight–observer 2 and click into Items
        Model: Alpha (default)
        Click Statistics
Reliability Analysis: Statistics
        Tick Intraclass correlation coefficient,
        Model: Two-Way Mixed (default)
        Type: Absolute Agreement
        Confidence Interval: 95% (default), Test Value: 0 (default), click Continue
Reliability Analysis
        Click OK

In the Reliability Statistics table, the Cronbach's alpha is reported. This is a test of reliability that can be used to assess the internal consistency of a scale. This statistic measures whether the items of a tool are measuring the same constructs. An acceptable value for Cronbach's alpha is 0.7 or 0.8.[7] The value of the Cronbach's alpha is identical to the ICC Average Measures when the ICC is calculated using either the two-way mixed consistency or two-way random consistency models.

Reliability

Reliability Statistics

Cronbach's alpha	N of items
0.996	2

In this example, there are two raters and as shown in the Intraclass Correlation Coefficient table, the ICC (2,1) is 0.992. That is, less than 1% of the variance is explained by rater differences. The 95% confidence interval around an ICC can be reported but the significance of the ICC is of little importance because it is expected that two measurements taken from the same person are highly related.

Intra-class Correlation Coefficient

| | Intra-class correlation[b] | 95% confidence interval | | F test with true Value 0 | | | |
		Lower bound	Upper bound	Value	df1	df2	Sig.
Single measures	0.992[a]	0.984	0.996	255.480	31	31	0.000
Average measures	0.996[c]	0.992	0.998	255.480	31	31	0.000

Two-way mixed effects model where people effects are random and measures effects are fixed.
[a] The estimator is the same, whether the interaction effect is present or not.
[b] Type A intra-class correlation coefficients using an absolute agreement definition.
[c] This estimate is computed assuming the interaction effect is absent, because it is not estimable otherwise.

10.4.3   *Reporting the results of ICC*

When reporting the results of ICC is important to identify which ICC was conducted and report other relevant results so that detailed information is available.[1] Where appropriate, measures of agreement can also be reported such as the measurement error or error range (discussed later in this chapter). The results of the above example can be reported as 'The inter-rater reliability was assessed using a two-way mixed, absolute agreement, single measures ICC to assess the degree of reliability between nurses when weighing babies. The ICC value was high (ICC = 0.99, 95 CI% 0.98, 1.00, $P < 0.001$) indicating a high degree of reliability and suggesting that weight was measured similarly by the nurses'.

10.5   Measures of agreement

When comparing agreement between continuous measurements, it is not appropriate to use a correlation coefficient such as Pearson's correlation coefficient (see Chapter 7) to measure the strength or linear relationship between two variables because it does not make sense to test the hypothesis that two measurements taken from the same babies using the same equipment are related to one another.[8] A second measurement that is, for example, twice as large as the first measurement would have perfect correlation but there would be very poor agreement. In addition, the size of the correlation coefficient value is influenced by the range of the variable.

The statistics that are used to assess agreement between measurements are shown in Table 10.2 and are the measurement error, error range, limits of agreement, and differences versus means (Bland and Altman) plot.

10.5.1   *Limits of agreement*

Assuming that the difference scores between two measurements are normally distributed it is expected that the 95% of the scores will lie within the interval calculate as the mean difference $+/- 1.96$ standard deviation of the differences (see Chapter 2). When measuring agreement, this range is called the 95% limits of agreement.

Research question

The file **observer-weights.sav** contains data from 32 babies who had their weight measured by two nurses who had no knowledge of each other's measurements.

Question: Do nurses measurements of babies weight have a high level of agreement?

Null hypothesis: There is no agreement between nurses' measurements.

To visually examine the data, the weights measured by both nurses could be plotted against each other in a scatter plot. To assess the level of agreement between the two measurements the limits of agreement can be calculated. Using the following SPSS commands *Transform → Compute Variable* to first calculate the mean of the two measurements for each baby using the *Mean* function located in *Functions and Special Variables*. Then the difference between the two measurements is calculated as a simple subtraction, that is measurement 1 – measurement 2. The subtraction can be in either direction but the direction must be indicated in the summary results and graphs. The two new variables are created at the end of the SPSS Data View spreadsheet and should be labelled as 'mean' and 'differences', respectively.

The size of the error can then be calculated from the standard deviation around the differences, which can be obtained using the *Analyze → Descriptive Statistics → Descriptives* commands with the 'differences' variable entered as the *Variable(s)*.

Descriptives

Descriptive statistics

	N	Minimum	Maximum	Mean	Std. deviation
Differences	32	−0.10	0.15	0.0125	0.06792
Valid N (listwise)	32				

The mean of the differences is 0.0125 and gives an estimate of the amount of bias between the two measurements. In this case, the measurements taken by nurse 1 are on average 0.0125 kg higher than nurse 2, which is a small difference. A problem with using the mean of the differences is that large positive difference values and large negative difference values are balanced out by one another and therefore negated. However, the mean ± 1.96SD can also be calculated from the Descriptive Statistics table. This range is calculated as $0.0125 \pm (1.96 \times 0.0679)$, or -0.12 to 0.15 and is called the limits of agreement.[9] The limits of agreement indicate that 95% of the differences between nurses lie in the range of -0.12 kg to 0.15 kg.

10.5.2   Differences-vs-means plot

The mean and difference values can be plotted as a differences-vs-means plot to show whether there is any systematic bias, that is whether the differences are related to the size of the measurement as estimated by the mean.[10] The shape of the scatter conveys important information about the agreement between the measurements. A scatter that is evenly distributed above and below the zero line of no difference indicates that there is no systematic bias between the two raters. A scatter that is largely above or largely below the zero line of no difference or a scatter that increases or decreases with the mean value indicates a systematic bias between raters.[11]

The values for the means and differences can be copied and pasted from SPSS to SigmaPlot and the figure can be created using the commands shown in Box 10.4. A recommendation for the axes of differences-vs-means plots is that the y-axis should be approximately one-third to one-half of the range of the x-axis.[10]

The lines for the mean difference and limits of agreement can be added by typing the x coordinates in column 3 and y coordinates of the lines into columns 4−6 and adding three line plots by using the SigmaPlot commands *Line → Simple Straight Line in Line*

Group → XY Pair options with *x* as column 3 each time and each *y* column. The columns for the coordinate data are as follows:

Column 3	Column 4	Column 5	Column 6
3.5	0.0125	−0.12	0.15
6.0	0.0125	−0.12	0.15

Box 10.4 SigmaPlot commands to create a differences-vs-means plot

SigmaPlot Commands

Data 1*

 Click on Create Graph tab at top of the screen
 Click on Scatter in sub-menu
 Click on Simple Scatter in Scatter Group
Create Graph – Data Format
 Under Data format, highlight XY pair, click Next
Create Graph – Select Data
 Highlight Column 1, click into Data for X
 Highlight Column 2, click into Data for Y
 Click Finish

Figure 10.1 shows that there is only a small amount of random error that is evenly scattered around the line of no difference. The figure also shows that most of the differences are within 0.1 kg. A wide scatter would indicate a large amount of measurement error.

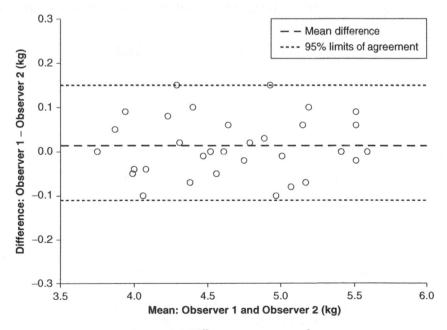

Figure 10.1 Differences-vs-means plot.

To determine whether there is systematic error, a Kendall's correlation coefficient between the means and the differences can be obtained since the variables are not normally distributed. The commands shown in Box 7.3 can be used to obtain the correlations shown below. This will show whether the differences are related to the means of the measurements.

Non-parametric Correlations

Correlations

			Differences	Mean
Kendall's tau_b	Differences	Correlation coefficient	1.000	0.045
		Sig. (two-tailed)	–	0.721
		N	32	32
	Mean	Correlation coefficient	0.045	1.000
		Sig. (two-tailed)	0.721	–
		N	32	32

The almost negligible correlation of 0.045 with a *P* value of 0.721 confirms the uniformity of variance in the repeated measurements. A systematic bias between the two measurements could also be inspected using a paired *t*-test or a non-parametric rank sums test, depending upon the distribution of the data.

10.5.3   *Measurement error*

A more useful statistic to describe agreement is to calculate the measurement error from the standard deviation of the differences of observations in the same participant.[8] This is calculated as follows:

$$\text{Measurement error} = \frac{\text{SD of differences}}{\sqrt{2}}$$

$$= \frac{0.06792}{1.414}$$

$$= 0.048\,\text{kg}$$

This error can then be converted to a range by multiplying by a critical value of 1.96.

$$\text{Error range} = \text{measurement error} \times \text{critical value}$$

$$= 0.048 \times 1.96$$

$$= 0.09\,\text{kg}$$

The error range indicates that the average of all possible measurements of a baby's weight is within the range of 0.09 kg above and 0.09 kg below the actual measurement taken. Thus for a baby with a measured weight of 4.01 kg, the average of all possible weights, which is expected to be close to the true weight, would be within the range 3.92 to 4.10 kg. This range can be taken to indicate the range in which the true weight of the baby lies.

10.5.4 *Reporting measures of agreement*

When reporting the results, the differences-vs-means plot gives the most informative description of agreement with the limits of agreement shown. Additional information of the mean difference and the error range are direct measures of agreement between two continuous measurements. The information can be reported as shown in Table 10.6.

Table 10.6 Reliability for weight measured by two different nurses

	Mean difference	Limits of agreement	Error range	ICC
Weight (kg)	0.013	−0.12, 0.15	0.09	0.99

10.6 Notes for critical appraisal

Paired measurements to estimate agreement must be treated appropriately when analysing the data. When critically appraising an article that presents these types of statistics, it is important to ask the questions shown in Box 10.5.

Box 10.5 Questions for critical appraisal

The following questions should be asked when appraising published results from paired categorical follow-up data or data collected to estimate the reliability of questionnaire responses or continuous measurements:
• Is the sample size large enough to have confidence in the summary estimates?
For reliability of categorical data:
• Is the percentage of positive or negative responses and proportion in agreement included in addition to kappa?
• Are kappa values inappropriately compared?
For reliability of continuous measurements:
• Have a differences-vs-means plot, the limits of agreement, a 95% range and the intra-class correlation been reported?
• Is Pearson's correlation used appropriately?

References

1. Kottner J, Audigé L, Brorson S *et al.*, Guidelines for reporting reliability and agreement studies (GRRAS) were proposed. *J Clin Epidemol* 2011; **64**: 96–106.
2. de Vet HCW, Terwee CB, Knol DL, Bouter LM. When to use agreement vs reliability measures. *J Clin Epidemol* 2006; **59**: 1033–1039.
3. Gisev N, Bell JS, Chen TF. Interrater agreement and interrater reliability: key concepts, approaches and applications. *Res Social Adm Pharm* 2013; **9**: 330–338.
4. Landis JR, Koch GG. The measurement of observer agreement for categorical data. *Biometrics* 1977; **33**: 159–174.

5. Donner A, Eliasziw. A goodness of fit approach to inference procedures for the kappa statistic: confidence interval construction, significance-testing and sample size estimation. *Stat Med* 1992: **11**:1511–1519.

6. Shrout PE, Fleiss JL. Intraclass correlations: uses in assessing rater reliability. *Psychol Bull* 1979;**86**:420–4277.

7. Bland JM, Altman DG. Cronbach's alpha. *BMJ* 1997; **314**:572.

8. Bland JM, Altman DG. Measurement error and correlation coefficients. *BMJ* 1996; **313**: 41–42.

9. Bland JM, Altman DG. Measurement error. *BMJ* 1996; **313**:744.

10. Bland JM, Altman DG. Statistical methods for assessing agreement between two methods of clinical measurement. *Lancet* 1986; **1**: 307–310.

11. Peat JK, Mellis CM, Williams K, Xuan W. *Health science research: a handbook of quantitative methods*. Allen and Unwin: Crows Nest, Australia, 2002.

CHAPTER 11

Diagnostic statistics

Like dreams, statistics are a form of wish fulfilment.
JEAN BAUDRILLARD (b. 1929), FRENCH SEMIOLOGIST

Objectives

The objectives of the chapter are to explain how to:
- compute sensitivity, specificity and likelihood ratios
- understand the limitations of positive and negative predictive values
- select cut-off points for screening and diagnostic tests
- critically appraise studies that use or evaluate diagnostic tests

In clinical practice it is important to know how well diagnostic tests, such as X-rays, biopsies or blood and urine tests, can predict that a patient has a certain condition or disease. The statistics positive predictive value (PPV), negative predictive value (NPV), sensitivity and specificity are all used to estimate the utility of a test in predicting the presence or absence of a condition or a disease. A statistic that combines the utility of sensitivity and specificity is the likelihood ratio (LR). If the outcome of the diagnostic test is binary, a likelihood ratio can be calculated directly. If the test result is on a continuous scale, a receiver operating characteristic (ROC) curve is used to determine the cut-off point that maximizes the LR.

Diagnostic statistics are part of a group of statistics that are used to describe agreement between two measurements. However, these statistics should be calculated only when there is a 'gold standard' to measure the presence or absence of disease against which the test can be compared. If a gold diagnostic standard does not exist, a proxy gold standard may need to be justified.[1] In this situation, the test being evaluated must not be included in the definition of the gold standard.[1] In measuring the diagnostic utility of a test, the person interpreting the test measurement must be blinded to the disease status of the patient.

11.1 Coding for diagnostic statistics

For diagnostic statistics, it is best to code the variable indicating disease status as 1 for disease present as measured by the gold standard or test positive and 2 for disease absent

Medical Statistics: A Guide to SPSS, Data Analysis and Critical Appraisal, Second Edition.
Belinda Barton and Jennifer Peat.
© 2014 John Wiley & Sons, Ltd. Published 2014 by John Wiley & Sons, Ltd.
Companion website: www.wiley.com/go/barton/medicalstatistics2e

Table 11.1   Coding for diagnostic statistics

	Disease present	Disease absent	Total
Test positive	a	b	a + b
Test negative	c	d	c + d
Total	a + c	b + d	N

or test negative. This coding will produce a table with the rows and columns in the order shown in Table 11.1. In this table, the row and column order is the reverse of that used to calculate an odds ratio from a 2×2 crosstabulation but is identical to the coding shown in Table 9.1 in Chapter 9, which is frequently used in clinical epidemiology textbooks.

11.2   Positive and negative predictive values

In estimating the utility of a test, PPV is the proportion of patients who are test positive and in whom the disease is present and NPV is the proportion of patients who are test negative and in whom the disease is absent. These statistics indicate the probability that the test will make a correct diagnosis.[2] Both PPV and NPV are statistics that predict from the test to the disease and indicate the probability that patients will or will not have a disease if they have a positive or negative diagnostic test. Intuitively, it would seem that PPV and NPV would be the most useful statistics; however, they have limitations in their interpretations.[2]

The statistics PPV and NPV should only be calculated if the study sample is selected randomly from a population and not if groups of patients and healthy people are recruited independently, which is often the case. From Table 11.1, the PPV and NPV can be calculated as follows:

$$PPV = \frac{a}{(a + b)}$$

$$NPV = \frac{d}{(c + d)}$$

Research question

The file **xray.sav** contains the data from 150 patients who had an X-ray for a bone fracture. A positive X-ray means that a fracture appears to be present on the X-ray, and a negative X-ray means that there is no indication of a fracture on the X-ray. The presence or absence of a fracture was later confirmed during surgery. Thus surgery is the 'gold standard' for deciding whether or not a fracture was present. The research aim is to measure how accurate X-rays are in predicting fractures in people with symptoms of a bone break. In computing diagnostic statistics, a hypothesis is not being tested so that the P value for the crosstabulation has little meaning.

Diagnostic statistics of PPV and NPV are computed using the SPSS commands shown in Box 11.1 with row percentages requested because PPV and NPV are calculated as proportions of the test positive patients and test negative patients who have the disease.

In SPSS, PPV and NPV are not produced directly or labelled as such but can be simply derived from the row percentages. Although the figures are given in percentages, diagnostic statistics are more commonly reported as proportions, that is, in decimal form.

Box 11.1 SPSS commands to compute diagnostic statistics

SPSS Commands

xray.sav - IBM SPSS Statistics Data Editor
> *Analyze → Descriptive Statistics → Crosstabs*

Crosstabs
> *Highlight X-ray results (test) and click into Row(s)*
> *Highlight Fracture detected by surgery (disease) and click into Column(s)*

Crosstabs
> *Click on Cells*

Crosstabs: Cell Display
> *Counts: tick Observed, Percentages: tick Row, Noninteger Weights: tick Round cell counts (default), click Continue*
> *Click OK*

X-ray results (test)* Fracture detected by surgery (disease) Crosstabulation

			Fracture detected by surgery (disease)		Total
			Present	Absent	
X-ray results (test)	Positive	Count	36	24	60
		% within X-ray results	60.0%	40.0%	100.0%
	Negative	Count	8	82	90
		% within X-ray results	8.9%	91.1%	100.0%
Total		Count	44	106	150
		% within X-ray results	29.3%	70.7%	100.0%

From the crosstabulation the row percentages are used and are simply converted to a proportion by dividing by 100.

$$\text{Positive predictive value} = 0.60 \left(\text{i.e. } \frac{36}{60} \right)$$

$$\text{Negative predictive value} = 0.91 \left(\text{i.e. } \frac{82}{90} \right)$$

This indicates that 0.60 of patients who had a positive X-ray had a fracture and 0.91 who had a negative X-ray did not have a fracture.

11.2.1   95% confidence intervals for PPV and NPV

To measure the certainty of diagnostic statistics, 95% confidence intervals for PPV and NPV can be calculated as for any proportion. If the confidence interval around a proportion contains a value less than zero, exact confidence intervals based on the

Table 11.2 Excel spreadsheet to calculate 95% confidence intervals

	Proportion	N	SE	Width	CI lower	CI upper
PPV	0.6	60	0.063	0.124	0.476	0.724
NPV	0.91	90	0.030	0.059	0.851	0.969

binomial distribution should be used. These can be calculated at StatPages on the web (see Useful Websites) rather than asymptotic statistics based on a normal distribution.[3] The formula for calculating the standard error around a proportion was shown in Chapter 8. The Excel spreadsheet shown in Table 11.2 can be used to calculate 95% confidence intervals for PPV and NPV. The confidence interval for PPV is based on the total number of patients who have a positive test result and the confidence interval for NPV is based on the total number of patients who have a negative test result.

The interpretation of the 95% confidence interval for PPV is that with 95% confidence, 47.6%–72.4% of patients with a positive X-ray will have a fracture. The interpretation of the 95% confidence interval for NPV is that with 95% confidence, 85.1–96.9% of patients with a negative X-ray will not have a fracture. Confidence intervals should be interpreted taking the sample size into account. The larger the sample size, the narrower the confidence intervals will be.

11.2.2 Limitations of PPV and NPV

Although PPV and NPV seem intuitive to interpret, both statistics vary with changes in the proportion of patients in the sample who are disease positive simply because they are based on row percentages. Thus, these statistics can only be applied to the study sample or to a sample with the same proportion of disease-positive and disease-negative patients. For this reason, PPV and NPV are not commonly used in clinical practice. Box 11.2 shows why these statistics are limited in their interpretation.

Box 11.2 Limitations in the interpretation of positive and negative predictive values

Positive and negative predictive values:
- are strongly influenced by the proportion of patients who are disease positive
- increase when the per cent of patients who have the disease in the sample is high and decrease when the per cent who have the disease is small
- cannot be applied or generalized to other clinical settings with different patient profiles
- cannot be compared between different diagnostic tests

In practice, the statistics PPV and NPV are only useful in settings in which the per cent of patients who have the disease present is the same as the prevalence of the disease in the population. This naturally rules out most clinical settings.

11.3   Sensitivity and specificity

The statistics that are most often used to describe the utility of diagnostic tests in clinical settings are sensitivity, specificity and likelihood ratio.[4,5] These diagnostic statistics can be computed from Table 11.1 as follows:

$$\text{Sensitivity} = \frac{a}{(a+c)}$$

$$\text{Specificity} = \frac{d}{(b+d)}$$

$$\text{Likelihood ratio} = \frac{\text{sensitivity}}{(1-\text{specificity})}$$

Sensitivity indicates how likely patients are to have a positive test if they have the disease and specificity indicates how likely the patients are to have a negative test if they do not have the disease. In this sense, these two statistics describe the proportion of patients in each disease category who are test positive or negative. Although the usefulness of these statistics is not as intuitive, sensitivity and specificity have advantages over PPV and NPV as shown in Box 11.3.

Box 11.3 Advantages of using sensitivity and specificity to describe the application of diagnostic tests

The advantages of using sensitivity and specificity to describe diagnostic tests are that these statistics:
- do not alter if the prevalence of disease is different between clinical populations
- can be applied in different clinical populations and settings
- can be compared between studies with different inclusion criteria
- can be used to compare the diagnostic potential of different tests

---

The interpretation of sensitivity and specificity is not intuitive and therefore to calculate these statistics it is recommended that the notations of true positives (TP), false positives (FP), true negatives (TN) and false negatives (FN) are written in each quadrant of the crosstabulation as shown in Table 11.3. The false negative group is the proportion of patients who have the disease and who have a negative test result, that is, $c/(a+c)$. The false positive group is the proportion of patients who do not have the disease and who have a positive test result, that is, $b/(b+d)$.

Thus, sensitivity is the rate of TP in the disease-present group $(a/a+c)$ and specificity is the rate of TN in the disease-absent group $(d/b+d)$.

Ideally, a diagnostic test would have high levels of sensitivity and specificity. However, this is not possible since there is a trade-off between sensitivity and specificity. As specificity increases, sensitivity is decreased, and vice versa. ROC curves, which are discussed later in this chapter, can be used to identify a cut-off value in a continuous measurement that maximizes the sensitivity and specificity.

Table 11.3   Terms used in diagnostic statistics

	Disease present	Disease absent	Total
Test positive	a TP (sensitivity) (true +ve)	b FP (false +ve)	
Test negative	c FN (false −ve)	d TN (specificity) (true −ve)	
Total	a + c	b + d	N

The 'opposites' rule applies to remembering the meaning of the terms sensitivity and specificity because: sensitivity has an 'n' in it and this applies to the TP, which includes a P in the name and specificity has a 'p' in it and this applies to the TN, which has an N in the name.

Is this logical? Well no, but the terminology is well established and this reverse code helps in remembering which term indicates the TN or TP. Reading vertically from Table 11.3 it can be seen that the rate of false negatives is the complement of the TP for patients who have the disease. Similarly, the rate of FP is the complement of the TN for patients who do not have the disease.

11.3.1   SpPin and SnNout

SpPin and SnNout are two clinical epidemiology terms that are commonly used to aid in the interpretation of sensitivity and specificity in clinical settings.[6] Although these rules are used as guides in clinical practice, to rule a disease in or out, both the sensitivity and specificity must be taken into account.

SpPin stands for **Sp**ecificity-**P**ositive-**in,** which means that if a test has a high specificity (TN) and therefore a low 1 − specificity (FP), a positive result rules the disease in. A test that is used to diagnose an illness in patients with symptoms of the illness needs to have a low false positive rate because it will then identify most of the people who do not have the disease. Although specificity needs to be high for a diagnostic test to rule the disease in, it is calculated solely from the group of patients without the disease.

SnNout stands for **Sn**sitivity-**N**egative-**out,** which means that if the test has a high sensitivity (TP) and a low 1 − sensitivity (FN), a negative test result rules the disease out. A test that is used to screen a population in which many people will not have the disease needs to have high sensitivity because it will then identify most of the people with the disease. Although sensitivity needs to be high in a screening test to rule the disease out, it is calculated solely from the group of patients with the disease.

The SPSS commands shown in Box 11.1 can be used to compute sensitivity and specificity but the column percentages rather than the row percentages are requested because sensitivity is a proportion of the disease-positive group and specificity is a proportion of the disease-negative group.

X-ray results (test)* Fracture detected by surgery (disease) Crosstabulation

| | | | Fracture detected by surgery (disease) | | Total |
			Present	Absent	
X-ray results (test)	Positive	Count	36	24	60
		% within fracture detected by surgery	81.8%	22.6%	40.0%
	Negative	Count	8	82	90
		% within fracture detected by surgery	18.2%	77.4%	60.0%
Total		Count	44	106	150
		% within fracture detected by surgery	100.0%	100.0%	100.0%

The column percentages can be simply changed into proportions by dividing by 100. Thus, from the above table:

$$\text{Sensitivity} = \text{TP} = 0.82$$

$$1 - \text{sensitivity} = \text{FN} = 0.18$$

$$\text{Specificity} = \text{TN} = 0.77$$

$$1 - \text{specificity} = \text{FP} = 0.23$$

The sensitivity of the test indicates that 82% of patients with a fracture will have a positive X-ray and the specificity of the test indicates that 77% of patients with no fracture will have a negative X-ray.

11.3.2 *95% Confidence intervals for sensitivity and specificity*

The confidence intervals for sensitivity and specificity can be calculated using the spreadsheet shown in Table 11.2. This produces the intervals shown in Table 11.4. Again, if the confidence interval of a proportion contains a value less than zero, exact confidence intervals should be used (e.g. StatPages shown in the Useful Websites).[3]

The 95% confidence intervals are based on the number of patients with the disease present for sensitivity and the number of patients with the disease absent for specificity. Because each 95% confidence interval is based only on a subset of the sample rather

Table 11.4 Excel spreadsheet for calculating confidence intervals around a proportion

Proportion	*N*	SE	Width	CI lower	CI upper
0.82	44	0.058	0.114	0.706	0.934
0.18	44	0.058	0.114	0.066	0.294
0.77	106	0.041	0.080	0.690	0.850
0.23	106	0.041	0.080	0.150	0.310

than on the total sample size, the confidence intervals can be surprisingly wide if the number in the group is quite small.

The interpretation of the intervals for sensitivity is that with 95% confidence between 70.6% and 93.4% of patients with a fracture will have a positive X-ray. Similarly, the interpretation for specificity is that with 95% confidence between 69.0% and 85.0% of patients without a fracture will have a negative X-ray.

11.3.3 Sample size

In calculating the required sample size to estimate sensitivity and specificity, it is important to have an adequate number of people with and without the disease. A high sensitivity rules the disease out; therefore, it is essential to enrol a large number of people with disease present to calculate the proportion of TP with precision. A high specificity rules the disease in, so it is essential to enrol a large number of people with the disease absent to calculate the proportion of TN with precision.

It is not always understood that to show that a test can rule a disease out, a large number of people with the disease present must be enrolled and that to show that a test is useful in ruling a disease in, a large number of people without the disease must be enrolled. For most tests, a large number of people with the disease present and with the disease absent must be enrolled to provide tighter confidence intervals, that is, more precision around both sensitivity and specificity.

In studies when both the new diagnostic test and the gold standard result in a binary variable (e.g. test positive and test absent), and an estimation of the disease prevalence is available, the sample size required for estimating sensitivity and specificity (with 95% confidence intervals) can be calculated using a nomogram.[7] A nomogram is a graphical tool with three or more lines or curves that can be read to estimate a variable, in this case, the sample size.

11.4   Likelihood ratio

Both sensitivity and specificity can be thought of as statistics that 'look backwards' in that they show the probability that a person with a disease will have a positive test rather than looking 'forwards' and showing the probability that the person who tests positive has the disease. Also, sensitivity and specificity should not be used in isolation because each is calculated from separate parts of the data. To be useful in clinical practice, these statistics need to be converted to a likelihood ratio that uses data from the total sample to estimate the relative predictive value of the test. The LR is calculated as follows:

$$LR = \frac{\text{Likelihood of a positive result in people with disease}}{\text{Likelihood of a positive result in people without disease}}$$

$$= \frac{\text{Sensitivity}}{1 - \text{specificity}}$$

$$= \frac{\text{TP}}{\text{FP}}$$

The LR is simply the ratio of the TP to the FP and indicates how likely a positive result will be found in a person with the disease than in a person without the disease.[1] This statistic provides clinical information about an individual because it indicates how likely a positive result will be found in a person with the disease compared to a person without the disease. A positive likelihood ratio greater than 1 indicates that a positive test result is associated with the presence of the disease, whereas a positive likelihood ratio of less than 1 indicates that a positive test result is associated with the absence of a disease.

From the previous calculation:

$$LR = \frac{0.82}{(1 - 0.77)} = 3.56$$

Confidence intervals around LR are best generated using dedicated programs (see the Diagnostic calculator website in Useful Websites). The LR indicates how much a positive test will alter the pre-test probability that a patient will have the illness. The pre-test probability is the probability of the disease in the clinic setting where the test is being used. The post-test probability is the probability that the disease is present when the test is positive. To interpret the LR, a likelihood ratio nomogram can be used to convert pre-test probability of disease into post-test probability.[3,8] Alternatively, the following formula can be used to convert the pre-test probability (Pre-TP) into a post-test probability (Post-TP):

$$Post\text{-}TP = \frac{(Pre\text{-}TP \times LR)}{(1 + Pre\text{-}TP \times (LR - 1))}$$

The size of the LR indicates the utility of the test in diagnosing an illness. As a rule, an LR greater than 10 is large and means a conclusive change from pre-test to post test probability. On the other hand, an LR between 5 and 10 results in only a moderate shift between pre- and post-test probability, an LR between 2 and 5 results in a small shift but sometimes reflects an important shift, and an LR below 2 is small and rarely important.[4]

The advantages of using a likelihood ratio to interpret the results of diagnostic tests are shown in Box 11.4.

Box 11.4 Advantages of using likelihood ratio as a predictive statistic for diagnostic tests

The advantages of likelihood ratio are that this predictive statistic:
- allows valid comparisons of diagnostic statistics between studies
- the diagnostic value can be applied in different clinical settings
- provides the certainty of a positive diagnosis

11.5   Receiver Operating Characteristic (ROC) Curves

ROC curves are an invaluable tool for finding the cut-off point in a continuously distributed measurement that best predicts whether a condition is present, for example whether patients are disease positive or disease negative.[9] ROC curves are used to find a cut-off value that delineates a 'normal' from an 'abnormal' test result when the test result is a continuously distributed measurement. ROC curves are plotted by calculating the sensitivity and specificity of the test in predicting the diagnosis for each value of the measurement. The curve makes it possible to determine a cut-off point for the measurement that maximizes the rate of TP (sensitivity) and minimizes the rate of FP (1 − specificity), and thus maximizes the likelihood ratio.

Research question

The file **xray.sav,** which was used in the previous research question, also contains data for the results of three different biochemical tests and a variable that indicates whether the disease was later confirmed by surgery. ROC curves are used to assess which test is most useful in predicting that patients will be disease positive. The null hypothesis is that the area under the ROC curve equals 0.5, that is, the test's ability to identify positive and negative cases is that expected by chance.

Before constructing an ROC curve, the amount of overlap in the distribution of the continuous biochemical test measurement in both the disease-positive and disease-negative groups can be explored using the SPSS commands shown in Box 11.5.

Box 11.5 SPSS commands to obtain scatter plots

SPSS Commands

xray.sav - IBM SPSS Statistics Data Editor
      Graphs → Legacy Dialogs → Scatter/Dot
Scatter/Dot
      Click on Simple Scatter, click on Define
Simple Scatterplot
      Highlight BiochemA and click into the Y Axis
      Highlight Disease positive and click into the X Axis
      Click OK

These SPSS commands can be repeated to obtain scatter plots for the test BiochemB and BiochemC as shown in Figure 11.1. In the plots, the values and labels on the *x*- and *y*-axes are automatically assigned by SPSS and are not selected labels. For example, in Figure 11.1 the group labels of 1 for 'disease present' and 2 for 'disease absent' on the *x*-axis are not displayed. Although the scatter plots are useful for understanding the discriminatory value of each continuous variable, they would not be reported in a journal article.

In the first plot shown in Figure 11.1, it is clear that the values for BiochemA in the disease-positive group (coded 1) overlap almost completely with the values for BiochemA in the disease-negative group (coded 2). With complete overlap such as this, there will never be a cut-off point that effectively delineates between the two groups.

In the plots for BiochemB and BiochemC as shown in Figure 11.1, there is more separation of the test measurements between the groups, particularly for BiochemC. The value of the tests in distinguishing between the disease-positive and disease-negative groups can be quantified by plotting ROC curves using the commands shown in Box 11.6 to produce Figure 11.2. In the data set, disease positive is coded as 1 and this value is entered into the State Variable box.

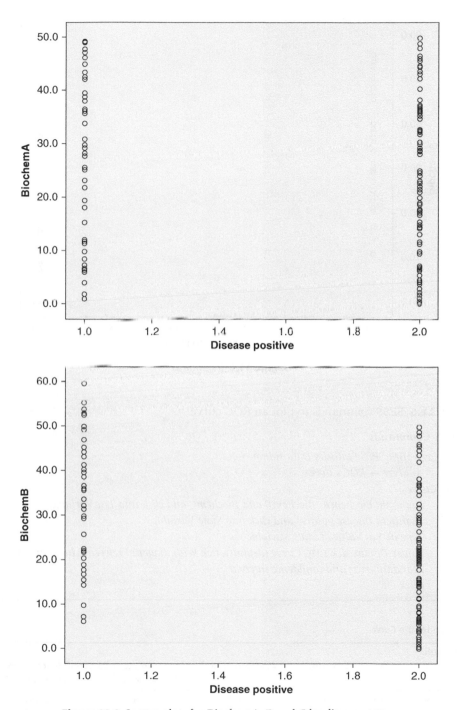

Figure 11.1 Scatter plots for BiochemA, B and C by disease status.

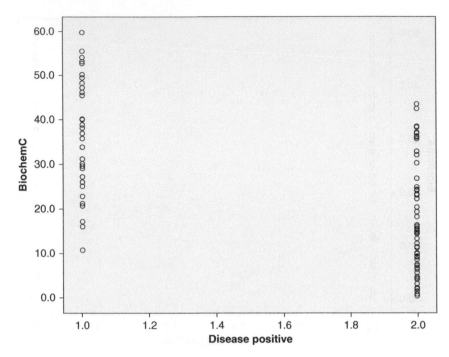

Figure 11.1 (*continued*)

Box 11.6 SPSS commands to plot an ROC curve

SPSS Commands

xray.sav - IBM SPSS Statistics Data Editor
     Analyze → ROC Curve
ROC Curve
     Highlight BiochemA, BiochemB and BiochemC and click into Test Variable
     Highlight Disease positive and click into State Variable
     Type in 1 as Value of State Variable
     Under Display tick ROC Curve (default), tick With diagonal reference line, and tick
     Standard error and confidence interval
     Click OK

Area Under the Curve

Test result variable(s)	Area	Std. error[a]	Asymptotic sig.[b]	Asymptotic 95% confidence interval	
				Lower bound	Upper bound
BiochemA	0.580	0.051	0.114	0.479	0.681
BoichemB	0.755	0.042	0.000	0.673	0.837
BiochemC	0.886	0.028	0.000	0.832	0.940

[a]Under the non-parametric assumption.
[b]Null hypothesis: true area = 0.5.

11.5.1   Interpretation of ROC curves

In an ROC curve, sensitivity is calculated using every value of BiochemA in the data set as a cut-off point and is plotted against the corresponding 1 – specificity at that point, as shown in Figure 11.2. Thus, the curve is the TP plotted against the FP calculated using each value of the test as a cut-off point. In Figure 11.2, the diagonal line indicates where the test would fall if the results were no better than chance at predicting the presence of a disease; that is no better than tossing a coin. BiochemA lies close to this line confirming that the test is poor at discriminating between disease-positive and disease-negative patients.

The area under the diagonal line is 0.5 of the total area. The greater the area under the ROC curve, the more useful the measurement is in predicting the patients who have the disease. A curve that falls substantially below the diagonal line indicates that the test is useful for predicting patients who do not have the disease.

When the measurement of interest cannot distinguish between two groups (e.g. disease positive or disease absent), that is, where there is no difference between the two distributions, the area under the ROC curve will be equal to 0.5 (the ROC curve will coincide with the diagonal). When there is a perfect separation of the values of the two groups, that is, no overlapping of the distributions, the area under the ROC curve equals 1 (the ROC curve will reach the upper left corner of the plot). The area under a ROC curve is less than 0.5 when the measurement predicts a negative test.

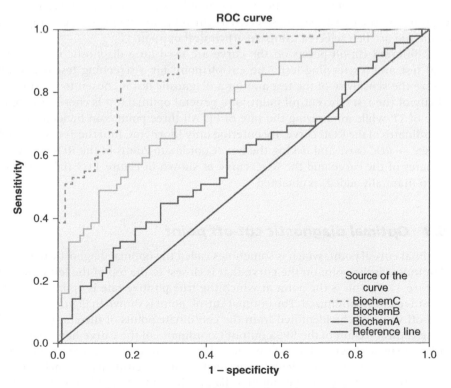

Figure 11.2 ROC curves for Biochem A, B and C.

The Area Under the Curve table indicates that the area under the curve for BiochemA is 0.580 with a non-significant *P* value (asymptotic significance) of 0.114, which shows that the area is not significantly different from 0.5. The 95% confidence intervals contain the value 0.5 confirming the *P* value that shows that this test is not a significant predictor of disease status.

The ROC curves in Figure 11.2 show that, as expected from the previous scatter plots, the tests BiochemB and BiochemC detect the disease-positive patients more effectively than BiochemA. In the Area under the Curve table, BiochemC is the superior test because the area under its ROC curve is the largest at 0.886. Both BiochemB and BiochemC have an area under the curve that is significantly greater than 0.5 and in both cases, the *P* value is < 0.0001. The very small amount of overlap of confidence intervals between BiochemB and BiochemC suggests that BiochemC is a significantly better diagnostic test than BiochemB, even though the *P* values are identical.

11.5.2   Calculating cut-off points

To make a choice of the cut-off point that optimizes the utility of the test is often an expert decision, considering factors such as the sensitivity, specificity, cost and purpose of the test. In diagnosing a disease, the gold standard test may be a biopsy or surgery, which is invasive, expensive and carries a degree of risk, for example the risk of undergoing an anaesthetic. Tests that are markers of the presence or absence of disease are often used to reduce the number of patients who require such invasive interventions. The exact points on the curve that are selected as cut-off points will vary according to each situation and are best selected using expert clinical opinion.

Three different cut-off points on the curve are used for a diagnostic test, a general optimal test and a screening test. The cut-off point for a screening test is chosen to maximize the sensitivity of the test and for a diagnostic test is chosen to maximize the specificity of the test. The cut-off point for a general optimal test is chosen to optimize the rate of TP while minimizing the rate of FP. All three points can be identified from the coordinates of the ROC curve. By entering only BiochemC into the Test Variable box of *Analyze → ROC Curve* and ticking the box 'Coordinate Points of the ROC Curve', the coordinates of the curve and the ROC curve as shown in Figure 11.3 (label for points has been manually added) is obtained.

11.5.3   Optimal diagnostic cut-off point

The optimal cut-off point, which is sometimes called the optimal diagnostic point or the Youden Index, is the point on the curve that is closest to the top of the left hand *y*-axis (see Figure 11.3). This is the point at which the true positive rate is optimized and the false positive rate is minimized. The optimal cut-off point is shown in Figure 11.3 and the test cut-off value can be identified from the coordinate points of the curve. The points from the central section of the SPSS output Coordinates of the Curve have been copied to an Excel spreadsheet and are shown in Table 11.5. In the table, the Excel function option has been used to also calculate Specificity and 1 − sensitivity for each point.

To find the coordinates of the optimal diagnostic point, a simple method is to use a ruler to calculate the coordinate value for 1 − specificity of the optimal cut-off point.

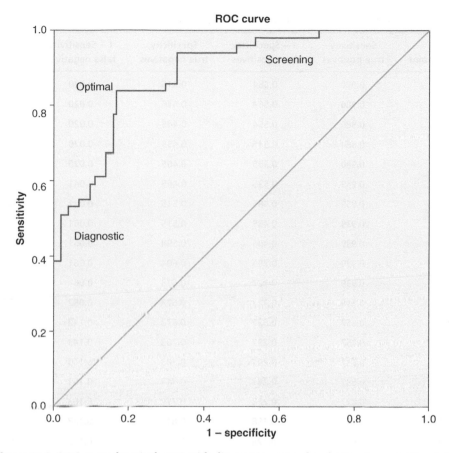

Figure 11.3 ROC curve for BiochemC with diagnostic, optimal and screening cut-off points.

Once the point is identified on the graph as being the closest point to the top of the y-axis on the ROC curve, a line can be drawn vertically down to the x-axis. The value for 1 − specificity is then calculated as the ratio of the distance of the point from the y-axis to the total length of the x-axis. Using this method, this value is estimated to be 0.167. In the '1 − specificity' column of Table 11.5, there are three values of 0.168, which are closest to 0.167. For the first value of 0.168, sensitivity equals 0.837 after which it begins to fall to 0.796 and 0.776. Thus, of the three points, the first point optimizes sensitivity, while 1 − specificity remains constant at 0.168. At this value, specificity is 1 − 0.168 or 0.832. The value of BiochemC at this coordinate is 24.8, which is the optimal cut-off point.

An alternative method to identify the cut-off point from the Excel spreadsheet is to use the following arithmetic expression, which uses Pythagoras' theorem, to identify the distance of each point from the top of the y-axis. In this calculation, the 'distance' has no units but is a relative measure:

$$\text{Distance} = (1 - \text{sensitivity})^2 + (1 - \text{specificity})^2$$

This value was calculated for all points in Table 11.5 using the function option in Excel. The minimum distance value is 0.055 for the cut-off point 24.8. Above and below this

Table 11.5   Excel spreadsheet to identify clinical cut-off points

Cut-off point	Sensitivity true positives	1 – Specificity false positives	Specificity true negatives	1 – Sensitivity false negatives	Distance
14.950	0.980	0.584	0.416	0.020	0.342
15.150	0.980	0.564	0.436	0.020	0.319
15.350	0.980	0.554	0.446	0.020	0.308
15.550	0.980	0.545	0.455	0.020	0.297
15.750	**0.980**	**0.535**	**0.465**	**0.020**	**0.286**
15.900	0.959	0.535	0.465	0.041	0.288
16.500	0.959	0.485	0.515	0.041	0.237
17.500	0.939	0.485	0.515	0.061	0.239
18.450	0.939	0.406	0.594	0.061	0.169
19.450	0.939	0.396	0.604	0.061	0.161
20.200	0.939	0.327	0.673	0.061	0.111
20.700	0.918	0.327	0.673	0.082	0.113
21.500	0.857	0.327	0.673	0.143	0.127
22.300	0.857	0.297	0.703	0.143	0.109
22.650	0.837	0.297	0.703	0.163	0.115
22.850	0.837	0.287	0.713	0.163	0.109
23.500	0.837	0.228	0.772	0.163	0.079
24.050	0.837	0.188	0.812	0.163	0.062
24.350	0.837	0.178	0.822	0.163	0.058
24.800	**0.837**	**0.168**	**0.832**	**0.163**	**0.055**
25.400	0.796	0.168	0.832	0.204	0.070
26.150	0.776	0.168	0.832	0.224	0.079
26.750	0.776	0.158	0.842	0.224	0.075
28.000	0.735	0.158	0.842	0.265	0.095
29.200	0.714	0.158	0.842	0.286	0.107
29.650	0.694	0.158	0.842	0.306	0.119
29.950	0.673	0.158	0.842	0.327	0.132
30.500	0.673	0.139	0.861	0.327	0.126
31.400	0.612	0.139	0.861	0.388	0.170
31.850	0.612	0.129	0.871	0.388	0.167
32.300	0.612	0.119	0.881	0.388	0.164
33.200	0.612	0.109	0.891	0.388	0.162
34.600	0.592	0.109	0.891	0.408	0.178
35.550	0.592	0.099	0.901	0.408	0.176

Table 11.5 (*continued*)

Cut-off point	Sensitivity true positives	1 – Specificity false positives	Specificity true negatives	1 – Sensitivity false negatives	Distance
35.650	0.571	0.099	0.901	0.429	0.193
35.900	0.551	0.099	0.901	0.449	0.211
36.350	0.551	0.079	0.921	0.449	0.208
36.650	0.551	0.069	0.931	0.449	0.206
36.800	0.531	0.069	0.931	0.469	0.225
37.050	0.531	0.050	0.950	0.469	0.223
37.600	0.531	0.040	0.960	0.469	0.222
38.100	0.510	0.040	0.960	0.490	0.241
38.500	**0.510**	**0.020**	**0.980**	**0.490**	**0.240**
38.250	0.510	0.030	0.970	0.490	0.241
39.200	0.490	0.020	0.980	0.510	0.261
39.850	0.469	0.020	0.980	0.531	0.282
41.100	0.388	0.020	0.980	0.612	0.375
42.700	0.388	0.010	0.990	0.612	0.375
44.250	0.388	0.000	1.000	0.612	0.375

Figures in bold represent cut-off points for screening, optimal and diagnostic test of Biochem C.

value, the distance increases indicating that the points are further from the optimal diagnostic point. When the point closest to the top of the y-axis is not readily identified from the ROC curve, this method is useful for identifying the cut-off value.

11.5.4 Cut-off points for diagnostic and screening tests

The cut-off points that would be used for diagnostic and screening tests can also be read from the ROC curve coordinates. For a diagnostic test, it is important to maximize specificity while optimizing sensitivity. From the ROC curve figure, the value that would be used for a *diagnostic test* is where the curve is close to the left hand axis, that is where the rate of FP (1 – specificity) is low and thus the rate of TN (specificity) is high. At the cut-off point where the test value is 38.5, there is a sensitivity of 0.510 and a low 1 – specificity of 0.02. At this test value, specificity is high at 0.98 which is a requirement for a diagnostic test. Ideally, specificity should be 1.0 but this has to be balanced against the rate of TP. At the three test values that have the same sensitivity of 0.510, the rate of false positive is higher for the cut-off points of 38.1 and 38.25 than for the cut-off point of 38.5, which maximizes specificity while optimizing sensitivity. At the cut-off points below 38.5 where specificity is also 0.98, a significant reduction in TP would occur if the cut-off point of 41.10 with a sensitivity of 0.388 was selected.

The value that would be used for a *screening test* is where the curve is close to the top axis where the rate of TP (sensitivity) is maximized. For a screening test, it is important to maximize sensitivity while optimizing specificity. At the cut-off point where the test value is 15.75, a high sensitivity of 0.98 is attained for a specificity of 0.465 (Table 11.5). At this point the false negative rate (1 − sensitivity) is low at 0.02 which is a requirement of a screening test. Ideally, sensitivity should be 1.0 but this has to be balanced against the rate of FP. The original SPSS output (not shown here) indicates that there are 13 test values below 15.75 at which sensitivity remains constant at 0.980 but there is a large gain in the rate of FP across these cut-off points from 0.535 to 0.703. Thus, at several cut-off values below 15.75, specificity decreases for no change in sensitivity.

For all three cut-off points, the choice of a cut-off value needs to be made using expert opinion in addition to the ROC curve. In this, the decision needs to be made about how important it is to minimize the occurrence of false negative or false positive results.

11.5.5   Reporting the ROC curve results

The results from the above analyses could be reported as shown in Table 11.6. The positive likelihood ratio is computed for each cut-off point as sensitivity/1 − specificity. A high positive likelihood ratio is more important for a diagnostic test than for a screening test. The 95% confidence intervals for sensitivity and specificity are calculated using the Excel spreadsheet in Table 11.2 with the numbers of disease-positive (49) and disease-negative (101) patients respectively used as the sample sizes.

Table 11.6   Cut-off points and diagnostic utility of test BiochemC for identifying disease-positive patients

Purpose	Cut-off value	Sensitivity (95% CI)	Specificity (95% CI)	Positive likelihood ratio
Screening	15.8	0.98 (0.94, 1.02)	0.47 (0.37, 0.57)	1.8
Optimal	24.8	0.84 (0.74, 0.94)	0.83 (0.76–0.90)	4.9
Diagnostic	38.5	0.51 (0.37, 0.65)	0.98 (0.95, 1.0)	25.5

11.6   Notes for critical appraisal

When critically appraising an article that presents information about diagnostic tests, it is important to ask the questions shown in Box 11.7. In diagnostic tests, 95% confidence intervals are rarely reported but knowledge of the precision around measurements of sensitivity and specificity is important for applying the test in clinical practice. In addition, estimating sample size in the disease-positive and disease-negative groups is of paramount importance in designing studies to measure diagnostic statistics with accuracy.

Box 11.7 Questions for critical appraisal

The following questions should be asked when appraising studies from which diagnostic statistics are reported:

- Was a standard protocol used for deciding whether the diagnosis and the test were classified as positive or negative?
- Was a gold standard used to classify the diagnosis?
- Was knowledge of the results of the test withheld from the people who classified patients as having a disease and vice versa?
- How long was the time interval between the test and the diagnosis? Could the condition have changed through medication use, natural progression, etc., during this time?
- Are there sufficient disease-positive and disease-negative people in the sample to calculate both sensitivity and specificity accurately?
- Have confidence intervals been calculated for sensitivity and specificity?

References

1. Greenhalgh T. How to read a paper: papers that report diagnostic or screening tests. *BMJ* 1997; **315**: 540–543.
2. Altman DG, Bland JM. Diagnostic tests 2: predictive values. *BMJ* 1994; **309**: 102.
3. Deeks JJ, Altman DG. Sensitivity and specificity and their confidence intervals cannot exceed 100%. *BMJ* 1999; **318**: 193.
4. Altman DG, Bland JM. Diagnostic tests 1: sensitivity and specificity. *BMJ* 1994; **308**: 1552.
5. Sackett DL, Richardson WS, Rosenberg W, Haynes RB. *How to practice and teach evidence-based medicine*. Churchill Livingstone: New York, 1997.
6. Sackett DL. On some clinically useful measures of the effects of treatment. *Evid Based Med* 1996; **1**: 37–38.
7. Malhotra RK, Indrayan A. A simple nomogram for sample size for estimating sensitivity and specificity of medical tests. *Indian J Opthamol* 2010; **58**: 519–522.
8. Fagan TJ. Nomogram for Bayes' theorem. *New Engl J Med* 1975; **293**:257.
9. Altman DG, Bland JM. Diagnostic tests 3: receiver operating characteristics plots. *BMJ* 1994; **309**: 188.

CHAPTER 12
Survival analyses

The individual source of the statistics may easily be the weakest link. Harold Cox tells a story of his life as a young man in India. He quoted some statistics to a judge who was an Englishman. The judge said, Cox, when you are a bit older, you will not quote Indian statistics with that assurance. The Government are very keen on amassing statistics – they collect them, add them, raise them to the nth power, take the cube root and prepare wonderful diagrams. But what you must never forget is that every one of those figures comes in the first instance from the chowkidar (village watchman), who just puts down whatever he pleases.

JOSIAH CHARLES STAMP (1880–1941)

Objectives

The objectives of the chapter are to explain how to:
- decide when survival analyses are appropriate
- obtain and interpret the results of survival analyses
- ensure that the assumptions for survival analyses are met
- report results in a graph or a table
- critically appraise the survival analyses reported in the literature

Survival analyses are used to investigate the time between entry into a study and the subsequent occurrence of an event. Although survival analyses were designed to measure differences in the time to death between study groups, they are frequently used for time to other events including discharge from hospital; disease onset; disease relapse or treatment failure; or cessation of an activity such as breastfeeding or use of contraception.

The time between the starting point of the study and the occurrence of the event is called the 'time to event' or 'survival time'. With data relating to time, a number of problems occur. The time to an event is often not normally distributed and follow-up times for patients enrolled in longitudinal studies may vary, especially when it is impractical to wait until the event has occurred in all patients. In addition, patients who leave the study early or who have had less opportunity for the event to occur need to be taken into account. Survival analyses circumvent these problems by taking advantage of the longitudinal nature of the data to compare event rates over the study period and not at an arbitrary time point.[1]

Medical Statistics: A Guide to SPSS, Data Analysis and Critical Appraisal, Second Edition.
Belinda Barton and Jennifer Peat.
© 2014 John Wiley & Sons, Ltd. Published 2014 by John Wiley & Sons, Ltd.
Companion website: www.wiley.com/go/barton/medicalstatistics2e

12.1   Study design

Survival analyses are ideal for analyzing event data from prospective cohort studies and from randomized controlled trials in which patients are enrolled in the study over long time periods. The advantages of using survival analyses rather than logistic regression for measuring the risk of the event occurring are that the time to the event is used in the analysis and that the different length of follow-up for each patient is taken into account. This is important because a patient in one group who has been enrolled for only 12 months does not have an equal chance for the event to occur as a patient in another group who has been enrolled for 24 months. Survival analyses also have an advantage over logistic regression in that the event rate over time does not have to be constant.

12.2   Censored observations

In survival analyses, patients who leave the study or do not experience the event are called 'censored' observations. The term *censoring* is used because, in addition to patients who survive, the censored group includes patients who are lost to follow-up, who withdraw from the study or who die without the investigators' knowledge. Classifying patients who do not experience the event for whatever reason as 'censored' allows them to be included in the analysis.

There are three types of censoring: right, left and interval. Right censoring occurs when participants leave the study or the study ends before the event occurs, if the event has occurred at all. Therefore participants who do not experience the event during the study, or withdraw from the study or were lost to follow-up are considered to be right censored. Right censoring occurs most frequently in medical research.[2] Left censoring occurs when the event has already occurred before enrolment or before a study examination has occurred. This type of censoring rarely occurs.[2] Interval censoring is when the event occurs in the interval between two study examinations; for example, if observations are only taken every 6 months. In this situation, it is not possible to precisely measure when the event actually occurred and the survival probabilities will be biased upwards.[3] Left and interval censoring commonly occur when study examinations of participants are infrequent.

12.3   Kaplan–Meier survival method

The Kaplan–Meier survival method is a non-parametric estimator of survival function and is appropriate to use when some of the data are censored.[3] The survival function is the probability of surviving to at least a certain time point and the graph of this probability is the survival curve. The Kaplan–Meier survival method can be used to compare the survival curves of two or more groups such as comparing a treated group to an untreated (placebo) group, or males compared to females. With this method, for each time interval, the probability of the patient surviving at the end of that time interval given that the patient survived at the start of the interval is calculated.[3] Thus, a conditional probability of patients surviving each time interval is calculated. In addition, data that are censored are also included in the calculation and reduce the number of patients at risk at the start of the next time interval. These conditional probabilities for each time interval are multiplied together to provide an overall or cumulative survival probability.

12.3.1 Assumptions of the Kaplan–Meier survival method

The assumptions for using Kaplan–Meier survival method are shown in Box 12.1. This method is a non-parametric test and thus no assumptions are made about the distributions of the variables.

Box 12.1 Assumptions for using survival analysis

The assumptions for using survival analysis are that:
- the participants must be independent, that is, each participant appears only once in their group
- the groups must be independent, that is, each participant is only in one group
- all participants are event free when they enrol in the study
- the measurement of time to the event is precise
- the start point and the event are clearly defined
- participants' survival prospects remain constant, that is, participants enrolled early or late in the study should have the same survival prospects
- the probability of censoring is not related to the probability of the event

---

In survival analyses, it is essential that the time to the event is measured accurately. For this, regular observations need to be conducted rather than, for example, surmising that the event occurred between two routine examinations.[3]

Both the start point, that is, entry into the study, the inclusion criteria and the event must be well defined to avoid bias in the analyses. This is especially important when using survival analyses to describe the natural history of a condition.[4] Using start points that are prone to bias, such as patient recall of a diagnosis or attendance at a doctor surgery to define the presence of an illness, will result in unreliable survival probabilities.

The reason for the event must also be clearly defined. When an event occurs that is not due to the condition being investigated, careful consideration needs to be given to whether it is treated as an event or as a withdrawal. In clinical trials, composite endpoints, for example, an event that combines death, acute myocardial infarction or cardiac arrest, are often used to test the effectiveness of interventions.[5]

Patients who are censored must have the same survival prospects as patients who continue in the study, that is, the risk of the event should not be related to the reasons for censoring or loss to follow-up.[3] The factors that influence patients' survival prospects, such as different treatment options, should not change over the study period and patients who experience more sickness in one treatment group should not be preferentially lost to follow-up compared with patients who experience less sickness in another treatment group. Secular trends in survival can also occur if patients enrolled early have a different underlying prognosis from those enrolled towards the end of the study. This would bias estimates of risk of survival in a cohort study but is not so important in clinical trials in which randomization balances important prognostic factors between the groups.

12.3.2   Sample size and data coding

As with all analyses, if the total number of patients in any group is small, say less than 30 participants in each group, the standard errors around the summary statistics will be large and therefore the survival estimates will be imprecise.

Plotting survival curves is not problematic when the study sample is large and the follow-up time is short. However, when the number of patients who remain at the end of the study is small, survival estimates are poor. Thus, it is important to end plots when the number in follow-up has not become too small.

When conducting a Kaplan–Meier survival analysis, the time variable must be continuous such as days, weeks or months; the event variable must be a binary or categorical variable and the factor variable categorical such as treatment type (treatment/placebo). Also, the data need to be entered with one binary variable indicating whether or not the event occurred and a continuous variable indicating the time to the event or the time to follow-up. The event is usually coded as '1' and censored cases coded as '0', although other coding such as '1' and '2' could be used.

Research question

The file **survival.sav** contains the data from 56 patients enrolled in a randomized clinical trial of two treatments in which 30 patients received the new treatment and 26 patients received the standard treatment. Patients were monitored daily and a total of 17 patients died. In this data set, the event is coded as 1 and censored cases are coded 0.

Question: Is the survival rate in the new treatment group higher than in the standard treatment group?

Null hypothesis: That there is no difference in survival rates between treatment groups.

Variables: Outcome variable = death (binary event)
                     Explanatory variables = time of follow-up (continuous), treatment group (categorical, two levels)

The commands shown in Box 12.2 can be used to obtain a Kaplan–Meier statistic to assess whether the survival times between the two treatment groups are significantly different.

The Case Processing Summary table shows summary statistics of the number in each group, the number of events and the number and per cent censored. These statistics show that there were fewer events but more patients who were censored in the new treatment group.

Box 12.2 SPSS commands to conduct a Kaplan–Meier survival analysis

SPSS Commands

survival.sav – IBM SPSS Statistics Data Editor
      Analyze → Survival → Kaplan-Meier
Kaplan-Meier
      Highlight days and click into Time
      Highlight event and click into Status
      Click on Define Event
Kaplan-Meier: Define Event for Status Variable
      Type 1 in Single value box, click Continue
Kaplan-Meier
      Highlight Treatment group and click into Factor
      Click Compare Factor
Kaplan-Meier: Compare Factor Levels
      Test Statistics: tick Log rank, Breslow, Tarone Ware,
      Select Pooled over Strata (default), click Continue
Kaplan-Meier
      Click Options
Kaplan-Meier: Options
      Statistics: tick Survival table(s) (default) and tick Mean and median survival
          (default); Plots: tick Survival
      Click Continue
Kaplan-Meier
      Click OK

Case Processing Summary

Treatment group	Total *N*	*N* of events	Censored	
			N	Per cent
New treatment	30	6	24	80.0
Standard treatment	26	11	15	57.7
Overall	56	17	39	69.6

The Survival Table is a descriptive table with the column labelled 'Time' indicating the day the event or censoring occurred. 'Status' indicates whether the patient experienced the event or was censored. 'Cumulative Proportion Surviving at the Time' indicates the proportion of patients surviving from the start of the study until that point in time. For example, the cumulative survival is 0.7111 at 36 days in group 1 (new treatment) and 0.5630 at 21 days in group 2 (standard treatment). The column labelled '*N* of Cumulative Events' indicates the total number of patients who have experienced the event from the start of the study until this time point. For example, in the new treatment group on day 16, 4 patients had died. The column labelled '*N* of Remaining Cases' indicates the number of patients remaining at that time who have not experienced the event or been censored.

In the Survival Table, it can be seen that the survival probabilities displayed in the column the 'Cumulative Proportion Surviving at the Time' are only calculated when an event occurs. As mentioned previously (Section 12.3), conditional probabilities at each event are used to generate the cumulative survival probability. For example, in the new treatment group, the conditional probability of surviving past day 9 is the number of patients who were alive at day 9 (end of interval) divided by the number of the patients who were at risk at the start of the interval (day 8); here this is $26/27 = 0.963$, which is shown in the Estimate column of the Survival Table. In the same treatment group, the conditional probability of surviving past day 12 is $24/25 = 0.96$ (not displayed in SPSS output). Here the number of cases at risk excludes those who are censored or have experienced the event. The cumulative survival probability of surviving past day 12 is $0.936 \times 0.96 = 0.924$, which is shown in the Estimate column of the Survival Table.

Survival Table

| Treatment group | | Time | Status | Cumulative proportion surviving at the time | | N of cumulative events | N of remaining cases |
				Estimate	Std. Error		
New treatment	1	5.000	0	.		0	29
	2	7.000	0	.	.	0	28
	3	8.000	0	.	.	0	27
	4	9.000	1	0.963	0.036	1	26
	5	9.000	0	.	.	1	25
	6	12.000	1	0.924	0.051	2	24
	7	15.000	1	0.886	0.062	3	23
	8	16.000	1	0.847	0.070	4	22
	9	16.000	0	.	.	4	21
	10	16.000	0	.	.	4	20
	11	19.000	0	.	.	4	19
	12	20.000	0	.	.	4	18
	13	23.000	0	.	.	4	17
	14	24.000	0	.	.	4	16
	15	25.000	0	.	.	4	15
	16	29.000	0	.	.	4	14
	17	31.000	0	.	.	4	13
	18	32.000	1	0.782	0.090	5	12
	19	32.000	0	.	.	5	11
	20	36.000	1	0.711	0.106	6	10
	21	38.000	0	.	.	6	9
	22	40.000	0	.	.	6	8
	23	41.000	0	.	.	6	7
	24	41.000	0	.	.	6	6
	25	42.000	0	.	.	6	5
	26	43.000	0	.	.	6	4
	27	48.000	0	.	.	6	3
	28	49.000	0	.	.	6	2
	29	58.000	0	.	.	6	1
	30	59.000	0	.	.	6	0

(Continued)

Treatment group		Time	Status	Cumulative proportion surviving at the time		*N* of cumulative events	*N* of remaining cases
				Estimate	Std. Error		
Standard treatment	1	1.000	1	.	.	1	25
	2	1.000	1	.	.	2	24
	3	1.000	1	0.885	0.063	3	23
	4	2.000	1	0.846	0.071	4	22
	5	3.000	1	0.808	0.077	5	21
	6	4.000	1	.	.	6	20
	7	4.000	1	0.731	0.087	7	19
	8	6.000	0	.	.	7	18
	9	7.000	1	0.690	0.091	8	17
	10	17.000	1	0.650	0.094	9	16
	11	20.000	0	.	.	9	15
	12	21.000	1	.	.	10	14
	13	21.000	1	0.563	.100	11	13
	14	31.000	0	.	.	11	12
	15	31.000	0	.	.	11	11
	16	32.000	0	.	.	11	10
	17	33.000	0	.	.	11	9
	18	33.000	0	.	.	11	8
	19	36.000	0	.	.	11	7
	20	39.000	0	.	.	11	6
	21	40.000	0	.	.	11	5
	22	40.000	0	.	.	11	4
	23	41.000	0	.	.	11	3
	24	43.000	0	.	.	11	2
	25	50.000	0	.	.	11	1
	26	65.000	0	.	.	11	0

Means and Medians for Survival Time

Treatment group	Mean[a]				Median			
			95% Confidence interval				95% Confidence interval	
	Estimate	Std. error	Lower bound	Upper bound	Estimate	Std. error	Lower bound	Upper bound
New treatment	48.591	3.686	41.367	55.816	.	.	.	.
Standard treatment	40.001	5.750	28.732	51.270	.	.	.	.
Overall	46.922	3.621	39.825	54.019	.	.	.	.

[a]Estimation is limited to the largest survival time if it is censored.

The Kaplan–Meier method produces a single summary statistic of survival time, that is, the mean or median. The mean survival time is estimated from the observed times and is shown for each group in the Means and Medians for Survival Time table. Mean survival is calculated as the summation of time divided by the number of patients who remain uncensored. This statistic can be taken to indicate the length of time that a patient can be expected to survive. Examination of the overlap of 95% confidence intervals for the new treatment and standard treatment groups suggests that possibly the difference between the curves is statistically significant (see Table 3.5 in Chapter 3).

The median survival time is the point at which half the patients have experienced the event. If the survival curve does not fall to 0.5 (i.e. survival probability of 50%), the median survival time cannot be calculated. In the above example, since both survival curves are above 0.5, the median values are not calculated.

12.3.3   Survival statistics

To examine whether there is a statistically significant difference between the survival curves of two or more groups, there are three tests that are calculated by SPSS, which are the Log Rank, Breslow and Tarone–Ware tests. The null hypothesis of these tests is that there is an equal risk of the event in all groups. That is, there is no difference in the probability of an event at any time between the populations. These tests are similar to chi-square tests in that the number of observed events is compared with the number of expected events. All three tests have low power for detecting differences when the survival curves cross one another.

The Log Rank test weights all time points equally and is the most commonly reported survival statistic.[6] This test is most likely to identify a difference when the risk of an event is constantly higher or lower for one group compared to another.[6,7] The assumptions of this test are the same as for the Kaplan–Meier method.[6] The assumption that the risk of an event in one group compared to the other group does not change over time is referred to as proportional hazards (see Section 12.4.2). If the survival curves cross one another, this suggests that the hazards are not proportional. In this situation, the log rank test will be less powerful and an alternative test should be considered.

The Breslow and Tarone–Ware tests are both weighted variants of the Log Rank test in that different weightings are given to particular points of the survival curve.[7] The Breslow test weights time points by the number of cases at risk at each time point. Thus, this test gives greater weight to early observations when the sample size is large and is less sensitive to later observations when the sample size is small. This test is appropriate when there are few ties in the data, that is, patients with equal survival times. The Tarone–Ware test weights all time points by the square root of the number of cases at risk at each time point. This test is a compromise between the Log Rank and the Breslow tests but is rarely used.

The Overall Comparisons table for the example above and obtained using the commands in Box 12.2 shows how the three tests can lead to different conclusions about whether there is evidence of a significant difference in the survival rate between groups. The Log Rank test is not significant at $P = 0.0705$. However, this test is not appropriate in this situation in which the number of patients remaining after 33–36 days is small with less than 10 patients in each group.

The Breslow test is significant at $P = 0.021$ and is the most appropriate test to report because more weight is placed on earlier observations. In this example, the Breslow P value is more significant than the Log Rank P value because more weight has been placed on the early observations. If early observations were more similar between groups and later observations more different, the Log Rank P value would have been more significant than the Breslow P value.

Overall Comparisons

	Chi-square	df	Sig.
Log rank (Mantel–Cox)	3.271	1	0.070
Breslow (Generalized Wilcoxon)	5.316	1	0.021
Tarone–Ware	4.388	1	0.036

Test of equality of survival distributions for the different levels of Treatment group.

12.3.4 Reporting the results of Kaplan–Meier

When reporting data from survival analyses, the P values from the statistical analyses do not convey information about the size of the effect. In addition to P values, summary statistics such as the follow-up time of each group, the total number of events and the number of patients who remain event free are important for interpreting the data. This information can be reported as shown in Table 12.1.

Table 12.1 Survival characteristics of study sample

Group	Number of cases	Number of events	Number censored	Mean survival time in days (95% CI)
New treatment	30	6	24 (80.0%)	49 (41, 56)
Standard treatment	26	11	15 (57.7%)	40 (29, 51)

Alternatively, the results can be reported using the following written text 'The Kaplan–Meier estimates indicated that the survival rate for 30 patients given the new treatment was 71% and for the 26 patients given the standard treatment was 56%. The Breslow test indicated that there was a statistically significant difference between the two survival rates ($P = 0.02$). The mean survival time for the new treatment group was 48 days and for the standard treatment group was 40 days. Collectively, these results suggest that the new treatment is more effective than the standard treatment'. In addition to this text, the Kaplan–Meier curve (see Section 12.3.5) can also be included.

12.3.5 Survival plots

Survival plots of time to event data are frequently used to report the results of clinical trials.[5] One of the most common survival plots used are Kaplan–Meier curves.[5] In plotting these curves, the data are first ranked in ascending order according to time. A curve is then plotted for each group by calculating the proportion of patients who remain in the study and who are censored each time an event occurs. Thus, the curves do not change at the time of censoring but only when the next event occurs.

The survival plot shows the proportion of patients who are free of the event at each time point. The steps in the curves occur each time an event occurs and the bars on the curves indicate the times at which patients are censored. The plots show the survival time for a typical patient. In the survival plot shown in Figure 12.1 obtained from the

Survival functions

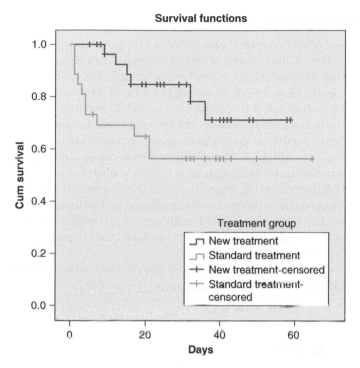

Figure 12.1 Survival curves for the two treatment groups.

commands in Box 12.2, the standard treatment group, which is the lower curve, has a poorer survival time than the new treatment group, which is the upper curve. The sections of the curves where the slope is steep, in this case the earlier parts, indicate the periods when patients are most at risk for experiencing the event. It is always advisable to plot survival curves before conducting the tests of significance.

There are several ways to plot survival curves and the debate about whether they should go up or down and how the y-axis should be scaled continues.[5] In SPSS, different presentations of the survival curve can be obtained by double clicking on the graph in SPSS Output View, the Chart Editor will be opened and the plot can be edited. Using the commands *Edit → Select X Axis* in the Chart Editor, the range of the x-axis and other properties of the plot such as chart size can be changed.

Plotting survival curves is not problematic when the study sample is large and the follow-up time is short. However, when the number of patients who remain at the end is small, survival estimates are poor. It is important to end plots when the number in follow-up has not become too small. Therefore, in the above example, the curves should be truncated to 31 days when the number in each group is 10 or more and should not be continued to 65 days when all patients in the standard treatment group have experienced the event or are censored.

The scaling of the y-axis is important because differences between groups can be visually magnified or reduced by shortening or lengthening the axis. In practice, a scale only slightly larger than the event rate is generally recommended to provide visual discrimination between groups rather than the full scale of 0–1. However, this can tend to make the differences between the curves seem larger than they actually are, for example in a plot in which the y-axis scale ranges from 0.5 to 1.0.

12.4 Cox regression

A Cox regression model (which is also called a Cox proportional hazards regression) provides an estimate of survival time while adjusting for the effects of other explanatory variables (referred to as covariates in this type of model). For example, in predicting an event such as death, factors such as age of the patient or number of years smoking cigarettes can be included in a Cox regression model. Compared to the Kaplan–Meier method where only categorical variables can be used to predict the event, with the Cox regression analysis a combination of categorical and/or continuous variables can be used to predict survival. In addition, Cox regression models can also manage censored data.

Cox regression is similar to other regression models such as linear regression or logistic regression (see Chapters 7 and 9, respectively), in that regression coefficients are generated, interaction between variables can be examined and adjustment for confounding factors can be made.[7] Where linear and logistic regressions models are used respectively to predict scores for a continuous and a binary variable, Cox regression models are used to predict the rate of an event.

A rule of thumb is that Cox models should have a minimum of 10 outcome events per predictor variable. However, there are some circumstances when this rule can be amended.[8]

12.4.1 Hazard ratio

Hazard is defined as the immediate risk of event occurrence.[9] The hazard rate or function is the probability that if the event has not occurred, it will occur in the next time interval, divided by the length of that interval.[10] If the time interval is small, the hazard function represents an instantaneous event rate among participants who have not experienced the event. In Cox regression analysis, the dependent variable is the hazard function at a given time.

With a Cox regression analysis, the effect of each covariate is reported as a hazard ratio. The hazard ratio is computed as the proportion of the rate (or function) of the hazard in the two groups. The hazard ratio can be used to estimate the hazard rate in a treatment group compared to the hazard rate in the control group. A hazard ratio of 2 indicates that, at any time point, twice as many patients in the one group experience an event compared with the other group. It is important to note that a hazard ratio of 2 does not mean that patients in the treated group improved or healed twice as quickly as patients in the control group. The correct interpretation of a hazard ratio of 2 is that a patient, who has been treated and has not improved by a certain time, has twice the chance of improving at the next time point compared to a patient in the control group.[10]

In Cox regression model, the hazard function at a given time is predicted by the baseline hazard function, which estimates the overall risk of the event where all explanatory variables equal zero. This term is similar to the constant term (i.e. the intercept) in linear regression. Regression coefficients are also generated for the explanatory variables or covariates that are included in the model. In building the Cox regression model, as in multiple linear regression (see Chapter 7), there are a number of different methods for including covariates in the model. In SPSS, the method options include enter, forward or backward. The enter option can be used to enter variables all at once or to sequentially add variables in blocks. With forward or backward method, there are three different criteria that can be used to determine whether variables are included: conditional, likelihood ratio (displayed as LR in SPSS) or Wald options. The inclusion or removal of variables is based on the corresponding statistics calculated. As with multiple linear regressions, it is important that both the clinical and statistical significance of variables be considered in building a parsimonious model.

The hazard ratio is sometimes used interchangeably to mean a relative risk (see Chapter 9); however, this interpretation is not correct. The hazard ratio incorporates the change over time, whereas the relative risk can only be computed at single time points, generally at the end of the study.

12.4.2   *Assumptions of Cox regression model*

The Cox regression model is a semi-parametric model and no assumptions are made about the distribution of survival. The assumptions shown in Box 12.1 should be met for Cox regression, as well as the assumption of proportional hazards. That is, the hazard (rate of the event) in one group should be a constant proportion of the hazard in the other study group over all time points. This assumption is important since the hazard ratio estimated by the model is for all time points [7] To test this assumption, when there are only two groups and no covariates, a simple test is to plot the Kaplan–Meier survival curves of the two groups together. If the curves are proportional and approximately parallel, then the assumption of proportional hazards is met. If the curves cross or if curves are not parallel and diverge they indicate that the rate of the event between the two groups is different (e.g. rate for one group increases constantly and the other group only slowly increases), and that the assumption of proportional hazards is not met. However, with small data sets the error around the survival curve is increased and therefore this test may not be accurate.[11] In addition, these plots are more complex to interpret with multivariable models. More appropriate methods are the log-minus-log plot[12] and examination of the partial residuals. The log-minus-log of the survival function, is the ln(−ln(survival)), versus the survival time. When the hazards are proportional, the curves should be approximately parallel. The residuals when plotted should be horizontal and close to zero (shown later in the chapter) if the hazards are proportional.

A statistical test can also be conducted to check for proportional hazards. The assumption of proportional hazards is similar to the assumption of homogeneity of regression in ANCOVA (see Chapter 5), which can be checked by assessing that there is no interaction between the covariate and factors (treatment levels).[12] In survival analysis, the assumption of proportional hazards can also be checked by assessing whether there is an interaction between time and treatment, as well as the covariates.[12] This is referred to an extended Cox regression model.[7]

Research question

Using the same file used earlier in this chapter, **survival.sav** which contains the data from 56 patients enrolled in a randomized clinical trial of two treatments in which 30 patients received the new treatment and 26 patients received the standard treatment. A total of 17 patients died.

Question: Are new treatment group or gender independent predictors of survival?

Null hypothesis: That there is no difference in survival rates between treatment groups or gender groups.

Variables: Outcome variable = death (binary event)
Explanatory variables = time of follow-up (continuous), treatment group (categorical, two levels), gender (categorical, two levels)

The commands shown in Box 12.3 can be used to obtain statistics to assess the independent effects of the predictor variables.

Box 12.3 SPSS commands to obtain a Cox regression

SPSS Commands

survival.sav – IBM SPSS Statistics Data Editor
     Analyze → Survival → Cox Regression
Cox Regression
     Highlight days and click into Time
     Highlight event and click into Status
     Click on Define Event
Cox Regression: Define Event for Status Variable
     Type 1 in Single value box, click Continue
Cox Regression
     Highlight Treatment group and click into Covariates
Cox Regression
     Click Next under Block 1 of 2
Cox Regression
     Highlight Gender and click into Covariates
     Click Categorical
Cox Regression: Define Categorical Covariates
     Click Gender into Categorical Covariates
     Change Contrast: select Indicator as Contrast and tick Change, select 'Last' as
         Reference Category and click Continue
Cox Regression
     Click Save
Cox Regression:Save
     Save Model Variables: tick Partial Residuals and click Continue
Cox Regression
     Click Options
     Cox Regression: Options
     Model Statistics: tick CI for Exp(B) 95%
     Display model information: select At each step (default), click Continue
Cox regression
     Click OK

Case Processing Summary

		N	Per cent
Cases available in analysis	Event[a]	17	30.4
	Censored	39	69.6
	Total	56	100.0
Cases dropped	Cases with missing values	0	0.0
	Cases with negative time	0	0.0
	Censored cases before the earliest event in a stratum	0	0.0
	Total	0	0.0
Total		56	100.0

[a] Dependent variable: days.

Categorical Variable Codings[a]

		Frequency	(1)
Gender[b]	1 = Male	25	1
	2 = Female	31	0

[a] Category variable: gender (gender).
[b] Indicator parameter coding.

The Case Processing table shows that 17 patients died and 39 were censored. The Categorical Variable Codings show the reference category is females as defined by the 'last reference category' in the SPSS commands and provides information on how to interpret the hazard ratios for gender.

Block 1: Method = Enter

Omnibus Tests of Model Coefficients[a]

−2 Log likelihood	Overall (score)			Change from previous step			Change from previous block		
	Chi-square	df	Sig.	Chi-square	df	Sig.	Chi-square	Df	Sig.
123.521	3.230	1	0.072	3.204	1	0.073	3.204	1	0.073

[a] Beginning Block Number 1. Method = Enter.

The Omnibus Tests of Model Coefficients tests the null hypothesis that all effects are equal to zero. The table reports the chi-square value for the overall model (a measure of goodness of fit), as well as the change from the previous model and the corresponding significance level. In this model, the comparison model is no predictors, with only the constant (intercept) included. The significance level for the overall score is not significant ($P = 0.072$), indicating that including the variable, treatment did not significantly improve the model.

Variables in the Equation

	B	SE	Wald	df	Sig.	Exp(B)	95.0% CI for Exp(B)	
							Lower	Upper
Group	0.885	0.508	3.029	1	0.082	2.422	0.894	6.558

The Variables in the Equation table shows the regression coefficient for treatment group which is 0.885. This is the logarithm of the hazard ratio for a patient given the new treatment (coded 1) compared with a patient given the standard treatment (coded 2). In this example, 11 patients died in the standard treatment group and six patients in the new treatment group. The exponential (anti-log) of this value is 2.422, which is shown on the column labelled Exp(B). This value indicates that the hazard (i.e. risk of dying) of a person receiving the new treatment is 2.422 compared to that of a person receiving the standard treatment. However, the significance level $P = 0.082$ is not significant and provides evidence that there is not a statistically significant difference in survival between the two groups.

Variables not in the Equation[a]

	Score	df	Sig.
Gender	5.428	1	0.020

[a]Residual Chi-square = 5.428 with 1 df
Sig. = 0.020.

The variables not in the equation estimate the change in the model fit if the variable gender is added to the model, the other two columns give the degrees of freedom, and P value for the estimated change. This table tells us that gender would improve the fit of the model, as confirmed in Block 2 below.

At Block 2, gender has been added to the model and the overall goodness of fit of the model has increased from the previous block, Block 1.

Block 2: Method = Enter

Omnibus tests of model coefficients[a]

-2 Log likelihood	Overall (score)			Change from previous step			Change from previous block		
	Chi-square	df	Sig.	Chi-square	df	Sig.	Chi-square	df	Sig.
118.102	8.657	2	0.013	5.418	1	0.020	5.418	1	0.020

[a]Beginning Block Number 2. Method = Enter.

Variables in the Equation

	B	SE	Wald	df	Sig.	Exp(B)	95.0% CI for Exp(B)	
							Lower	Upper
Group	0.882	0.508	3.011	1	0.083	2.416	0.892	6.545
Gender	1.173	0.533	4.850	1	0.028	3.233	1.138	9.186

Covariate Means

	Mean
Group	1.464
Gender	446

The Variables in the Equation table shows that the hazard ratio (Exp(B)) for the treatment group is 2.416 with a P value of 0.083 is not significant as it was in Block 1. The hazard ratio for gender is 3.233 with a significant P value of 0.028. The estimates shown in the column labelled Exp(B) are the adjusted hazard ratios for other variables included in the model. In this example, these estimates are the adjusted independent effects of treatment group and gender. The results indicate gender is an independent predictor of survival and that females are at a lower risk than males. Since the reference category was entered as 'last', the hazard ratio for being male relative to female is shown. The hazard ratio of 3.233 indicates that 3.2 times as many males experience a hazard at any time point compared to females.

To check the assumption of proportional hazards, the log–log plot and the residuals can be examined. To obtain a log–log plot, the categorical variable of treatment group needs to be defined as Strata in SPSS. Using the commands shown on Box 12.4 the log–log plot shown in Figure 12.2 is obtained. The log-minus-log plot shows that the curves are approximately parallel suggesting that the hazards are proportional.

Box 12.4 SPSS commands to obtain a log minus log plot

SPSS Commands

survival.sav – IBM SPSS Statistics Data Editor
   Analyze → Survival → Cox Regression
Cox Regression
   Highlight days and click into Time
   Highlight event and click into Status
   Click on Define Event
Cox Regression: Define Event for Status Variable
   Type 1 in Single value box, click Continue
Cox Regression
   Highlight Gender and click into Covariates
   Click Treatment group into Strata
Cox Regression
   Click Plots
Cox Regression: Plots
   Plot Type: select log minus log, click Continue
Cox Regression
   Click Continue

Partial residuals for each covariate can be generated and saved to the SPSS datasheet using the commands shown in Box 12.3. To check the residuals, the variables produced

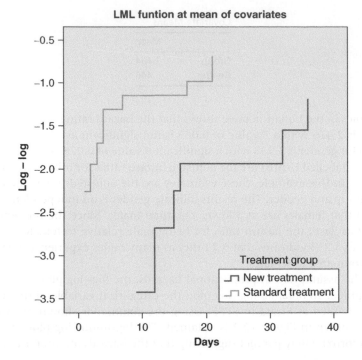

Figure 12.2 Log–log plot comparing standard treatment and new treatment.

at the end of the SPSS datasheet, partial residuals for group (PR1_1) and partial residual for gender (PR2_1) can be plotted against a time rank variable. To obtain a time rank variable the SPSS commands in Box 12.5 can be used. To obtain a scatterplot for each residual the SPSS commands shown in Box 7.2, with the ranked time variable (Rdays) plotted on the *x*-axis and each residual variable plotted separately on the *y*-axis to obtain the two residual plots as shown in Figure 12.3. It is also helpful for interpretation to plot the horizontal reference line at zero. To obtain the reference line, double click on the plot displayed in SPSS output and the Chart Builder will open, use the commands *Edit* → *Select Y Axis*, click on the *Scale* tab, tick *Display lie at origin* and click *Apply*. If the hazards are proportional, there should not be a clear trend over time (e.g. significantly increasing or decreasing over time) and the residuals should be centred close to zero. For the plots in Figure 12.3, although it is a small data set, there does not appear to be any trend and the residuals are close to zero. The results from the log-minus-log plot and the residuals suggest that the assumption of proportional hazards has been met.

Box 12.5 SPSS commands to obtain a rank time variable

SPSS Commands

survival.sav – IBM SPSS Statistics Data Editor
      Transform → Rank Cases
Rank Cases
      Highlight days and click into Variable(s), click OK

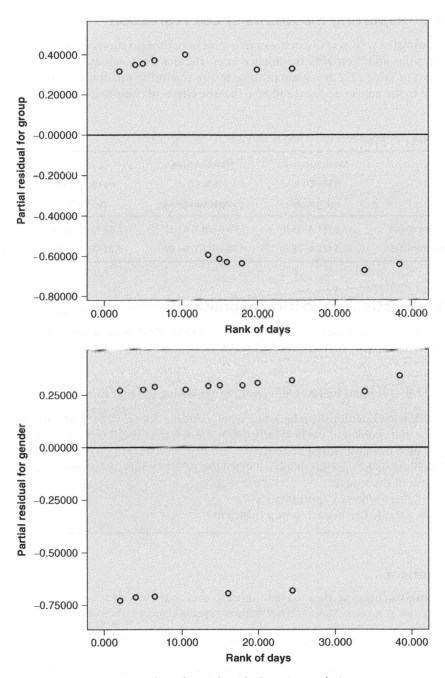

Figure 12.3 Plots of partial residuals against rank time.

12.4.3 Reporting the results of Cox regression

In reporting the results of Cox regression the mean or median survival time, the adjusted hazard ratios and their 95% confidence intervals, and the P values should be reported as shown in Table 12.2. It is good practice to also report the unadjusted hazard ratios in addition to the adjusted hazard ratios so that the effects of confounding can be judged.[13]

Table 12.2 Independent predictors of survival

Group	Mean survival (95% CI) in risk group	Mean survival (95% CI) in comparison group	Hazard ratio (95% CI)	P value
Treatment (new)	48.6 (41.4, 55.8)	40.0 (28.7, 51.3)	2.42 (0.89, 6.55)	0.08
Gender (female)	30.5 (22.8, 38.3)	55.1 (47.3, 63.0)	3.23 (1.14, 9.19)	0.03

12.5 Questions for critical appraisal

The questions that should be asked when critically appraising a journal article that reports a survival analysis are shown in Box 12.6.

Box 12.6 Questions to ask when critically appraising the literature

The following questions can be asked when critically appraising the literature:
• Is the start point and event clearly defined and free of recall or other bias?
• Has time been measured accurately?
• Have any factors preferentially changed the patient's survival prospects over the course of the study?
• Are figures reported appropriately?
• Is the sample size in each group sufficient?

References

1. Altman DG, Bland M. Time to event (survival) data. *BMJ* 1998; **317**: 468–469.
2. Sedgwick P. Kaplan–Meier survival analysis: types of censored observations. *BMJ* 2013; **347**: f4663.
3. Bland JM, Altman DG. Survival probabilities (the Kaplan–Meier method). *BMJ* 1998; **317**: 1572.
4. Norman GR, Streiner DL. *Biostatistics. The bare essentials*. Mosby Year Book Inc.: Missouri, USA, 1994.
5. Pocock SJ, Clayton TC, Altman DG. Survival plots of time-to-event outcomes in clinical trials: good practice and pitfalls. *Lancet* 2002; **359**: 1686–1689.
6. Bland JM, Altman DG. The logrank test. *BMJ* 2004; **328**: 1073.

7. Wright RE. Survival analysis. In: *Reading and understanding more multivariate statistics*, Grimm LG, Yarnold PR (editors). American Psychological Association: Washington, USA, 2000, 363–406.

8. Vittinghoff E, McCulloch CE. Relaxing the rule of ten events per variable in logistic and Cox regression. *Am J Epidemiol* 2006; **165**: 710–718.

9. Cox DR, Oates D. *Analysis of survival data*. Chapman & Hall: New York, 1984

10. Spruance SL, Reid JE, Grace M, Samore M. Hazard ratio in clinical trials. *Antimicrob Agents Chemother* 2004; **48**: 2787–2792.

11. Walters, SJ. Analyzing time to event outcomes with a Cox regression model. *WIREs Comput Stat* 2012; **4**: 310–315, doi: 10.1002/wics.1197.

12. Tabachnick BG, Fidell LS *Using multivariate statistics*, 4th edn. Allyn and Bacon: Boston, MA, 2001.

13. Sedgwick, P. Hazards and hazard ratios. *BMJ* 2012; **345**: e5980.

Glossary

Adjusted odds ratio Odds ratio which is adjusted for the effects of the other variables in the model.

Adjusted R square (R^2) R^2 is the square of the R value (i.e. $R \times R$) and is referred to as the coefficient of determination. The adjusted R^2 value is adjusted for the number of explanatory variables included in the regression model. This adjusted value can be used to compare regression models that have a different number of explanatory variables included.

Agreement Agreement is the degree to which scores are similar or different when two or more measurements are taken from the same participants on different occasions. Statistics that can be used to describe agreement include percent in agreement, differences-vs-means plot and limits of agreement.

Alternative hypothesis In hypothesis testing, a null and alternative hypothesis is specified. The alternative hypothesis states that there is a difference between the summary statistics of the populations from which the samples were drawn. The alternative hypothesis may be a one-sided or two-sided test.

Analysis of variance (ANOVA) A parametric test that can be used to compare differences in the mean values of three or more independent groups simultaneously. Thus, ANOVA is suitable when the outcome measurement is a continuous normally distributed variable and when the explanatory variable is categorical with three or more groups.

Analysis of covariance (ANCOVA) A parametric test that can be used to compare differences in the mean values of one or more groups after adjusting for a continuous variable, that is, a covariate.

Asymptotic method With this method, the significance levels for the statistical tests are calculated based on the assumption that the sample size is large and the data conform to a particular distribution, for example, normal distribution. When this assumption is not met, exact statistics should be used.

Balanced design Studies with a balanced design have an equal number of observations in each cell. This can be achieved only in experimental studies or by data selection. Most observational studies have an unbalanced design with unequal number of observations in the cells.

Bivariate statistics Tests in which the relationship between two variables is estimated, for example, an outcome and an explanatory variable.

Boxplot (box-whisker plot) A graphical representation of the data where the black horizontal line inside the box indicates the median and the inter-quartile range is the length of the box. The whiskers are the lines extending from the top and bottom of the box. The whiskers represent the minimum and maximum values when they are within 1.5 times above or below the inter-quartile range.

Medical Statistics: A Guide to SPSS, Data Analysis and Critical Appraisal, Second Edition.
Belinda Barton and Jennifer Peat.
© 2014 John Wiley & Sons, Ltd. Published 2014 by John Wiley & Sons, Ltd.
Companion website: www.wiley.com/go/barton/medicalstatistics2e

Case–control study A study design in which individuals with the disease of interest (cases) are selected and compared to a control or reference group of individuals without the disease.

Censored observation A term used to indicate that an event did not occur during the period of observation, in this, the survival time for an individual is censored. The reasons for censoring could be that the participant withdrew, was lost to follow-up or did not experience the event during the period of observation.

Centering To avoid collinearity in quadratic equations or when there is an interaction in a model, centering, that is, subtracting a constant (normally the group mean value) from the data values can be applied. Centering is commonly used in regression analysis.

Chi-square tests A statistic used to test whether the frequency of an outcome in two or more groups is significantly different, or that the rows and columns of a crosstabulation table are independent.

Coefficient of determination (R^2) Pearson correlation coefficient (r), can be squared to obtain the coefficient of determination, R^2, which indicates the percent of variance in one variable that can be explained by the other variable.

Collinearity A term used when there is a strong linear relationship between two explanatory variables.

Complete design A study design is complete when there are one or more observations in each cell and is incomplete when some cells are empty.

Confidence interval The 95% confidence interval is the interval in which there is 95% certainty that the true population value lies. Confidence intervals are calculated around summary statistics such as mean values or proportions. For samples with more than 30 cases, a 95% confidence is calculated as the summary statistic ± (SE × 1.96), where SE equals standard error. The confidence limits are the values at the ends of the confidence interval.

Confounder Confounders are nuisance variables that are related to the outcome and to the explanatory variables and whose effect needs to be minimized in the study design or analyses so that the results are not biased.

Cook's distance A measure of influence commonly used in multivariate models to detect influential observations. Influence measures the change in the model if the data point is removed. Values greater than $4/(n-k-1)$ are considered influential (n = sample size, k = number of variables in model).

Correlation A correlation coefficient describes how closely two variables are related, that is, the amount of variability in one measurement that is explained by another measurement. There are three types of bivariate correlations: Pearson's correlation coefficient (r), Spearman's ρ (rho) and Kendall's τ (tau).

Covariance structure In linear mixed models, within-subject correlations are modelled using the covariance structure. The covariance structure is built on the variance around the outcome measurement at each time point and on the correlations between measurements taken at different times from the same participant. The appropriate covariance structure (e.g. autoregressive first order, unstructured) which describes the structure of the correlation among data points must be determined before analysis.

Cox regression Provides an estimate of survival time while adjusting for the effects of one or more explanatory variables (referred to as covariates). For example, in predicting death, factors such as age of the patient or number of years smoking cigarettes can be included.

Cross tabulation (or contingency) table A table used to display the frequency of cases for two or more categorical variables. The data for chi-square tests are summarized using crosstabulation tables.

Differences-vs-means plots The means and differences between two measurments can be plotted as a differences-vs-means plot to show whether there is systematic bias, that is whether the differences are related to the size of the measurement as estimated by the mean. The plot is used assess agreement between measurements.

Discrepancy A measure of how much a case is in line with other cases in a multivariate model.

Dummy (or indicator) variables A series of binary variables typically with values 1 and 0 that have been derived from a multi-level ordinal variable. These variables are used to identify subgroups or represent an attribute such as a smoker or non-smoker. Dummy variables are commonly used in regression models.

Effect size A term used to describe the magnitude or strength of the difference, typically between two groups. Measures of effect size include Cohen's d, Cohen's f, eta squared, and omega squared.

Explanatory variable (independent or predictor variable) A variable that is hypothesized to influence the outcome variable.

Error term See Residual.

Estimated marginal means The estimated mean value of a factor adjusted (averaged) for all other factors in the model, that is, the predicted mean values.

Eta squared (η^2) A measure of the strength of association between the outcome and the explanatory factor. As such, eta squared is an approximation to R squared. Eta squared is calculated as the ratio of the factor variance to the total variance. Values range from 0 to 1 with larger values indicating a stronger association.

Exact statistics With these statistics, the significance levels are calculated based on the exact distribution of the test statistic. Exact tests are used when the numbers in a cell or group are small or unbalanced or the data are skewed and therefore the assumptions for asymptotic statistical tests are violated.

Explanatory variable A variable that is a measured characteristic or an exposure and that is hypothesized to influence an event or a disease status (i.e. outcome variable). In cross-sectional and cohort studies, explanatory variables are often exposure variables.

F value An F value is a ratio of variances. For one-way ANOVA, the F value is calculated as the mean between-group variance divided by the mean within-group variance, that is, the unexplained variance divided by the explained variance. For factorial ANOVA, the F value is the within-group mean square divided by the error (residual) mean square. For regression, the F value is the ratio of the mean regression sum of squares divided by the mean error sum of squares.

Factorial ANOVA A factorial ANOVA is used to examine the effects of two or more factors, or explanatory variables, on a single outcome variable. When there are two explanatory factors, the model is described as a two-way ANOVA, when there are three factors as a three-way ANOVA, and so on.

Fixed factor A fixed factor is a factor in which all possible groups or all levels of the factor are included in the model, for example, males and females or number of siblings.

Hazard ratio In survival analysis, the hazard ratio is the ratio of the hazard rates in two levels of an explanatory variable. For example, in a clinical trial, the treated population may die at half the rate per unit time as the control population. The hazard ratio would be 0.5 indicating that a patient, who has been treated and has not improved by a certain time, has half the chance of improving at the next time point compared to a patient in the control group.

Heteroscedasticity Heteroscedasticity indicates that the residuals at each level of the explanatory variable have unequal variances.

Histogram A graphical representation of the distribution of a continuous variable which indicates how frequently data points occur in certain intervals.

Homogeneity of variance When the population variances are equal, homogeneity of variance exists. That is, the variance of one variable is stable at all levels of another variable. Levene's test can be used to check for homogeneity of variance, which is an assumption of two sample t-test and ANOVA.

Homoscedasticity Homoscedasticity indicates that the residuals at each level of the explanatory variable have equal or similar variances. To test for homoscedasticity, a plot of the standardized residuals by the regression standardized predicted value can be examined. Homoscedasticity is an assumption of regression analysis.

Incidence Rate of new cases with a condition occurring in a random population sample in a specified time period, for example, 1 year.

Influence Influence is calculated as leverage multiplied by discrepancy and is used to assess the change in a regression coefficient when a case is deleted. Cook's distance is a measure of influence.

Interaction An interaction occurs when the effects of an explanatory variable on the outcome variable changes depending upon the level of another explanatory variable.

Inter-quartile range A measure of spread, that is, the width of the band that contains the middle half of the data that lies between the 25th and 75th percentiles. That is, the range in which the central 25–75% (50%) of the data points lie.

Interval scale variable A variable with values where differences in intervals or points along the scale can be made, for example, the difference between 5 and 10 is the same as the difference between 85 and 90.

Intervening variable A variable that acts on the pathway between an outcome and an exposure variable.

Intra-class correlation (ICC) ICC describes the relative extent to which two continuous measurements taken by different raters or two measurements taken by the same rater on different occasions are reliable. ICC values range from 0 to 1, with a value of 1 indicating perfect concordance between measurements.

Kaplan-Meier survival method This method is a non-parametric estimator of survival function and is appropriate to use when some data are censored. The survival function is the probability of surviving to at least a certain time point and the graph of this probability is the survival curve. The Kaplan–Meier survival method can be used to compare the survival curves of two or more groups.

Kappa statistic This statistic can be used to assess the concordance of responses for two or more raters or between two or more occasions after taking account of chance agreement. Kappa is an estimate of the proportion in agreement between raters in excess of the agreement that would occur by chance.

Kurtosis A measure of whether the distribution of a variable is peaked or flat. Measures of kurtosis between -1 and 1 indicate that the distribution has an approximately normal bell-shaped curve and values around -2 to $+2$ are a warning of some degree of kurtosis. Values below -3 or above $+3$ indicate that there is significant peakedness or flatness and therefore that the data are not normally distributed.

Leverage Leverage indicates the influence of a data point on the fit of a regression. Leverage is a measure of how far a data point is from the mean of that predictor variable. Leverage values can range from 0 (no influence) to $n-1/n$, where n equals the sample size, with values close to 1 highly influential.

Likelihood ratio The likelihood ratio is calculated as the probability of a test result in people with the disease divided by the probability of the same test result in people without the disease. A ratio greater than 1 indicates that the test result is associated with the presence of the disease. Likelihood ratios are commonly used to assess the utility of a diagnostic test. When the diagnostic test only has two outcomes, sensitivity and specificity can be used to calculate the likelihood ratios.

Limits of agreement Assuming that the difference scores between two measurements are normally distributed it is expected that the 95% of the scores will lie within the interval calculated as the mean difference $+/-$ 1.96 standard deviation of the differences. When measuring agreement, this range is called the 95% limits of agreement.

Linear-by-linear (or trend) test A statistic used to test for trends in crosstabulations where one variable is an ordered variable. This test is used to examine whether there is a trend for an outcome to increase or decrease across the categories of the ordered variable. This association is equivalent to testing whether the slope of a regression through the estimates is different from zero.

Linear mixed model A statistical model that includes both fixed and random effects. This model is commonly used to analyse data when there are repeated or multiple measurements on participants.

Log rank test This test can be used to examine whether there is a statistically significant difference between the survival curves of two or more groups. This tests that there is no difference in the probability of an event at any time between the groups.

Logistic regression Logistic regression is used to predict a categorical outcome variable from a set of explanatory variables. When the outcome variable is binary, this is referred to as binary logistic regression. In logistic regression, the odds ratio for an explanatory variable is adjusted for the other variables in the model.

Mahalanobis distance This is the distance between a case and the centroid of the remaining cases, where the centroid is the point where the means of the explanatory variables intersect. Mahalanobis distance is used to identify multivariate outliers in regression analyses. A case with a Mahalanobis distance above the chi-squared critical value at $P < 0.001$ with degrees of freedom equal to the number of explanatory variables in the model is considered to be a multivariate outlier.

Mann–Whitney U test A non-parametric test which is based on ranking the measurements from two samples to estimate whether the samples are from the same population. This test is non-parametric equivalent of a two-sample t-test.

Maximum value The largest numerical value of a variable.

McNemar's chi-square test (paired data) Paired categorical measurements taken from the same participants on two occasions or categorical data collected in matched case–control studies can be analysed using this test.

Mean A measure of the centre or the average value of the data.

Mean square Mean squares are estimates of variance used in analysis of variance and regression. The mean square is calculated as the sum of the squares divided by their degrees of freedom.

Measurement error The difference between the true value of the measurement and the actual value of the measurement. Measurement errors may be due to bias (systematic errors) and/or random variation. The measurement error can be calculated using the standard deviation of the differences of observations in the same participant and is used to describe the level of agreement between observations.

Median The point at which half the measurements lie above and below this value, that is, the point that marks the centre of the data.

Minimum value The smallest numerical value of a variable.

Multicollinearity Multicollinearity refers to when two or more explanatory variables are significantly related to one other. Multicollinearity between explanatory variables inflates the standard errors and causes imprecision because the variation is shared. Thus, the model becomes unstable (i.e. unreliable).

Multiple linear regression A linear model used to measure the extent to which two or more explanatory variables predict a continuous outcome variable.

Multivariate statistics Tests in which the relationship between more than two variables are examined simultaneously.

Negative predictive value The proportion of individuals who have a negative diagnostic test result and who do not have the disease.

Nominal variable A variable with values that do not have any ordering or meaningful ranking and are generally categories, for example, values to indicate that participants are retired, employed or unemployed.

Non-parametric tests Statistical tests that have no assumptions about the distribution of the data.

Normal distribution A probability distribution that describes the likelihood of a value occurring in the population. A normal distribution is symmetrical about its mean. The mean and median of a normal distribution are equal.

Null hypothesis A null hypothesis states that there is no difference between the summary statistics of the populations from which the samples were drawn, that is group statistics are equal or that there is no relationship between two or more variables. If the null hypothesis is accepted, this does not necessarily mean that the null hypothesis is true but can suggest that there is not sufficient or strong enough evidence to reject it.

Number needed to be exposed for one additional person to be harmed (NNEH) NNEH is the number of people who need to be exposed to the risk factor of interest to cause harm to one additional person. NNEH is calculated from the absolute risk increase (ARI), which is the difference in the proportion of participants with the outcome of interest in the exposed and unexposed groups.

Number needed to treat (NNT) NNT is the number of patients need to be administered a treatment to prevent one adverse event. NNT are commonly used to assess the effectiveness of treatments. If a treatment had an NNT value equal to 5, this means that five patients would have to be treated with the drug to prevent one adverse event.

Odds ratio The odds ratio is the odds of a person having a disease if exposed to a risk factor divided by the odds of a person having a disease if not exposed to the risk factor. An odds ratio of 2 can be interpreted as the odds that an exposed person has the disease present are twice that of the odds that a non-exposed person has the disease present. Odds ratios are commonly reported in case-control studies.

One sample *t*-test A parametric test that can be used to test if the sample mean is equal to a specified value.

One sided (or one tailed) tests When the direction of the effect is specified by the alternate hypothesis, for example, $\mu > 50$, a one-tailed test is used. The tail refers to the end of the probability curve. The critical region for a one signed test is located in only one tail of the probability distribution. One-sided tests are more powerful than two-sided tests for showing a significant difference because the critical value for significance is lower and are rarely used in health care research.

Optimal diagnostic cut-off point (or Youden Index) This is the point on a ROC curve at which the true positive rate is optimized and the false positive rate is minimized.

Ordinal variable A variable with values that indicate a logical order such as codes to indicate socioeconomic or educational status.

Outcome (dependent) variable The outcome of interest in a study, that is the variable that is dependent on or is influenced by other variables (explanatory variables) such as exposures and risk factors.

Outliers There are two types of outliers: univariate and multivariate. Univariate outliers are defined as data points that have an absolute z score greater than 3. This term is used to describe values that are at the extremities of the range of data points or are separated from the normal range of the data. For small sample sizes, data points that have an absolute z score greater than 2.5 are considered to be univariate outliers. Multivariate outliers are data values that have an extreme value on a combination of explanatory variables and exert too much leverage and/or discrepancy.

***P* value** A P value is the probability of a test statistic occurring if the null hypothesis is true. P values that are large are consistent with the null hypothesis. On the other hand, P values that are small, say less than 0.05, lead to rejection of the null hypothesis because there is a small probability that the null hypothesis is true. P values are also called significance levels. In SPSS output, P value columns are often labelled 'Sig.'

Paired *t*-test A parametric test that is used to estimate whether the means of two continuous related measurements are significantly different from one another. This test is used when two measurements are related because they are collected from the same participant at different times, from different sites on the same person at the same time or from cases and their matched controls.

Parametric tests Statistical tests which assume that the continuous variables being analysed has a normal distribution. Parametric tests are preferable to non-parametric tests because they have more statistical power.

Partial correlation The correlation between two variables after the effects of a third or confounding variable has been removed.

Planned (*a priori*) contrasts Specific group differences can be assessed using planned contrasts, which are decided before data collection commences. The number of planned contrasts should be limited and have a theoretical and/or empirical basis. Planned contrasts generally have more statistical power than post-hoc tests.

Population A collection of individuals to whom the researcher is interested in making an inference, for example, all people residing in a specific region or in an entire country, or all people with a specific disease.

Positive predictive value The proportion of individuals with a positive diagnostic test result who have the disease.

Post-hoc tests After a statistically significant difference is found overall between groups, post-hoc tests are conducted to identify where particular group differences exist. Post-hoc testing occurs during the data analyses and typically involves all possible comparisons between groups.

Power The ability of the study to demonstrate an effect or association if one exists, that is to avoid type II errors. Statistical power can be influenced by many factors including the frequency of the outcome, the size of the effect, the sample size and the statistical tests used.

Prevalence Rate of total cases with a condition in a random population sample In a specified time, for example 1 year.

Proportional hazards The hazard (rate of the event) in one group should be a constant proportion of the hazard in the other study group over all time points. Proportional hazards are an assumption of Cox's regression.

Protective odds ratio If An odds ratio which is less than 1.0 indicates that the risk of disease in the exposed group is less than the risk in the non-exposed group. This suggests that exposure has a protective effect.

Quartiles Obtained by placing observations in an increasing order and then dividing into four groups so that 25% of the observations are in each group. The cut-off points are called quartiles. The four groups formed by the three quartiles are called 'fourths' or 'quarters'

Quintiles Obtained by placing observations in an increasing order and then dividing into five groups so that 20% of the observations are in each group. The cut-off points are called quintiles.

R square (R^2) See coefficient of determination.

r value Pearson's correlation coefficient that measures the linear relationship between two continuous normally distributed variables.

R Multiple correlation coefficient, that is, the correlation between the observed and predicted values of the outcome variable.

Random factor Factors are considered to be random when only a sample of a wider range of groups or all possible levels is included. For example, factors may be classified as having random effects when only three or four ethnic groups are represented in the sample but the results will be generalized to all ethnic groups in the community.

Range The difference between the lowest and the highest numerical values of a variable, that is, the maximum value subtracted from the minimum value. The term range is also often used to describe the values that are the limits of the range, that is, the minimum and the maximum values, for example, range 0–100.

Rank sum tests Non-parametric tests, which are used when the data do not conform to a normal distribution, are used to compare distributions of two or more groups by ranking their measurements as scores, for example, the Mann–Whitney U test.

Ratio scale variable An interval scale variable with a true zero value so that the ratio between two values on the scale can be calculated, for example, age in years is a ratio scale variable but calendar year of birth is not.

Receiver operating characteristic (ROC) curve These curves can be used to identify the cut-off point in a continuously distributed measurement that best predicts whether a condition is present, for example whether patients are disease positive or disease negative. ROC curves are plotted by calculating the sensitivity and specificity of the test in predicting the diagnosis for each value of the measurement.

Relative risk The ratio of the probability of the outcome occurring in the exposed group compared to the probability of the outcome occurring in the non-exposed group. Relative risk can only be used when the sample is randomly selected from the population. A relative risk of 2 indicates that the prevalence of the outcome in the exposed group is twice as high as the prevalence of the outcome in the non-exposed group.

Reliability Reliability is used to measure the ratio of the variability between the same participants (for example, by different raters or at different times) to the total variability of all participants in the sample. Measures of reliability include the statistics kappa and ICC.

Repeated measures An analysis of variance where multiple measurements of the same outcome variable has been obtained using the same participants. This may occur over a time period or under different conditions. For example, the blood pressure of patients is collected at three time points – baseline, post-treatment, and follow-up or the blood pressure of participants is measured when they are off medication and measured again when they are on medication.

Residual The difference between a participant's value and the predicted value, or mean value, for the group. This term is often called the error term.

Risk The probability that any individual will develop a disease. Risk is calculated as the number of individuals who have the disease divided by the total number of individuals in the sample or population.

Risk factor An aspect of behaviour or lifestyle or an environmental exposure that is associated with a health-related condition.

Sample Selected and representative part of a population that is used to make inferences about the total population from which it is drawn.

Sensitivity Proportion of disease-positive individuals who are correctly diagnosed by a positive diagnostic test result.

Significance level See *P* value.

Simple linear regression A linear model used to measure the extent to which one explanatory variable predicts a continuous outcome variable.

Skewness A measure of whether the distribution of a variable has a tail to the left- or right-hand side. Skewness values between -1 and $+1$ indicate very little skewness and values around -2 and $+2$ are a warning of a reasonable degree of skewness but possibly still acceptable. Values below -3 or above $+3$ indicate that there is significant skewness and that the data are not normally distributed.

SnNout This term is the acronym for **Se**nsitivity-**N**egative-**out,** which means that if the test has a high sensitivity (true positives) and a low 1 − sensitivity (false negatives), a negative test result rules the disease out.

Specificity The proportion of disease-negative individuals who are correctly identified as disease free by a negative diagnostic test result.

Sphericity An assumption of repeated measures ANOVA when there are three or more repeated measures conditions. Sphericity requires that the variances of the differences for all pairs of repeated measures are constant. The assumption of sphericity can be tested using Mauchly's test which gives an estimate of epsilon (ϵ). This statistic has a value of 1 when sphericity is met.

SpPin This term is the acronym for **Sp**ecificity-**P**ositive-**in**, which means that if a test has a high specificity (true negatives) and therefore a low 1 − specificity (false positives), a positive result rules the disease in.

Standard deviation (SD) A measure of spread such that it is expected that 95% of the measurements lie within 1.96 standard deviations above and below the mean. The standard deviation is the square root of the variance.

Standardized coefficients Partial regression coefficients that indicate the relative importance of each variable in the regression equation. These coefficients are in standardized units similar to z scores and their dimension allows them to be compared with one another.

Standard error (SE) A measure of precision that is the size of the error around a a summary statistic. For continuous variables, the standard error around a mean value is calculated as $SD/\sqrt{n}$. For other statistics such as proportions and regression estimates, different formulae are used. For all statistics, the SE will become smaller as the sample size increases for data with the same spread or characteristics.

SE of the estimate This is the approximate standard deviation of the residuals around a regression line. This statistic is a measure of the variation that is not accounted for by the regression line. In general, the better the fit, the smaller the standard error of the estimate.

String variable A variable that generally consists of words or characters but may include some numbers. This type of variable is also known as an alphanumeric variable.

Survival plot A survival plot such as Kaplan–Meier curves shows the proportion of patients who are free of the event at each time interval. The steps in the curves occur each time an event occurs and the bars on the curves indicate the times at which patients are censored.

t-value A t-distribution is closely related to a normal distribution but depends on the number of cases in a sample. A t-value, which is calculated by dividing a mean value by its standard error, gives a number from which the probability of an event occurring is estimated from a t-table.

Tolerance A measure of multicollinearity. Tolerance has an inverse relationship to VIF in that VIF = 1/tolerance. VIF values less than 0.2 indicate multicollinearity.

Transformation If the data do not follow a normal distribution, for example, the distribution is skewed then a transformation can be applied such as taking the logarithm of the data so that the data follows a normal distribution and parametric tests can be used.

Trimmed mean The 5% trimmed mean is the mean calculated after 5% of the data (i.e. outliers) are removed. This method is sometimes used in sports competitions, for example, skating, when several judges rate performance on a scale.

Two sample t-test (Student's t-test or an independent samples t-test) A parametric test used to estimate whether the mean value of a normally distributed outcome variable is significantly different between two groups of participants.

Two-sided (or two-tailed) tests When the direction of the effect is not specified by the alternate hypothesis, for example, $\mu \neq 50$, a two-sided test is used. The tail refers to the end of the probability curve. The critical region for a two-sided test is located in both tails of the probability distribution. Two-sided tests are used in most research studies.

Type I error A term used when a statistically significant difference between two study groups is found although the null hypothesis is true. Thus, the null hypothesis is rejected in error.

Type II error A term used when a clinically important difference between two study groups does not reach statistical significance. Thus, the null hypothesis is not rejected when it is false. Type II errors typically occur when the sample size is small.

Type sum of squares (SS) Type III SS are used in ANOVA for unbalanced study designs when all cells have equal importance but no cells are empty. This is the most common type of study design in health research. Type I SS are used when all cell numbers are equal, type II is used when some cells have equal importance and type IV is used when some cells are empty.

Univariate tests Descriptive tests in which the distribution or summary statistics for only one variable are reported.

Unstandardized coefficients These are the regression coefficients in the equation $y = a + bx$, where 'a' is the constant and 'b' is the coefficient for explanatory variable.

Variance A measure of spread that is calculated from the sum of the deviations from the mean, which have been squared to remove negative values.

Variance inflation factor (VIF) A measure of multicollinearity which is calculated as $1/(1 - R^2)$ where R^2 is the squared multiple correlation coefficient. A VIF ≥ 4 is a sign of multicollinearity.

Wilcoxon signed rank (or matched pairs) test A non-parametric equivalent of the paired t-test that tests whether the median of the differences between pairs of observations is equal to zero.

z Score This is the number of standard deviations of a value from the mean. z scores, which are also known as normal scores, have a mean of zero and a standard deviation of one unit. Values can be converted to z scores for variables with a normal or non-normal distribution; however, conversion to z scores does not transform the shape of the distribution.

Useful websites

A New View of Statistics

http://www.sportsci.org/

A peer-reviewed website that includes comprehensive explanations and discussion of many statistical techniques including confidence intervals, chi-squared and ANOVA, plus some Excel spreadsheets to calculate summary statistics that are not available from commonly used statistical packages.

Binomial confidence intervals

http://statpages.org/confint.html

Website that provides a calculator for computing exact confidence intervals for samples from the Binomial and Poisson distributions.

CONSORT (CONsolidated Standards of Reporting Trials) statement

http://www.consort-statement.org/consort-statement/

Guide to the analysis, interpretation and reporting of randomized controlled trials.

Diagnostic test calculator

http://araw.mede.uic.edu/cgi-bin/testcalc.pl

Online program for calculating statistics related to diagnostic tests such as sensitivity, specificity and likelihood ratio.

Effect size calculator

http://www.uccs.edu/~lbecker/

Calculates Cohen's effect size using means and standard deviations, or t values and degrees of freedom. Also has detailed information on different effect sizes measures and how they are calculated.

Effect size illustrator

http://esi.medicine.dal.ca/

An interactive tool that helps with the calculation and practical interpretation of effect sizes.

Medical Statistics: A Guide to SPSS, Data Analysis and Critical Appraisal, Second Edition.
Belinda Barton and Jennifer Peat.
© 2014 John Wiley & Sons, Ltd. Published 2014 by John Wiley & Sons, Ltd.
Companion website: www.wiley.com/go/barton/medicalstatistics2e

Epi Info

http://www.cdc.gov/epiinfo/downloads.htm

With Epi Info, a questionnaire or form can be developed, the data entry process can be customized and data can be entered and analysed. Epidemiologic statistics, tables, graphs, maps and sample size calculations confidence intervals around a proportion can be produced. Epi Info can be downloaded free.

Gpower

http://www.gpower.hhu.de/

A comprehensive sample size calculation program for t-test, F test, chi-square test, z test, and some exact tests.

GraphPad Quickcalcs

http://www.graphpad.com/quickcalcs

Online program for calculating many statistical tests for continuous and categorical data including McNemars, number need to treat (NNT), kappa, and so on.

Help service

http://www.stat-help.com/index.html

A free online statistics help service. The site also has links to education notes, calculation spreadsheets and statistical software.

HyperStat Online Textbook

http://davidmlane.com/hyperstat/

Provides information on a variety of statistical procedures, with links to other related Web sites, recommended books and statistician jokes.

IBM SPSS

http://www-947.ibm.com/support/entry/portal/product/spss/spss_statistics?product
Context=1478422152

Download product manuals and troubleshooting documentation for SPSS.

Kappa statistics

http://www.vassarstats.net/kappa.html

This program allows you to calculate Cohen's kappa and weighted kappa statistics by entering the numbers into a contingency table.

Martin Bland Web page

http://www-users.york.ac.uk/~mb55/

Web page with links to talks on agreement, cluster designs, and so on, statistics advice and access to free statistical software. There is a section on the site that shows how to compute 95% confidence intervals around a median values. The site also includes an index to all BMJ statistical notes that are online, a statistics guide for research grant applicants and a directory of randomization software.

Public Health Archives

http://www.jiscmail.ac.uk/archives/public-health.html
   Mailbase to search for information or post queries about statistics, study design issues, and so on. This site also has details of international courses, and so on.

Quick-R

http://www.statmethods.net/index.html
   Useful website on how to use *R* including how to calculate power using *R*.

R program

http://www.r-project.org/
   R program can be downloaded for free and can be used to conduct a range of statistical techniques including linear and nonlinear modelling, classical statistical tests, time-series analysis, classification and clustering. It can also be used to calculate power for proportions, ANOVA, chi-square, correlations, *t*-tests, linear models (e.g. regression) and repeated measures.

Random number generator

http://www1.assumption.edu/users/avadum/applets/applets.html
   Generates random number sequences for various clinical scenarios.

Raynald's SPSS Tools

http://www.spsstools.net/
   Website with syntax, macros and online tutorials on how to use SPSS and with links to other statistical websites.

ROC curve calculator

http://www.rad.jhmi.edu/jeng/javarad/roc/JROCFITi.html
   This website calculates a ROC curve from data with 95% intervals around the curve.

Running a linear mixed model in SPSS

http://www.ats.ucla.edu/stat/spss/library/spssmixed/mixed/mixed_diet_intro.htm
   A website that shows how to run a linear mixed model in SPSS and interpret the output.

Russ Lenth's power and sample size page

http://www.stat.uiowa.edu/~rlenth/Power/

A graphical interface for studying the power of one or more tests including the comparison of two proportions, *t*-tests and balanced ANOVA.

Sample size estimation

https://www.statstodo.com/StatsToDoIndex.php
Provides a sample size calculator for many analysis situations including survival analyses and also provides a statistics calculator for many statistical tests.

Sample size estimation for regression equations

http://danielsoper.com/statcalc3/calc.aspx?id=1
Provides a sample size calculator for linear regression analyses with one or more predictor variables in the equation.

Sealed envelope

https://www.sealedenvelope.com/power/
Provides a sample size calculator for superiority, non-inferiority and equivalence randomized controlled trials.

Simple Interactive Statistical Analysis (SISA)

http://www.quantitativeskills.com/sisa/
Simple interactive program that provides tables to conduct statistical analysis such as chi-square and *t* tests from summary data.

Statistics pages

http://www.statpages.org/
A comprehensive website with educational material, information of free statistical packages, many statistical calculators and much more.

Stats Calculator

https://www.mccallum-layton.co.uk/tools/statistic-calculators/sample-size-calculator/
A website that allows you to make sample size calculations, estimate confidence intervals around proportions and mean values and conduct some statistical tests.

STROBE (STrengthening the Reporting of OBservational studies in Epidemiology)

http://www.strobe-statement.org/
A website that provides guidelines for the reporting of results from observational studies.

Index

Note: Page numbers in *italic* refer to figures, those in **bold** refer to tables

---

Medical Statistics: A Guide to SPSS, Data Analysis and Critical Appraisal, Second Edition.
Belinda Barton and Jennifer Peat.
© 2014 John Wiley & Sons, Ltd. Published 2014 by John Wiley & Sons, Ltd.
Companion website: www.wiley.com/go/barton/medicalstatistics2e

Printed and bound by CPI Group (UK) Ltd, Croydon, CR0 4YY

27/10/2024

14580171-0003